17✓

D1478930

Creating Happy Healthy Babies

A Holistic Midwife's Approach to
Pregnancy, Labour and Birth

Vicki Delpero

BALBOA.
PRESS
A DIVISION OF HAY HOUSE

Balboa Press books may be ordered through booksellers or by contacting:

Balboa Press
A Division of Hay House
1663 Liberty Drive
Bloomington, IN 47403
www.balboapress.com
1 (877) 407-4847

Because of the dynamic nature of the Internet, any web addresses or
links contained in this book may have changed since publication and may
no longer be valid. The views expressed in this work are solely those
of the author and do not necessarily reflect the views of the publisher,
and the publisher hereby disclaims any responsibility for them.

The author of this book does not dispense medical advice or prescribe the use
of any technique as a form of treatment for physical, emotional, or medical
problems without the advice of a physician, either directly or indirectly. The
intent of the author is only to offer information of a general nature to help
you in your quest for emotional and spiritual well-being. In the event you use
any of the information in this book for yourself, which is your constitutional
right, the author and the publisher assume no responsibility for your actions.

Any people depicted in stock imagery provided by Thinkstock are models,
and such images are being used for illustrative purposes only.
Certain stock imagery © Thinkstock.

Print information available on the last page.

ISBN: 978-1-4525-2636-2 (sc)
ISBN: 978-1-4525-2637-9 (hc)
ISBN: 978-1-4525-2638-6 (e)

Library of Congress Control Number: 2014918738

Balboa Press rev. date: 02/04/2015

Disclaimer

Information provided in this book is based on a range of research sources and antipodal evidence gained through clinical experience and intended for general information and guidance. Procedures, suggestions and ideas are not intended to replace professional medical advice, rather to supplement and work synergistically in conjunction with professionals trained in the field of conception and pregnancy. Consult your medical practitioner for conditions needing diagnosis or attention. Advise them of any suggestions you may wish to adopt from this book.

Children

And a woman who held a babe against her bosom said, 'Speak to us of Children.'

And he said:

Your children are not your children.

They are the sons and daughters of Life's longing for itself.

They come through you but not from you,

And though they are with you, yet they belong not to you.

You may give them your love but not your thoughts.

For they have their own thoughts.

You may house their bodies but not their souls,

For their souls dwell in the house of tomorrow, which you cannot visit, not even in your dreams.

You may strive to be like them, but seek not to make them like you.

For life goes not backward nor tarries with yesterday.

You are the bows from which your children as living arrows are sent forth.

The archer sees the mark upon the path of the infinite, and He bends you with His might that His arrows may go swift and far.

Let your bending in the archer's hand be for gladness;

For even as he loves the arrow that flies, so He loves also the bow that is stable.

Khalil Gibran 1883 - 1931

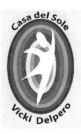

Natural Fertility
& Maternity Care

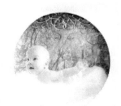

Email: wellness@casadelsole.com.au
Text: 0419 532 286
www.casadelsole.com.au

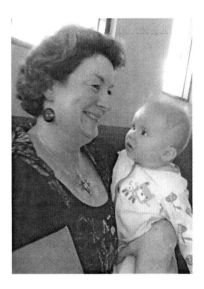

Vicki Delpero
Registered Midwife,
Registered Nurse,
Teaching Diploma of
Psychosomatic Therapy,
Neuro-Emotional Technique
Therapist (NETT),
THETA Practitioner,
Professional Reflexology Practitioner,
The Liquid Crystals Practitioner,
Certificates in Nutrition and
Herbal Medicine,
BA Vocational Education,
Reiki Master.

Founding Board Member 1998-2006,
Reflexology Association of Australia.
Executive Member 2012-Current, International
Association of Psychosomatic Therapists.

To my children, Justin, Martin and Vanessa and their partners,
that they may have beautiful, blissful pregnancies and experience
a labour of love in the birthing of their own children.

Foreword

In 'Creating Happy Healthy Babies' Vicki Delpero presents a wealth of knowledge beautifully reflecting her twenty plus years midwifery experience. The med-wyf, coming from the original Anglo Saxon, was also known as the wise woman and she has been a traditional source of information and support for women and their families throughout the history of our race. It is only recently that we have seen her stature reduced by the rise of a patriarchal system that, while presenting many advantages that we all enjoy, has in its wake overseen the destruction of important life affirming values and practices. The loss of these has rendered most women afraid of and ignorant about their own bodies, at a time when they have the opportunity to experience the power and triumph that is rightfully theirs as women giving birth. The Newtonian framework within which this model has operated needs to be exposed for the deeply flawed one that it is. Vicki does this and presents an expanded, rich alternative for women and their families.

Vicki's voice is authoritative and compelling. Those who are fortunate to have a copy of this book will benefit from the wisdom and knowledge that she presents. Understanding the interplay between the body, mind and emotions puts us in a position of power and we can become most effective in bringing about desired changes for ourselves and for those we care for. The time-honoured practices that Vicki introduces will require a paradigm shift for many. This is both necessary and exciting and marks a crucial point in our evolution. Cultures vary, however the act of a baby making its way out of its mother's body does not. Our mammalian inheritance that we have acquired on our way to becoming human works (circumstances support the process). The biological intelligence that conceives and gestates the baby will continue into birth and lactation when Mother Nature's divine design is understood, respected and supported.

We live in a time of revolution in the place of birth in our culture that began about 40 years ago. After generations of being anaesthetized, separated from their babies, ignored and overridden many women world wide are demanding change, and like Vicki Delpero are asserting and reclaiming their appropriate place as the authorities and creators of the future. They are demanding that their and their babies' basic human rights are observed during pregnancy and birth. Enjoy this remarkable book.

Shivam Rachana, International College of Spiritual Midwifery
http://www.womenofspirit.asn.au/ www.lotusbirth.net

Contents

Preface

There is no doubt that advances in medical and obstetric care have contributed greatly to the improvement of women's maternal health care and lowered infant mortality rates, especially for women in high risk categories. However this medicalisation of pregnancy and birth has led to a loss of personal power for the healthy birthing woman. With such a strong emphasis on the 'need' for medical care many women have lost faith in their ability to give birth without medical assistance. This is compounded by lower birth rates and more nuclear families meaning women have less contact with other pregnant women and less experience of natural birth and newborn babies. Some women have never held a baby before giving birth to their own.

The majority of pregnancies require little if any medical intervention, particularly when soon to be parents are well informed and learn to work *with* their bodies rather than in conflict with the changes that are occurring. At the end of this book I share with you my own personal journey of pregnancy and birth as a testimony to how the choices we make can have profound effects on the outcome of births.

The objective of this book is to present information and choices, based on my professional experiences and research, that may not be readily available in the modern day maternity system. It is not that this system is inadequate, but with resources stretched to the limit, the focus has become prevention of complications and detection of abnormalities. This system is challenged to address the individual needs of women, so

I encourage you to take responsibility, ask questions and do your own research.

My Professional Journey

I first trained as a midwife in 1986 at the time that Active birth and Natural birth were becoming the 'catch cry' of maternity carers world wide. I read and was educated in the styles of natural birth gurus such as Sheila Kitzinger, Ida May Gaskin, Janet Balaskas and Shivam Rachana, Spiritual Midwife. Thus my own midwifery experiences became firmly grounded in the belief that birth is a natural event requiring support and love, not intervention.

Eighteen months before I began training as a midwife I had given birth to my first child, Justin. As a registered nurse, I held strong beliefs in the Western model of maternity care and unconsciously carried quite a lot of fear about birth. Although I experienced a loving pregnancy, the birth was intrusive and involved a good deal of medical intervention, resulting in a difficult and traumatic birth for my eldest son.

At the time I had thought this a normal birthing experience. During midwifery training I discovered that what had happened to me was not necessary, but a result of medical mismanagement, and that I had been the victim of my own naivety and of giving my power to the system. I felt violated by what had happened, and as my training continued I also began to understand how the experience could have been so very different.

Seven months into midwifery training I found myself pregnant again. At first I was very confused about what direction to take in order to have a better experience of birth this time. I was taking the oral contraceptive pill (unaware at the time how detrimental this could be to my health) and had decided to stop taking it in anticipation of creating another child, only to find I was already pregnant. He had decided he was coming and that was that. He often brags that if he can get through 'the pill' he can do anything.

From the moment I was consciously aware of his conception my life changed. I began to look at life differently. I chose different healthy eating patterns, began researching alternative health care and seeking out more aligned natural maternity health care givers. I just knew at some level this pregnancy was different and that the birth had to be different. People who no longer supported my ideas dropped away and a totally new circle of friends developed who aligned with my philosophies. I became the healthiest I'd ever been, and as a consequence an advocate for health.

One day a homebirth midwife came to present to our student group about the benefits of homebirth. Martin (in utero at the time) did not stop kicking me from the moment she arrived until she left. I felt myself getting excited at the prospect of having a home birth. I declared to my friend sitting with me that this was the option I'd been looking for. When I told my husband he was elated. After the awful hospital experience with our first son he was relieved that it would be a private experience at home. He had every faith in me. I found myself connecting and talking to my baby every day. We developed a strong bond of trust. There was not a doubt within me that this was the right path.

I was less fearful and trusted totally in the natural process. Because I'd had such an awful experience the first time I spent a lot of time visualising and affirmating to prepare myself mentally for this birth. Martin continued to direct me to the right midwife. He would let me know when not to speak to certain people or when to spend more time with an enlightened being that had experienced a positive birth. This was my first experience of Baby Whispering (intuitive listening to the baby in utero). When Martin chose to come into the world it was a gentle three hour birth without drama. I was quite shocked by the difference in the two birth experiences! I kept saying 'this is not hurting like last time?' The feeling I had was of total elation and achievement, I knew there was a different way to the fearful dramatic births that are often portrayed by the media.

From that moment forward I dedicated my life to assisting and improving the experience of conception, pregnancy and birth for anyone willing to listen and change. I believe my shift in confidence and state of mind had a direct effect on Martin in utero, instilling trust and confidence at a cellular level. So who chose who? Who directed who for their higher purpose? The full story is included later in this book.

I became a most passionate advocate, promoting homebirth as a viable option and assisting with organisation of the 1989 National Homebirth conference in Hobart. I began teaching natural birth classes with the homebirth group and eventually set up a class through adult education with another passionate advocate. We stirred the pot and vowed to improve maternity services for women in Tasmania. I continued to work as a midwife in the hospital doing what I could to make a difference until the birth of my daughter, Vanessa. I apologise to all my colleagues from that time as I know I drove them crazy with my passionate obsession to want to change the maternity system.

Eventually our small homebirth advocacy group decided that homebirth was too exclusive. It was time to take the principles of a homebirth into the hospital setting. We felt it was very important to include all women no matter what their choice of birth setting. Every woman deserved the opportunity to birth naturally whether at home or in hospital and the setting should have no bearing on the outcome. The Natural Birth Association came into being with the aim of acting as advocates for women. The association instigated many changes to maternity services in Tasmania over the next ten years. It was during this time that the Hobart birth centre and The Know Your Midwife scheme (KYM) were first established, with more acceptance of homebirth as a safe alternative. Birthing was revolutionised in Tasmania and women began to have a choice.

In 1993 the Natural Birth Association Tasmania Incorporated was granted funding for a resource centre and a free homebirth program under the commonwealth government's Alternative Birthing Services Program. This was a great achievement and a testimony to the hard work that had been undertaken to change the attitudes of key players in local maternity services. In 1994 I was offered the position of Midwife Coordinator to the Homebirth Program and to run the Childbirth Information Service, thus embarking on one of the most incredible learning curves of my life over the next three years. The program was very successful with over 200 women receiving free homebirths, until Federal policy changed and funding cuts to national women's services resulted in the closure of the Homebirth

Program. However by this time a credible service had been established that was then able to continue on as a private business for the midwives to run.

Couples began tracking me down asking to attend childbirth classes, having heard positive recommendations from those who had attended previous classes. These classes were well attended and whilst I felt they were making a difference there seemed to be something missing. I was working at the local private maternity hospital, often caring for women with pregnancy or labour complications. Through the research and study I had undertaken over past years I knew that many of these complications could have been prevented, or at least assisted, through maternity reflexology, natural therapies and specific nutrition.

Following training in maternity reflexology (1995) with Suzanne Enzer, I went on to become a professional reflexologist. I was drawn to many seminars on reproductive health, fertility and pre-conceptual care. As my interest and knowledge continued to grow I began to specialise in maternity reflexology and natural fertility care, whilst continuing to work as an independent midwife. During this time I developed a working relationship with another therapist, creating a practice focused on a wide range of reproductive health issues relating to pregnancy and labour. In 1998 we were asked to present our success story at the National Reflexology Association of Australia conference in Brisbane. What a surprise, we hadn't even written a book yet! We were greeted with a standing ovation in recognition of the work we had been doing. It was a natural progression following this to conduct and teach natural fertility and maternity care workshops across Australia.

The practice naturally evolved and in May 2000 a healing and teaching practice was formalized under the name Stream of Life (SOL), specialising in preconception, infertility, maternity care, childbirth education and maternity reflexology. Also during this time, being very passionate about reflexology as a modality, as a founding Board Member of the Reflexology Association of Australia I was instrumental in assisting its growth professionally. I maintained this role for several years. The Stream of Life practice continued successfully for many years and I have tremendous gratitude for this amazing time of fun, learning and personal growth. As with all things, change is inevitable and in 2008 I moved to working independently from my current practice, Casa del Sole 'House of the Sun' (Soul).

A key focus for my practice is continual learning and experience, using a range of healing modalities to achieve results by providing a holistic approach that combines spirit, mind and body. Since 2008 Psychosomatic Therapy has become a key component of my work. I now have the greatest pleasure in teaching this nationally accredited Certificate III training within Australia and overseas.

My Philosophy

I believe that balance must occur between our spirit, mind and physical body and when all three are in unison the human body works in harmony. My philosophy is that we are here to experience life to its fullest, encompassing all emotions.

Just working in the physical sense, such as undergoing surgery and taking prescription drugs, does not necessarily resolve the actual issue behind the symptoms. Unless we deal with the underlying emotional/ spiritual issue, treating just the physical symptoms is likely to provide only temporary relief, thus merely delaying for the short term symptoms that will likely recur. Hermann Müller, Psychosomatic Therapy Founder and Director, relates to this concept as 'Issues in the Tissues', the issues (source) being the emotions that have been stored in your cellular memory.

Thoughts attached to emotions are picked up by the body and locked in for future reference. Thoughts and ideas accumulate, creating belief systems that dictate our behaviour. The body functions and reacts from these subconscious beliefs. This is known as body language, and explains why we often see people's actions not matching what they say. Our body language tells far more about who we are than what we say. This is the basis of Psychosomatic Therapy body-mind communication.

Actions are imbedded more deeply than thoughts or words, because actions are based on feelings. If you want to change your behaviour, first think the thought in a constructive way. Then deliberately change your behaviour to match the thought. Repetition makes it part of your life.

In other words think it, feel it, become it.

Choose how you want to behave
Consciously choose your actions and reactions moment to moment.
Fine tune your mind and body by saying to yourself:
'At this moment I am choosing to feel...'
Feel the feeling, express it and let it go.

Choose your words
The words you speak have psychological and physiological effects. Choose to speak kindly, use language that is pro-health.
Ask yourself:
'Is what I am speaking coming from my heart or from my negative mind?'

Choose actions
State out loud your intention.
'I am choosing to...'
This brings awareness and communication between your body and mind.
'I choose to smile because I can.'

Notice automatic behaviours
Become aware of your daily habitual behaviours:

- are those behaviours pro-health?
- slow down, speak and walk with intention and choice.

This then becomes self awareness.

Choose responsibility (the ability to respond)
Self-awareness brings responsibility and the ability to respond from the heart rather than react from the ego. Your body responds to the way that

you think and feel. For example, rigid thoughts can create rigid areas in the body whereas soft, nurturing, caring thoughts and feelings create a softer toned body.

Women who believe pregnancy is a natural and healthy state, and labour a beautiful transitional experience, are more likely to create healthy pregnancies and easier births. This is because they are able to work intuitively with their body rather than living in a state of fear. We all have an inner knowing or 'gut feeling' about what feels right for us, known as our intuition, inner tutor or wise voice. Unfortunately busy lifestyles create stress, often resulting in an inability to truly be in touch with our feelings. As our minds are busy doing rather than allowing us to be still and feel, it is easy to get caught up in the 'shoulds' and 'have tos'.

It is these 'shoulds', 'have tos' and doing the 'right thing' due to perceived ideas about what is expected of us that appear to cause more disharmony and chaos in our lives than anything else. The body and mind become conflicted. The body feels, the mind thinks. This conflict makes life a struggle, resulting in energy burnout and imbalance within the body. You make decisions and choices every single moment. These choices can be positive or result in a struggle. Fear and control are a negative form of dealing with things whereas love and surrender are the positive. The mind appears to have an innate tendency to find the negative thought first or to find fault or judgement before searching for the positive. Ultimately everyone is right in their own mind, and through training we can learn to accept and allow it to be what it is. Each person has their own perceptions and experiences to draw from that are different to yours and mine. Unless you can walk in another's shoes you cannot judge whether that person is right or not.

Learning to surrender can be one of the greatest assets towards a relaxed pregnancy and birth. Allow yourself to let go of unnecessary controls so that you can get in touch with your inner knowing. Peace will come when you learn to accept and flow.

Thoughts Are Powerful

Every action is the result of a thought in the form of a decision. The decision can be made with wisdom and deliberation or from spontaneous, mindless reaction. This is why affirming statements and creative visualisations are such powerful healing tools.

Positive thoughts yield positive results. As a wise sage once said "nothing is ever that bad, it is just the way you view it". If we come from truth, integrity and the best for all concerned, in other words, acting from our higher self and heart centre, then balance can be achieved.

Like a river, the spirit, mind and body will flow smoothly and freely, creating their own path. This involves consciousness, the healing process and time to resolve the negative input and cellular memories from our past. To get to this point involves a major surrender of negative thoughts, inferiority feelings, agitation, worry and anxiety and the idea that we are not worthy of the best in life.

The Dalai Lama discusses this consistently throughout 'The Art of Happiness'. He challenges the reader to decide whether an action will give us pleasure or ultimate happiness. For example taking drugs or smoking may bring immediate pleasure, but is likely to eventually bring disease and unhappiness, therefore the preferred choice is not to smoke in anticipation of future happiness.

Natural health care comes from this belief system, recognising every person as an individual with a completely different journey to another. A holistic approach to healing believes that the human spirit, mind and body work in unison and together has its own intelligence which requires emotional and physical nurturing to achieve its goal of perfect health.

Natural health care is simplistic in nature and gentle in action.

Is your health a commodity you are allowing to waste and whittle away? Or do you respect your health and view it as an investment? Investing time, money and effort into the maintenance of your health is like investing money in a good superannuation scheme, you will reap the rewards tenfold in the future. You probably understand the importance of maintaining your car, but how often do you consider the importance of maintenance or service of your body?

Do you take for granted that your body will keep on going, ignoring the warning lights for so long that when one day it just breaks down the damage is almost irreparable? The effort to repair the damage can be costly, requiring a huge commitment, and is often much harder than preventative care. Does lack of information or misinformation stop you from seeking out preventative health care or adopting a healthier lifestyle? Or do you believe 'it won't happen to me'?

Western medicine has become a multi-million dollar industry reliant on technological advances and pharmacology. There is little promotion of and hardly any reference to the importance of preventative health care and the connection between spirit, mind and body. By contrast, traditional doctors from places such as India or China treat the balance between the spirit, mind and body as the basis of health. For these doctors prevention of illness is the standard practice and they are paid for preventing rather than for treating illness.

This focus on the physical has never been more evident than it is now in maternity care and obstetrics, with ever growing trends towards encouraging Caesarean Section (C/S) for birth. Some Australian hospitals have a C/S rate as high as seventy percent.

The physiological and spiritual needs of a natural birth for future generations will be forgotten unless we commit to making a difference by helping women understand why it is important to keep birth normal. Michel Odent (renowned French obstetrician) has created a research database, Primal Health, in order to provide evidence as to why we need to keep birth normal for the sake of future generations.

http://www.primalhealthresearch.com/

This is not to say that modern medicine is bad, but that balance is essential in all things. By combining the wisdom of traditional medicine with modern technology the health care provided is far more holistic and sound. At the individual level it is essential that you seek out a practitioner who views health from this holistic approach and has the time to listen to your needs. Cultivating a sense of happiness, peace and wellbeing within ourselves by relaxing and letting go can be far more effective than taking any form of medicinal drug.

Prevention is better than seeking a cure. Prevention relies on keeping balance. Knowledge is empowerment, giving you the ability to make changes where necessary. Enjoying full health means honouring and respecting who you are. Your body is a highly tuned organism capable of miracle after miracle when its needs are met. Ultimately healing and re-balancing rely upon you. When you embrace change, working in alignment with your soul's journey, a balanced state of well being can occur. There are two questions to ask on a moment-by-moment basis 'is this who I am?' and 'what would love do now?'

Blooming Pregnancy

According to the World Health Organisation pregnant women have the right to:

1. Choose the type of care they and their baby will have.
2. Information about their health and options of care.
3. Information about the intervention rates of local maternity services.
4. Demand that they be treated with care, respect and intelligence.
5. Expect and ask for information about pregnancy, labour, birth and feeding.
6. Speak up if they don't understand what they've been told.
7. Find out what are all the options, not just listening to one opinion. Maternity care is loaded with one sided views.
8. Hospital care. No hospital can refuse treatment in Australia.
9. Know what drugs are prescribed and why, what they are for and what are the side effects?
10. Not take or do anything that does not feel right, no matter how much the 'experts' are pushing their ideals. To be informed first before making a decision.
11. Fully understand their doctor or midwife's status on such things as water birth, inductions, epidurals, episiotomies, forceps, caesareans, natural birth, Syntometrine for the delivery of placenta, Vitamin K injections, immunisation, circumcision.
12. To seek another care giver that suits their needs.
13. Not compromise their experience for any one else except for the health of self or their baby.
14. Make sure they have the right people with them at the birth, this includes as many as they feel comfortable with.
15. The birthing area to be private and conducive to their comfort and ease of birth not the doctor or midwife.
16. Refuse any hospital routine or policy. Policy is only a generalised way of doing things, it is not law. The baby belongs to the parents not the hospital medical staff.
17. Refuse students, researchers or doctors.

18. Refuse any treatment they have not given their consent to first.
19. See their hospital and doctors' records.
20. Check the bill and request an itemised account.
21. A second opinion.

Remember who is paying for the service - as with any other service ensure you get what you pay for.

http://www.who.int/publications/en/

Making a Decision

Making choices is part of everyday life, some as simple as where to sit or what to wear. Often decisions involve some risk. If your decision creates a situation you had not planned on, then you have to face the consequences of your actions. But if you don't try you will never know either. Is there such a thing as a bad decision? Isn't life about experience anyway? Are we meant to have the experience for the learning involved? Whatever the outcome the experience is not a 'failure', it is just an experience.

Creating and raising children involves making lots of decisions. Making decisions on behalf of another person is one of the major stresses faced by new parents. It is no longer just about you, the individual, but you the mother, partner, siblings and baby. People used to taking responsibility and making decisions in other areas of their lives can find they struggle in this new territory. When we become emotionally involved in the situation our judgement can be clouded.

Sometimes the barrage of risk factors are overwhelming to you as decision maker, so you avoid making a decision, hoping someone else will do it for you. Many love to do this for you, they are called rescuers. In the long run being rescued doesn't help you grow, it only serves to take your power away. I often say to parents to beware of this trait. If you take the hurdle away from your child hoping to make it easier for them, then the next hurdle may possibly be bigger in order for the lesson to be learnt anyway.

4

Some maternity carers become rescuers, wanting to take the intense experience of labour away. This may be due to their own need to nurture or their fear around birth, especially if their faith in the birth process is not strong. If we remove the experience then we take away a rite of passage - the important experience of transition to motherhood. They may offer all types of analgesia and interventions in an attempt to make the birthing woman's road easier but in the long run this may make the whole situation longer and more complicated, doing mother and baby a disservice.

For instance, I had a client come to me stating that her blood pressure (BP) was high and her obstetrician had suggested she be induced at the end of the week. This client wanted to birth naturally and was terrified by the thought of induction. She promptly burst into tears. I checked her BP reading - 140/80. As an experienced midwife, this did not set off any alarm bells.

I reassured her and showed her the research around maternity BP. I suggested there didn't seem to be any reason to induce, rather it seemed more logical for her to be monitored and observed. After a relaxing reflexology session her BP measured 110/60, extremely good. If there had been a problem the BP would have remained high. With the correct information on board she was able to make a clear choice, as she felt empowered, informed and strong. Refusing induction and the associated risks, she went on to birth naturally and beautifully two weeks later without any problems with her BP.

One of the single most important decisions you will make as a prospective parent, in terms of the outcome of the birth and the potential future health of your child, concerns the choice of caregiver for your pregnancy, labour and birth. Research clearly shows that the attitudes, philosophy and practices of the main caregiver during labour and birth will shape the management of the event and have a huge impact on the quality of the experience for both parents and baby.

> "... a midwife, with a training and philosophy centred on birth as a normal bodily process, approaches assisting a woman in labour differently from a doctor, who tends to view birth from his training

in the medical model of treating illness. A midwife is more likely to assume that the labour is going well unless it is demonstrably not the case, whereas a doctor is more likely to assume there will be a problem and demand proactive intervention, just in case problems occur later."

Exerpt from Robertson, A, 'Empowering Women, Teaching Active Birth in the 90's', 1994, p.64

The thing to know is that proactive intervention does not necessarily prevent problems, but can in fact create them.

Positive Steps to Decision Making

Define the problem by being clear about the nature of it:

- do your research, find out what is available, what information can help you make your decision more easily
- get the facts, don't assume, find reliable sources of advice
- be aware of the beliefs and background of the people you ask for assistance.

What do you want instead?

- once you have an idea of the outcome you want, it is easier to envisage possible pathways towards the goal
- list the pros and cons of your decision and weigh these up.

How can you achieve your goal?

- explore the various avenues available, look for choices, even those not so obvious.

What are your priorities?

- list the priorities that will be affected by this decision
- discuss the decision in depth with your partner, friend or midwife
- form a back up plan, look for the worst scenario and plot a contingency plan that can be used if needed, know what you are most afraid of and what your limitations are.

Let's take the plunge, feel the fear and do it anyway:

- did it work?
- evaluate the outcome - is this what you really want?

Everyone makes mistakes, don't be afraid to try again. Re-evaluate and move to plan B.

Remember Time:

- take time out, re-evaluate
- take time to change the scene
- take time to move
- take time to consider
- take time to seek counsel.

I was called one evening to assist in a labour ward. I wasn't rostered on, but I said yes. On arrival I noticed my clients Alex and Victoria were in one of the labour rooms. At handover the report was that there was foetal distress and the discussion centred on calling the obstetrician to do a caesarean section. I asked to be their primary midwife and to wait on any action until I had time to assess the situation.

Alex and Victoria were so relieved to see a familiar face. Their baby's heart rate was somewhat high and erratic. Having faith in my methods, they relaxed and we put plan B into action. Moving the bed we put Victoria on the floor on a mat, leaning over a ball. Alex was very familiar with natural therapies and homeopathy and pulled the appropriate tools from his bag.

I administered cell salts, massaged Victoria's feet with lavender oil, created a meditation visualisation and darkened the room, relaxing the energy. Baby Raphael's heart rate calmed and Victoria settled into a good labour rhythm. We laboured together as a team overnight and Raphael was born twelve hours later without intervention. Alex and Victoria had hoped I would be on roster. By taking time, re-evaluating, changing the environment and energy, a caesarean section was avoided.

Hormones

Whether your pregnancy was planned or is a complete surprise, the physical and emotional changes can come slowly or may be very strong and overwhelming. The complex hormonal changes alter many body systems to accommodate and nourish your baby and prepare your body for childbirth. High amounts of oestrogen may cause morning sickness. Increasing blood and fluid volumes can cause faintness. Exhaustion may manifest and then be interrupted by sudden bursts of energy.

The hormones that once configured themselves monthly now group together to create and maintain another human life. These hormones form a powerful concoction, resulting in the magnification of emotions and intense thoughts. These feelings are particularly meaningful and need to be explored rather than ignored as just 'moods' due to pregnancy. All these hormones have a role and help to build the bonding and attachment that must develop between the mother and child for the sake of the child's survival.

Pregnancy is probably the time of greatest emotional upheaval for a couple. It is a rite of passage that marks a woman's entrance into adulthood, regardless of age. Pregnancy comes with a myriad of changes, a change of career and perception of self, a change in the couple's relationship if there is a partner and a greater stress for those travelling the path alone.

Oestrogen and progesterone are produced by the corpus luteum until the placenta and the growing baby take over the role of producing these hormones. Levels of these hormones are much higher than in the non-pregnant state. Their role is to ensure the changing body's environment sustains a healthy pregnancy. They are also the main cause for some of the normal variables that occur in pregnancy, such as fluid retention.

Progesterone

Progesterone is a strong attachment hormone and extremely active during pregnancy. Responsible for maintaining the pregnancy and the commencement of labour, progesterone assists the production of the hormone relaxin. Aptly named, relaxin's role is the relaxing of ligaments and connective tissue and facilitating a more flexible pelvis and spine in order to accommodate the growing uterus and the needs required for birth. Relaxin also acts as a vasodilator (causes dilation of the walls of the blood vessels), which can result in feeling dizzy or light-headed in the first few months of pregnancy.

Progesterone assists other hormones including prolactin, which prepares the breasts for breastfeeding and peaks after birth to instigate milk production. Endorphins are produced along with cortisone in response to, as well as creating, emotional changes within the mother in a feedback mechanism. Progesterone also assists in the production of oxytocin (discussed in detail ahead).

Oestrogen

Oestrogen is responsible for the production of progesterone by the corpus luteum during the early weeks of pregnancy and acts as an immune inhibitor, protecting your baby from your immune system during the first trimester. Oestrogen increases and strengthens the lining of the womb so that it may cope with the expansion of pregnancy, support your growing baby and provides support for the strong contractions of labour. Oestrogen also increases the size of the nipples and assists in developing milk glands.

Human Chorionic Gonadotrophin (HCG)

This stimulates the thyroid gland to increase metabolism to assist the body in coping with the extra load of the changing and growing baby. HCG is also important in cell replication and proliferation.

The Role of Oxytocin – The Love Hormone

Increasing use of technology to interfere with the process of natural birth can result in natural hormones being suppressed, leading to long-term problems and risking the future emotional status of the next generation.

For some time there has been acknowledgement of the importance of keeping pregnancy and birth normal in order for the hormones to complete the role they were originally designed to do. Oxytocin is one of the most important hormones involved with the evolution of humanity, the unsung hero of reproduction. Without it we would not have the impetus to continue our species.

Oxytocin is the hormone that ensures our survival through creating the love, connection and unification as a community. No matter how singular we become as a race the deeper tribal urge to be with others is always present. It is the epitome of altruistic love. Any positive interaction with another human being creates oxytocin. When you meet an old friend in the street and feel that welcoming surge of warmth that is oxytocin.

Oxytocin is in full force when we gather to eat and socialise together. It creates that warm fuzzy feeling when you curl up with a loved one on the couch, or sit playing a game with a child. Oxytocin is activated from the moment of the first signs of attraction to another, to the deep connection of love-making. It is released by touch, stimulation of the breasts, vagina, clitoris, cervix and is the hormone of birth.

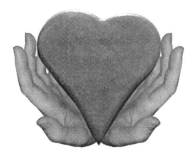

Oxytocin is Responsible For:

- the after glow following love-making and creating the feeling of well-being after an orgasm
- triggering bonding and care taking patterns in both men and women
- sperm and ovary production whilst ensuring the motility of the fallopian tubes for sperm transport
- the in-sucking of the uterus to catch the sperm
- assisting motility of the ovum to meet the sperm at conception
- keeping the cervix closed during pregnancy
- uterine contractions which help the uterus develop during pregnancy and then the more powerful expulsive contractions of labour
- expulsion of the placenta through contractions post-delivery
- initiating bonding between mother and baby
- involution of the uterus following birth to return it to normal size
- initiating milk ejection from the breasts for the initial feed following delivery
- maintaining breastfeeding and milk production.

Oxytocin Increases:

- at around 32 weeks when the baby moves into the lower uterine segment in preparation for labour

- as the baby moves further into the pelvis and onto the cervix
- when the membranes surrounding the baby break, increasing the intensity of labour to complete the first stage of labour
- at the end of first stage of labour (transition), clearing the way for the baby to be birthed by the stronger and more direct contractions of second stage
- when the baby's head stretches the perineum during crowning, increasing the intensity of contractions to help push the baby out
- following birth, signalling the placenta to begin to shutdown and to shear away, giving mum the urge to push so as to ensure strong contractions for delivery of the placenta
- helping mum become alert to ensure the bonding process begins.

Ways to Stimulate Oxytoxin Production:

- relaxation
- visualisation
- affirmations
- soft gentle words
- caressing massage, kissing, cuddling
- orgasm

- vaginal stretch
- clitoral stimulation
- pressure on the cervix
- stretching of the pelvic floor muscles
- perineal massage
- nipple stimulation

Inhibitors to Oxytocin Production:

- stressful thoughts
- worry/fear/anxiety
- external stimuli such as the environment and relationships around the woman
- internal stimuli such as fear, doubts, past experiences and memories

- anaesthetic injections numb the natural reflex of the perineum
- artificial induction or augmentation of labour
- episiotomy removes the stretch trigger of the perineum

- separation of mother and baby
- sexual abuse

- deep emotional conditioning or trauma
- anger

Lack of Oxytocin Can Cause:

- an inability to create warm loving relationships
- an inability to achieve orgasm
- slow labour
- slow dilation
- prolonged second stage of labour

- post-partum haemorrhage
- breastfeeding problems
- lack of bonding and parental protective behaviours
- isolative behaviour

Physical Changes

Uterus

Non-pregnant uterus	8 cm x 5 cm x 2.5 cm - 60 grams
Pregnant uterus	38 cm x 25 cm x 20 cm - 1000 grams

The uterus is a hollow, muscular organ of pregnancy, shaped like a pear with the narrow end pointing down. It starts to enlarge at around the sixth week. The first sixteen weeks of uterine growth is due to tissue enlargement stimulated by oestrogens. The uterus becomes thick walled and almost circular, constantly contracting from the moment of conception until a few weeks after birth. From twenty weeks tissue growth almost ceases and the increase in size is due to stretching of the uterine wall from the growth of the baby. As it enlarges the uterus rises up out of the pelvis. Towards the end of pregnancy the lower part softens (forming the lower uterine segment), helping to mould baby's head into a smaller size for birth and allowing baby to sink lower into the pelvis, eventually engaging at around 36 weeks. The number and size of blood vessels increases along with the size of the uterus. The cervix becomes softer and the glands secrete mucous which forms a plug to act as a barrier to infection. This plug comes away in the last few days before labour, often referred to as a 'show'.

Placenta
The placenta is the anchor that attaches the baby to the uterine wall. It is the transportation system for oxygen, carbon dioxide, nutrients, waste and hormone production. Acting as a barrier protecting the baby, the placenta is fully developed by 14 weeks and on average weighs 600grams at birth, or one sixth of the infant's weight.

Metabolism
In the first trimester you can become very tired as your metabolism works overtime adjusting your system to the new growth. Your baby is fully formed by twelve weeks so there is an incredible amount of change that occurs in that time. By the second trimester most women, if well nourished and rested, are physically and emotionally adjusted to pregnancy and usually enjoy a feeling of well being. Metabolism increases anywhere from ten to twenty percent in the second half of pregnancy due to the demands of your growing baby and maternal tissues. A section discussing nutritional needs has been included in this book.

Ovaries
Once conception has taken place ovulation ceases and the corpus luteum or 'yellow body' is now empty. The corpus luteum now produces the hormones to maintain pregnancy for the first six to ten weeks, until the placenta takes over the role of hormone secretion. The ovaries and tubes rise upwards as the uterus enlarges.

Vagina
The vagina becomes softer, more supple and sensitive and changes to a deep pink or even bluish purple colour. Blood supply and mucous secretion increase due to higher oestrogen production. Increased blood flow to the

area may increase the chances of vaginal varicose (unusually swollen or enlarged veins). The increase in vaginal secretions and a change in PH can create a higher risk of infection. Symptoms of infection aren't always apparent during pregnancy as the hormones of pregnancy can mask them. It is very important throughout your pregnancy to maintain good gut health to ward off unwanted bacteria as this is essential to maintaining good immune status. I suggest reduced sugar intake, eating healthy fermented foods such as yoghurt and taking high quality probiotics.

Clitoris

The clitoris can become highly sensitive, resulting in many women preferring a less direct approach during love-making.

Kidneys/Bladder

Throughout your pregnancy you can expect to wee more often than has been usual for you. This is due to the ever increasing load placed on your kidneys as your baby grows. This increase is particularly noticeable later in pregnancy.

Ligaments

The hormones of pregnancy allow softening of the ligaments to accommodate the growing baby and assist in delivery. Lack of exercise and tone may lead to the ligaments becoming over stretched and weakened, which can lead to back, hip and joint pain. Good posture, supportive shoes and regular exercise such as yoga, swimming and pilates can help.

Skin

Hormonal changes increase the melanin production of the skin and the sweat and sebaceous glands become more active. As your abdomen enlarges, you may find your skin itchy due to dryness. It is great to pamper yourself with massages, crèmes and oils, which may also prevent stretch marks.

I recommend coconut oil as it seems to help in preventing stretch marks. Pigmentation may appear, especially a dark line from the navel to the pubis known as the Linca Nigra. This pigmentation generally disappears after birth.

Blood Volume

From around week ten of pregnancy there is a surge of hormones to relax the arterial walls. This facilitates an increase in blood volume in order to supply the enlarging organs, placenta and especially the uterus. Blood pressure drops quite markedly, resulting in many women feeling light headed and some may even faint. From mid-pregnancy your uterus will use twenty five percent of your circulating blood.

As the blood supply increases blood pressure returns to normal. Iron is a very important component of this system. One third of your iron supply passes to your baby, so it is essential you replace this iron with nutritional iron from a good diet rather than taking iron supplements, as taking the supplement may actually create high blood pressure (the opposite effect).

See Anaemia in the 'Complimentary Therapies For Discomforts of Pregnancy' section for more suggestions. Also see Ferritin in 'Tests During Pregnancy'.

Circulation

The average pregnant body can retain at least an extra seven litres of water by the end of pregnancy. Many women find they suffer from circulation problems with Carpal Tunnel Syndrome being the most distressing. Varicose veins are common, especially with women who are on their feet all day. At night rest your legs by lying on the floor with the legs up the wall, support your back with a cushion, don't cross legs when sitting and wear support stockings. Women who have fortnightly reflexology treatments usually avoid circulation problems or varicose veins. I highly recommend Pure which contains 92 ionic minerals and trace elements essential to life (see Complimentary Therapies for Discomforts of Pregnancy for more details).

Breasts

Breast changes can be one of the first signs of pregnancy, with a sense of fullness, a tingling feeling and discomfort when touched. Breasts usually enlarge quickly and there does seem to be a sequence of changes common to most women.

Week 3-4	prickling and tingling
Week 6	breasts enlarged and tender, areola (the coloured circle around your nipple) develops
Week 8	surface veins are visible with little nodules (Montgomery's' tubercles) appearing in the areola. Sebaceous glands secrete sebum to keep nipples soft and supple.
Week 12	darkening of the areola, particularly in dark skinned women, often fluid can be expressed from the nipples and is an excellent thing to practice in preparation for breastfeeding
Week 16	colostrum can be expressed by some women and a secondary areola appears. It is thought that oestrogen is responsible for growth and progesterone for production and secretion.

Your breasts can become quite enlarged and heavy by the time of birth, usually returning to their normal size after a couple of months of feeding. In some cases breasts can even become smaller as fatty tissue is replaced with milk creating glands. Touching and exposing your breasts to fresh air helps you become familiar with them in readiness for breastfeeding.

Weight Gain

Weight Gain in pregnancy is expected and totally normal. On average, by the time you give birth you will likely way 12-13kg more than you did before pregnancy. A third of this weight gain is created from the baby, the placenta and amniotic fluid. The other two thirds comes from the extra blood volume, weight of the uterus, extra ligaments and muscle, overall increase in fluid and the extra weight of the breasts. You will naturally store extra fat in readiness for breastfeeding. So it stands to reason that breastfeeding is the best way to rid that extra fat gain - another great incentive to naturally feed your baby.

Emotional Changes

Pregnancy can be a time of great sensitivity and heightened emotions. Acknowledging and expressing your feelings is healthy for you and your baby. Through my work as a Psychosomatic Therapist I have come to understand that many long term emotional imbalances can stem from the time in the womb. When you acknowledge and express how you truly feel this allows emotion (energy in motion) to be released, creating a more harmonious environment for your growing baby.

There are large adjustments to be made - changing body image and shape, the impending responsibility of caring for a child and the role of parenting, financial burdens and fear about labour and birth.

Pregnancy is a time of emotional cleansing, renewing for the new life. You may find you are dealing with many emotional blocks from the parenting you received as a child. Pregnancy is a time when you need to be nurtured and cared for with a good support system from understanding women who listen to your concerns. A good midwife (meaning with women) or doula can provide this role.

You may experience changed feelings about sexuality, relationship, loss of libido, change of career - especially older mums with established lives. Whether your pregnancy was planned or not may affect your emotional state.

I encourage fortnightly sessions of Maternity Reflexology and Psychosomatic Therapy, which not only provides relaxation and detoxification but an opportunity to discuss any concerns or fears with your therapist in an open and caring environment. There are many reflexologists trained in pregnancy care http://www.reflexology.org.au/home2/

Partners also need to be nurtured as they are the closest to you, whilst experiencing their own insecurities and emotions. They are trying to support and understand you when you may be struggling to understand yourself. If there are relationship issues, now is a very important time to seek help and guidance.

Fear is a real issue for women during pregnancy as they face the concept of labour, birth and parenting - an unknown paradigm. The amount of information readily available can create confusion and unnecessary concerns. Sometimes I think the less women know the more instinctual and natural the pregnancy and birth.

It is so important not to dismiss your feelings of concern and fear, but to expand them and tease them out to get to the bottom of where they are coming from. Memories and feelings of relationships with your own mother and father will surface. Our parents or early carers are our first role models, and many women will judge their own expectant performance on these first role models.

Many feelings of pregnancy cannot be explained and in some ways this is preparation for the unexpected challenges of parenting. Some women express how out of control they feel as their body automatically goes about the development of their child. These feelings are to be expected and welcomed as they rise again and again as a mother copes with the spontaneous upheaval a child brings.

This is a time when as a woman you will become attuned to your body. Talking and communicating is a must for every woman. For couples it is important that you both invest some time clarifying whether your anxieties about having a child are motivated by a true readiness to bond with your little one. During the earliest stages of a baby's life in utero, a profound connection can be instilled between you and your child. Psychological and biological studies show that a first-trimester baby possesses enough self-awareness to sense their mother's emotions.

When emotions are locked up and pushed down, your body and in turn your baby, can feel stressed. This is discussed in greater detail in the section 'Complimentary Therapies and Remedies'.

Having a baby is a normal event in life - it is not an illness and it requires co-ordination of mind and body. As the mother your state of mind and sense of calmness and security is essential. Hopefully you will emerge from the experience joyful, full of pride and satisfaction.

Choosing Your
Place of Birth

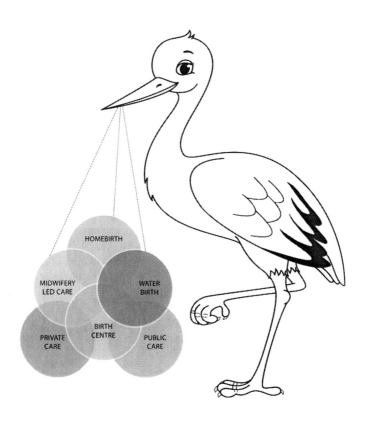

The antenatal care you choose will generally depend upon your choice of birth place. It is important to know what choices are available in your area. Homebirth is a viable choice in Australia, however finding a midwife who is willing to work with you may be a challenge in some locations. You can contact your local homebirth group, the local midwives, birth centre and private and public hospitals for information. I have provided a list of helpful <u>websites</u> at the back of this book.

The issues surrounding each birth choice are discussed in more detail in the <u>Labour and Birth</u> section where an outline is provided of what each option provides. Australia's federal government has moved to provide more choice for women to enlist an independent midwife as their main carer funded by Medicare. Not many midwives have taken up this option due to the high cost of insurance but still this is a great move forward for birthing women. The Australian College of Midwives has been working hard to give women the option to birth with a midwife, which is how it should be.

Thanks to the Foundation for the Advancement of Midwifery, funding is being provided for increasing numbers of women in the United States to have access to midwifery led care. Their website explains how they operate and why, and may provide a good model for increasing funding for Australian women who might otherwise miss out on the opportunity to experience midwifery led care.

http://www.foundationformidwifery.org/

Choosing Your Birth Carer

"Research is showing increasingly that the things that make the most difference to improving the outcome of labour are not technological advances, but feeling comfortable about the place in which you give birth and the human support you have at the time."

Nicky Wesson, 'Quote of the Week'.
Midwifery Today E-News 2(24).

Prior to the development of modern maternity units, homebirth was the norm. This was a place where women felt comfortable and safe. Birthing was primarily the responsibility of women hence the phrase 'women's business'.

Women surrounded themselves with the wise women of the community who provided encouragement, physical comfort, emotional support and most of all a belief in the ability of the woman to birth her baby as nature intended.

There was little medicalisation of birth but rather a strong connection with herbal lore, the mystery of life, connection to the lunar cycle and a faith and trust in the birthing process. New mothers were supported and honoured with the attending women remaining with the mother for several days following the birth, guiding and assisting her in her new role. From the moment girls began menstruating they celebrated their puberty and were taken into the circle of women, being then surrounded by birthing women and the talk of other women's experiences. There was no mystery or fear of a process so natural.

So what has happened in our society? The majority of women now give birth in a hospital, devoid of familiarity and intimacy. The wise, wondrous, patient midwife has been replaced by electronic equipment. Whilst there are still many traditional midwives available they are becoming less as the obstetric nurse takes her place.

Throughout her life a woman is subjected to media interpretations of birth. Instead of embracing the prospect of birth women are led to fear the experience, looking for easy ways to avoid it if possible. Women's knowledge has become based on what the experts have to say rather than trusting their own intuition.

The ancient wisdom of the generations of women gone before is lost. The fear of losing a child becomes so great that women hold the experts in awe as the ones to ensure the safety of their child. Although there is much knowledge and assistance available from wise women, birthing women tend to be so caught up in the medical system of birth that they are not aware of or do not seek out this knowledge. There is a trend towards intellectual thinking rather than a trust in the messages from their own body, a lack of trust in their own gut feelings (intuition or inner tutor).

Often childbirth classes are focused on information and the physical stages of birth, when what a woman really needs to know is how to connect with her body and her baby so that the two can work together in unison. Giving birth in hospital was instigated by male medics, supported by elite society as the intellectual human moved further away from their earth connections, trusting the mind and forgetting the body.

Misinformation is common and the majority of people believe birth away from a hospital is fraught with danger even though there is so much evidence supporting the safety of homebirth when attended by an experienced midwife.

During the postnatal period women are instructed and taught by strangers who often give conflicting advice. Frequently women are discharged and sent home within 48 hours of the birth with little support. The majority of women do not have the opportunity to witness another woman giving birth and have little contact with newborns to observe and learn mothering skills from others.

The developed countries that have the lowest mortality and morbidity statistics are those, such as the Netherlands, where the majority of births take place at home under midwife care. Although statistically fewer women die in childbirth today, there is much evidence to suggest the drop in mortality rates is due to many reasons including improved lifestyles and nutrition, not necessarily the move to hospital birth.

Why is it that people feel compelled to take away the experience of labour from a woman when it can be the most profound of her life? High level athletes and performers go through immense pain in perfecting their craft but spectators and supporters would never dream of stopping them and lending a hand. A birthing woman falls into the same category, she is running the marathon of her life and how she fares will impact upon her whole life as a parent. Natural birth advocates continue to etch away at the medical system, providing statistics that support natural birth and the need for one on one midwife centered care.

Worldwide statistics tell us that ninety percent of women are capable of birthing normally without complications. So why do women choose so much intervention? The experience is far more traumatic with higher levels of perineal damage, postnatal complications and, as Michel Odent is confirming through his research bank, long-term relationship problems for the next generation.

The Industrialisation of Birth

The practice of midwifery has a history as long as we have been reproducing. The word midwife means 'with woman'. Traditionally women gave birth with women and it was society's belief that women were more than capable of giving birth without assistance. The fact that humanity exists in the population numbers it does is testimony to this.

The midwife was a respected member of the community. She carried and used different tools to assist the process that worked in alignment with the natural ebb and flow of birth such as aromatherapy, reflexology, herbs, body movements and homeopathy. Most midwives were also the tribal medicine women who worked in attunement with Mother Nature and in traditional societies today still do. The downfall of the midwife came with the growth of the Christian and puritan religions who believed that women were evil temptresses.

During the industrial revolution around the 13th century midwives sadly were portrayed in a dim-light, often seen as drunken, slovenly, outcaste women struggling to make a living. The local surgeon became esteemed in the eyes of the people. The surgeon's knife was for males only and midwife's were viewed with a down the nose tolerance. As these tools of the trade became more prevalent the surgeons realized their potential to make money. The growth of intervention in obstetrics was inevitable. Around the 15th century surgeons began to teach the methods of extraction and version (turning the baby). Men were deemed to have the more intellectual and alert mind than women so things of this nature were left to the male to perform. Less and less midwives were called to the aid of birthing women throughout the aristocracy.

During the 16th century Peter Chamberlain developed the first set of forceps. Kept secret for almost a hundred years, these forceps became the tool of the male midwives in the 17th century. Many more women died at the hands of their misuse than fared well. Because male midwives charged a higher fee, their service became akin to the higher social status of societies rich. Interestingly it was also around this time that the need for intervention soared amongst birthing women. This was mainly due to too many pregnancies, lack of hygiene and low nutritional status. It was during this period that the refining of grains was introduced. With this invention came a major reduction in essential vitamins and minerals. Cities bulged at the seams with more and more people cramming into smaller housing with very poor sanitary conditions. Formal training of anatomy and physiology began around this time, leading to medical training at the exclusion of women.

The plot thickens. Following the introduction of anesthesia things changed immensely. Queen Victoria was the first woman to use chloroform for the birth of her child, increasing its attraction. As more and more women were given chloroform the need for forceps increased because they were lying down, not involved in the birth and unable to push. This led to the need for more medically trained men to be present at births. And so began the medical model of birthing. Three hundred years later we still face the challenge of medicalised birthing.

Over the next couple of centuries modern medicine spread and evolved, with increasing scientific involvement. Women became less in tune with the forces of nature. Strong religious beliefs added puritanical approaches to life. The feminine mystic was closeted away, no longer discussed. Women became the possessions of males to be adorned and displayed. Wet nurses and nannies were employed so women had less time to commit to mothering. It was the loss of an art in the aristocratic world.

The introduction of hospital birthing is a relatively new phenomena introduced around the 1920's to the industrialized world. But it wasn't until the 1950's that it became the norm. Following the Second World War a great materialistic wave took hold. Houses became decadent, bigger, crisp and clean with every conceivable modern appliance that could be found. There was almost an emphasis on sterility, anything natural was viewed with contempt as if plunging the onlooker back into a time of struggle.

Women were no longer deemed the expert in mothering and scientists discovered what was best for the next generation of children. Pregnancy and birth were seen through the eyes of the scientist, a state of medical attention. Then the introduction of stirrups gave the busy, efficient doctor full control. It was also around this time that artificial feeding became the norm as inaccurate scientific research canned the benefits of breast-feeding. Breastfeeding was not a fashionable thing to do. Further and further people moved away from skin to skin contact. The only way most experienced touch and caressing was during lovemaking. The demise of the midwife had occurred. She was now the handmaiden to the doctor, more a nurse than a midwife, and in some states of America was outlawed.

After the flamboyant and radical changes of the 1960's women began to take back their power and their body's. Many no longer listened to what the 'experts' had to say but found solicitude with like minded people and a chance to reconnect with the essence of their being. A rise in homebirths took place. Imagine the horror of the medical world who saw this as people being irresponsible. The hippie revolution took hold, swinging the pendulum back to the earth mother. Wonderful midwives appeared such as Ida May Gaskin, whose spiritual midwifery book is still in print some fifty years later, with her wonderful use of terms such as 'rush' for contraction, 'fanny' and the discovery of kissing for relaxation of the cervix.

Then the medical fraternity fought back. In the 1970's narcotics were introduced to stem the pain of labour. Little research was undertaken and the long-term side effects were not known, yet so began the intervention journey. Obstetricians are trained to focus their attention on the abnormalities that can occur, therefore when dealing with a normal healthy pregnancy may be more likely to rely on interventionist techniques. Midwives on the other hand are trained to see birth more as a natural event requiring no intervention in the majority of cases. Midwives' experience of birth is one of a delicate but strong spiritual connection between mother and baby.

"How can we expect a physician to handle the unusual delivery
when he has not been trained to allow the normal delivery?"
Maggie Banks, RM, *Breech Birth, Woman Wise*.
Hamilton, NZ (1998) Birth Spirit Books Ltd

The 1980's saw the introduction of the Active Birth concept as midwives such as Janet Balaskas and Sheila Kitzinger became strong advocates for the return of the natural birth. Women were encouraged to get up and get active to help themselves. More women began and continue to experience natural births under midwifery care. High levels of intervention still continue under obstetrical care. Higher numbers of inductions and caesarean sections are happening now than ever before as women are encouraged to choose these interventions by their obstetrician. Currently a woman holding private health insurance is more likely to seek out obstetric care and in some areas has up to an eighty percent higher chance of intervention during her birth experience. There are some obstetricians who are excellent midwives and women need to be informed so they can choose wisely who will care for them during their birth and labour.

Three Wise Women

Do you know what would have happened if it had been
three wise women instead of three wise men?
They would have asked for directions, arrived on time,
helped deliver the baby, cleaned the stable, made a casserole
and brought practical gifts.
Be bold, be proud.
Persist in spreading the word that midwives are not only experts
In normal birth but also expert at keeping birth normal.
Judy Edmunds CPM, *Midwifery Today* 2(2), 2000

Homebirth

When deciding whether a homebirth is right for you, you need to consider if you have enough support following the birth, such as a supportive partner, family or friends. Homebirth is still controversial in Australia due to ignorance and out-dated information, complicated by the inability of midwives to get adequate insurance. Most homebirth researchers state clearly that statistically homebirths are safer than hospital due to less use of intervention, a greater knowledge of the birthing woman's needs and the high level of experience homebirth midwives have.

Homebirth requires a trust in the natural process of birth and provides:

- the freedom to express yourself in your own environment without the disruption of moving to an alien environment
- freedom from hospital policy and restrictions
- continuity of care with a midwife of choice, who will stay with you if you do need to transfer to the hospital for delivery
- respect of your wishes, beliefs and cultural needs
- individual care with a highly skilled midwife
- privacy and intimacy
- safety with less likelihood of unnecessary interventions or staff you may not gel with
- close monitoring with a midwife who knows you and is able to assess changes to the normal progress of labour more efficiently than in a busy hospital labour ward where you may be one of many
- more rest - women express that they are able to rest more as there are less interruptions and noise at home than in hospital
- parents with an easier bonding time, with less distractions and less interference from many carers.

www.homebirthaustralia.org

30

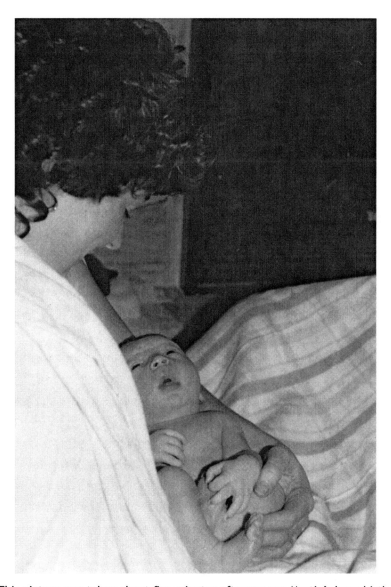

This picture was taken about five minutes after my son Martin's homebirth.

Water Birth

The benefits and safety of warm water as pain relief in labour and birth are well researched and documented. Hopefully we will see water birth become a common practice as it can considerably reduce the intensity of labour. When a labouring woman enters a bath at body temperature there is immediate pain relief, which is probably associated with a reduced level of endorphins and catecholamines. You only have to experience how a bath can make you feel when you have an aching back or limbs from doing too much vigorous exercise to understand how this can benefit you during labour.

It has been my experience that water is a key component in helping to relieve the intensity of contractions, whether it is in a shower, bath or water pool. The bath can be of great benefit depending on how large the bath and the birthing mum are. Most women need to submerge their whole body up to their arm pits to get good relief, but not all baths afford this luxury. If there is a separate portable shower head, I have found encouraging mum to run the water over her pubic bone during a contraction brings great relief.

Using a birth ball to sit on in the shower is an excellent way to take control of your labour, especially if you have a hand held shower head so you can direct the spray of water onto your body. Partners can join you in the shower and provide support and extra energy.

The Birth Pool is probably the absolute best option as it allows enough space for mother and partner to be in the bath together or for the mother to fully stretch out, allowing the water of the bath to take her weight. Most privately practicing midwives have access to birthing pools that can be hired by couples for their own birth. Alternatively, blow up pools of about waist high depth (when you are sitting) are a worthwhile purchase and can be used for the children to play in later. You will need to hire a submergence heater to maintain water heat otherwise you will use a lot of hot water.

Water is not an option in all birthing suites so it is important you explore what is available when deciding where you want to give birth and if the service is open to you bringing in your own water pool. Be sure to allow the necessary time it takes to fill the pool, as some women deliver before the pool is ready. Also find out what the birthing policies are in regard to water birth, as many units in Australia require that you leave the water for delivery, even though research supports the claim that birthing in water is very safe. Most of the women I have assisted tend to leave the water for the birth, or have semi squatted using the edges of the pool for leverage, as they have needed the added assistance of gravity by having their feet firmly on the ground to push.

Most water births happen at home, and whilst some birthing units are allowing the use of water pools others provide deep baths and water tanks within their units. Find out what's available by talking to your local Homebirth group or Independent Midwives group.

In Australia a good source of information is:

www.bellybelly.com.au/birth/waterbirth-in-australia

The risk of infection is an issue well discussed amongst water birth opponents. A study of 1385 women with premature rupture of membranes after 34 weeks of gestation evaluated the risk of infection in mothers and neonates, with 538 women in the first stage of labour taking a bath while 847 did not (Eriksson et al., 1996). These women were given 24-72 hours to establish labour before being induced with Oxytocin. Vaginal exam was avoided during this time until labour was well established. The study concluded that a tub bath did not increase the risk of maternal or neonatal infection even after premature rupture of the membranes and prolonged latency.

Twice as many first time mothers (57%) left the pool prior to delivery compared to multi-birth mothers (43%). The midwives did realise that the first time mums were often asking to leave during transition and after this they encouraged the mothers to stay in the water and they appeared to cope better. Sixty eight percent of the induced labours delivered in the pool, a high level considering this group is at a high risk of requiring pain relief.

The outcome of the study suggested that a woman should not enter the pool under 5cm dilated as entering prior to this has the opposite effect of slowing down the labour. Apgar scores were excellent in 99.7% of babies. Forty six percent of the women experienced intact perineum with the rest experiencing first and second degree tears that healed within a few days.

Timing is very important. When a woman has been in the pool for more than two hours it may slow labour and decrease the efficiency of contractions. Thus, as Michele Odent points out, the timing of immersion in the water during labour must be taken into account as it can make a big difference (Journal of Nurse-Midwifery, 1997).

Another earlier but very valid study looked at the outcomes of water births over a three-year period (1994-1996) at Good Hope, NHS Trust, Birmingham, England (Brown, 1998). 1082 women indicated antenatal that they wished to use the pool during labour. 541 actually entered the pool and 343 delivered in the pool, including 10 vaginal birth after caesarean section (VBAC). Mothers who chose to enter the water pools experienced good outcomes.

Overall this study indicated the great benefit of water in assisting mothers to have a less painful labour and a more gentle birth for their babies. Women expressed their pleasure in using the pool and how they felt in control of their birth experience. The British Journal of Midwifery concluded that water birth is a very safe option (April 1998, no.4, pp236-243).

August, 1999, the British Medical Journal published an unprecedented study about the perinatal mortality and morbidity among babies delivered in water (Gilbert & Tookey). This study is authoritative for several reasons:

1. conclusions are based on large numbers: the authors traced 4,032 babies born under water in England and Wales between April 1994 and March 1996
2. the authors belong to a prestigious department of epidemiology and public health (Institute of Child Health, London, United Kingdom)
3. the report has been published in a respected peer review medical journal.

The main recommendations of the study:

- women should enter the water after 5cm dilated; this will speed up labour and reduce the need for pain relief
- the water needs to be the same temperature as the women's body never above 37 degrees.

"At the dawn of a new phase in the history of childbirth one can anticipate that, if a small number of simple recommendations are taken into account, the use of water during labour will seriously compete with epidural anaesthesia. Then helping women to be patient enough and enter the pool at the right time will appear as a new aspect of the art of midwifery."

A Landmark in the History of Birthing Pools,
Michel Odent, MD, 2000 Midwifery Today, Inc.

Birth Centre

If you aren't comfortable with homebirth but the philosophy suits your needs, a birth centre is a good compromise. Most birth centres are conducted by midwives and can be free standing centres separate from but close to the local maternity unit, or run as a separate unit within the maternity unit. Because they are run by midwives they have a philosophy of natural birth principles and generally do not provide intervention. If women need medical intervention they are transferred to the closest labour ward for care.

Birth centres provide an apartment style or home style setting, providing furniture and queen size beds so that couples may live together for the duration of time they hire the centre, usually over a 24-48hr period. Partners are very welcome and stay with the birthing woman following the birth. Some Birth Centres can be hired by the couple along with the midwife of choice. Once the birth is over the midwives continue to provide postnatal home care for mother and baby for a week or two.

Other centres are managed by a team of midwives, which the couple meet throughout their pregnancy and the midwife who cares for them during the labour and birth will depend on who is on roster. The aim is still continuity of care but within a team focus. Care continues after the birth.

Most Birth Centres have restrictions and guidelines that the midwives and couple must comply with. Some common guidelines are as follows;

- birth must take place within 24hrs of admittance to the unit
- the woman must be low risk and under 35 years of age
- the woman must not have experienced a previous difficult labour, birth or caesarean
- any signs of complications, for example hypertension or foetal distress, requires transfer to a medically managed birth
- most birth centres do not allow water births but do use water in labour via showers to help mother manage her contractions.

Midwifery Led Care

Many Australian hospitals have started rolling out primary midwifery models of care. These are employed midwives who are assigned a case load, where they look after you as a primary care midwife. They provide antenatal care by visiting you at home throughout your pregnancy and early labour, providing birth care at the local hospital and then postnatal home care following the birth.

This is an excellent program, one that will hopefully take off and become the norm as it is in New Zealand, where the majority of woman are looked after by a primary care midwife whether birthing at home or in hospital. The Australian College of Midwives (ACM 2012) reported that an Australian study of 2314 women found that women who received care from a primary 'known' midwife rather than the fragmented standard care had better outcomes, including a 22% reduction in caesarean rate. The recommendation by Australian government ministers that the professional indemnity insurance exemption for privately practicing midwives be extended until June 2015 allows midwives to continue to collaborate with other health providers, thus providing a high degree of safety and quality of care for expectant mothers (ACM 2012).

The Know Your Midwife Scheme (KYM)

This is a team structured midwifery program in a hospital setting. The team of five midwives are the primary carers for you throughout your pregnancy under the guidance of the resident doctor, or in the private hospitals by your obstetrician of choice. Your labour and birth are conducted within the general labour/delivery suite. The main advantage is the provision of continuity of care by the team of midwives with one of them being on roster to look after the labouring woman during the birth. Again the midwives follow guidelines and restrictions created by the policies of the hospital they are working in. Once you have birthed, you will transfer to the general postnatal ward where you will be looked after by the postnatal staff or the KYM team will continue care, depending on the policy of the hospital.

Private Care

Privately insured women have a choice of obstetrician care during their pregnancy, choice of which private hospital they will give birth in, and once booked in will be cared for by the midwives rostered on duty that day. The obstetrician as the primary carer will drop in from time to time to check on progress and will be called for the birth.

It is generally the obstetrician who dictates the type of care the woman receives, with the delivery unit having guidelines regarding their preferences for procedures and care. The maternity unit midwives still do the majority of care during the labour whilst keeping in contact with the obstetrician. It is important to understand that research indicates that on average privately insured women are eighty percent more likely to undergo some form of medical intervention under obstetric care compared to midwifery led care.

This is one of the reasons I created my midwifery care practice with the focus on privately insured women. Years of working in private maternity units gave me insight into a missing component of care for these women. Even though they felt they were receiving an above average level of care, they tended to be less educated about options, therapies and techniques that could make pregnancy and birth easier, and so ran a higher risk of intervention and caesarean birth.

I provide comprehensive antenatal care alongside their obstetric care. Women receive nurturing, education and increased confidence, enhancing their experience and increasing their chances of a natural birth. My pregnant clients visit for an hour once a fortnight for reflexology and massage, which allows time for discussion and education. I also provide an intensive Childbirth Class focused on the partners. My aim is to ensure women are in the right frame of mind and body by the time they give birth so they are able to relax and let go, allowing nature to do what it knows how to do best. I am supported by several local obstetricians who send their clients to me as they realise it makes their work easier. I have had great success turning breech babies, which is discussed later.

Public Care

Generally women who do not hold private insurance are cared for by the local maternity unit. Mothers will likely be seen throughout pregnancy in the antenatal clinic by midwives and doctors on roster, so there is little continuity of care and you may only see a doctor during pregnancy for two or three regular checks. The birth takes place in the general labour ward under the care of the rostered midwives. Most are seen by the doctor on duty but mainly left to the care of the midwife. The resident doctor is kept informed of progress and most women have good birth outcomes because they are looked after by midwives.

Tests During Pregnancy

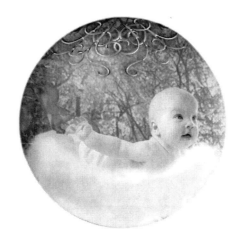

There are a number of tests that may be carried out during pregnancy. It is essential to understand that all must have your consent first. This section helps you to make an informed decision about these tests by providing a thorough understanding of their purpose and implications.

Antenatal Visit Assessments

Abdominal Palpation
Generally done at every visit, the skilled birth attendant can gather much information from this technique. The caregiver feels the outside of the abdomen, to assess the height of the fundus (uterus) and the position and size of the baby. Generally the abdomen will be measured to ensure your baby is progressing within normal growth range.

Weight
Routine weighing is no longer recommended. It was introduced into antenatal care in London during the Second World War to detect poor nutrition. Routine weighing is of less importance today, other than as part of an overall health assessment. Underweight women have increased risk of complications such as pre-term or low infant birth weight. Overweight women have a higher risk of gestational diabetes, hypertension and large babies causing birth complications. Maintaining a healthy lifestyle is more important to a healthy pregnancy outcome.

Urine
Your health care professional will be looking for three main things when doing a urine test:

Sugar to eliminate the risk of gestational diabetes. It can be quite normal to have traces of sugar in the urine but if sugar keeps testing positive then it is important to follow up with 24 hour glucose tolerance tests to check for Gestational Diabetes which can be harmful to you and your baby.

Protein can be a sign of a urine infection or kidney imbalances. Later in pregnancy may be a sign of pre-eclampsia if accompanied with high blood pressure or excess fluid retention.

Ketones are a by-product of energy metabolism from stored fats and can be an indication your diet is low in carbohydrates. This can occur if there is severe nausea and vomiting or dietary restrictions resulting in an excessive loss in weight. Maintaining good nutrition and energy in pregnancy is essential. Ketones in combination with sugar may indicate diabetes.

Blood Pressure (see <u>Hypertension</u> in the 'Complimentary Therapies For Discomforts of Pregnancy' section)

Blood pressure is of particular interest in pregnancy due to the increased volume of circulating blood that occurs by the end of the second trimester. The extra load on the body can create tension in the arterial walls, hence the name Hypertension. An average blood pressure for a healthy young woman is around 110/70 to 120/80. The blood pressure does drop during the second trimester due to the relaxation of the arterial walls to allow for the extra circulating blood. It is therefore expected that your blood pressure may be quite low during pregnancy.

Your maternity carer is most interested in the diastolic pressure, the lower of the two readings, as this indicates the pressure at rest within the artery. Having your blood pressure taken regularly indicates what is normal for you. If your blood pressure rises markedly above what would be normal for you then note is taken as this could indicate pre-eclampsia and measures are needed to decrease it. Most health professionals will tell you there is little you can do to reduce your blood pressure, but you will find as you read further into this book there are several well researched methods that have good results.

Foetal Heart

Foetal heart is monitored from around twelve weeks to assess foetal wellbeing. This is probably one of the most soothing sounds you will love hearing during your pregnancy as an indicator that all is well. A stethoscope or hand held Doppler instrument (from 24weeks by Pinards) is used to hear the baby's heartbeat. Don't be surprised by the sound - the normal foetal heart-rate is very fast, between 120 and 160 beats per minute. There is an old midwives' belief that a heart rate around 120 is a boy, above 150 is a girl.

Kick Charts

The American College of Obstetricians and Gynaecologists (ACOG 2013) recommends that you time how long it takes you to feel ten kicks, flutters, swishes or rolls. Ideally, you want to feel at least ten movements within two hours. Most likely you will feel ten movements in much less time. Kick charts are strongly recommended for high risk pregnancies, beginning at 28 weeks. However it is questionable whether it is beneficial or creates more concern for you, as your baby will normally have periods when it is asleep, sometimes lasting as long as four hours. Babies naturally become quieter closer to birth. If at any time you are concerned please check with your maternity carer. It is better to be sure rather than spending time worrying, which is detrimental to both you and your baby.

Pap Smear

This is done at booking in or at the postnatal visit to assess the health of the cervix. Pap smear is recommended as a routine check as the highest rates of cervical abnormalities occur in women of reproductive age and with early detection can be easily treated.

Cardiotocograph (CTG)

Assesses the heart rate and well being of the baby. Foetal heart and movements are monitored for approximately twenty minutes. It is often used twice weekly when the pregnancy is past forty one weeks. Also used throughout labour to assess how the baby is coping with contractions. It can be over used in labour, which can lessen the mother's ability to move about and cause positioning problems for the baby in labour. This is discussed in more detail in the 'Labour and Birth' section of this book.

Some Short Hand Abbreviations

Primagravida	First time pregnancy
Multigravida	Has been pregnant before
Para	Viable pregnancy
BP	Blood pressure
NAD	No abnormality detected
Hb	Haemoglobin levels in blood
Fe	Iron
FHH	Foetal heart heard
FHR	Foetal heart rate
FMF	Foetal movements felt
ROA/LOA	Right or left occipito anterior, baby head down in right or left position
ROP/LOP	Right or left occipito posterior, baby head down but facing backwards
VX	Vertex – means head facing downwards
Br	Breech
Eng/E	Engaged, baby has dropped into pelvis
EDD/EDC	Estimated date of delivery/confinement

Blood

Blood Group

This is precautionary to establish your group in case of the need of transfusion.

Rhesus Factor

Better known as the Rh-ve Blood Group System (Rh+ve and Rh-ve).

If a mother is Rh-ve and the father is Rh+ve there is a chance the baby could be Rh+ve, creating a possible conflict between mother and baby. If somehow the mother's blood is exposed to the baby's blood through the slightest of bleeds, then the mother will create antibodies against the Rh antigen. It will most likey not affect the current pregnancy, but exposes future pregnancies to an antigen-antibody attack which can be very detrimental to subsequent babies. If you are Rh-ve you will receive an injection of Anti-D after the birth of your baby to safeguard future pregnancies.

Full Blood Count

To measure the haemoglobin level, check for anaemia and the white and red cell counts. It is used as a base measurement in case complications arise and to establish if there are any health problems early in pregnancy. A test may also be done to detect sexually transmitted diseases as these can be carried in your body without any symptoms and may be detrimental to your growing baby.

Rubella

Ideally it is recommended that you are checked for Rubella antibodies before you become pregnant so that immunisation can be given as prevention if required. Rubella immunity will be checked in early pregnancy. If your test is negative, meaning you have no antibodies, you are at risk if you come into contact with Rubella and should keep away from people who might have Rubella. Once your baby is born you should be immunised to protect against Rubella in future pregnancies.

Ferritin

Is the protein used by your body to store and release iron in a controlled manner. The iron stored by ferritin is used to make the oxygen carrying component of your red blood cells (haemoglobin). If you have a tendency to have a high turnover of red blood cells, as indicated by high blood loss during menstruation, you may then require a higher than average intake of iron from your diet during pregnancy. Iron is required by your baby, otherwise your iron storage level (your ferritin level) will slowly decrease. If your ferritin level is low and you take supplements, it can take some time to slowly build up because the extra iron you take will probably be diverted by your body for immediate use and for intermediary stages. Only once your daily usage is being met will you start to store the excess iron in the ferritin protein as ferritin is the last-stage storage for excess iron. Despite this, you should feel better within a couple of weeks of taking supplements.

Iron Deficiency Happens in Stages

In early iron deficiency the ferritin level is low because your body has no excess iron to store. At this stage haemoglobin is normal so you are not anaemic. In latent iron deficiency your body starts to churn out more of an iron transport protein, hoping to catch whatever iron might be passing through your digestive system. The haemoglobin is still normal at this stage.

Only in late stage iron deficiency, where your body is very short of iron, does the haemoglobin start to fall. Red blood cells have a life span of about 120 days, so the haemoglobin drops and the onset of anaemia is gradual.

One of the key symptoms is tiredness. Early stage iron deficiency is very common in pregnancy. Avoid drinking tannins such as tea, coffee and wine as these will inhibit the absorption of iron. The type of supplement you take is very important. I have found liquid iron such as Fluradix to be the best, along with Hemagenics IC from Healthworld and Ferrum Phos cell salts. Natural iron supplements are better absorbed by the body.

It is important to note that if you have healthy iron levels taking iron supplements can create an overload, resulting in high viscosity and high blood pressure. A healthy, balanced diet is the best way to ensure a good intake of iron. See nutritional sources.

Antibodies

Antibody tests are done to find certain antibodies that attack red blood cells. Antibodies are proteins made by the immune system. Normally antibodies bind to foreign substances such as bacteria and viruses and cause them to be destroyed. A Coombes test can be undertaken to check for antibodies that may be attacking healthy blood cells. Generally this is done if you have a family history. Taken at booking-in 12wks, 24wks, 32wks and 36wks.

Triple Test / Alpha Feto Protein (AFP)

At fifteen to twenty weeks this test is offered to parents to test for neural tube defects in the baby such as Spina Bifida, which occurs in one in five hundred babies. Also tests for chromosomal disorders such as Down Syndrome which occur in one in six hundred babies, occurring more often in mothers over 35 years of age. The test shows the level of Alpha-Fetoprotein (AFP), Oestriol and Human chorionic gonadotropin (HCG) and detects around eighty five percent of all unborn babies who have neural tube defects and around sixty five percent of unborn babies with Down Syndrome. I have had clients come concerned with a positive Triple Test, meaning a one in two hundred chance they could be carrying a Down Syndrome baby. It is important to understand here that there is also a 199 chance in two hundred that they are not carrying a Down Syndrome baby, which puts a different perspective upon the result. This test does not detect the severity of the disability and is not conclusive, so requires follow up of an amniocentesis for confirmation and ultrasound. Further investigation usually allays any further concerns, but if you do choose to investigate further you need to consider what the results will mean to you and whether you intend to abort or just want to know. Sometimes it is important to know that everything is okay so that the rest of your pregnancy can be continued without concern or worry.

Human Placental Lactogen (HPL)

Assesses foetal well being from about thirty five weeks by assessing blood levels. Low levels may indicate foetal distress.

Chorionic Villus Sampling (CVS)

This test is used to rule out foetal abnormalities, sex-linked diseases and metabolic disorders. Performed at nine to eleven weeks into pregnancy, the accuracy of the procedure is quite valid but if further detail is required an amniocentesis may be requested.

Around three percent of women undergoing CVS will require an amniocentesis due to a failure to obtain good laboratory results. CVS early in pregnancy allows a termination to be performed (if requested) before the pregnancy is noticeable and before the mother feels the baby moving. This is safer for the mother at this stage than it is at a later point in the pregnancy and can be done in a Day Surgery Unit without requiring an overnight admission to a hospital.

CVS The Procedure

CVS can be performed via a needle through the abdomen (trans-abdominal) or by using a small plastic catheter through the cervix.

The trans-abdominal method is a similar experience to amniocentesis. Using a needle similar to that used for giving an injection, a tiny sample is taken from the developing placenta and then examined under a microscope to ensure enough cells have been gathered to give a valid result. The specialist undertaking the procedure observes positioning of the needle closely on an ultrasound.

The cervix method involves a biopsy of the tissue of the chorionic villus, the finger like projections in the lining of the uterus that grow to become the placenta. A catheter is passed into the vagina through the cervix and into the uterus. An ultrasound scan is performed to locate the position of the placenta and then biopsy is taken. Results are known within two weeks and if necessary termination can be carried out by curette at eleven to twelve weeks.

CVS Risk Factors

Four percent of women undergoing CVS experience a miscarriage following the test. The difficulty is whether this is a result of the test or as a result of spontaneous abortion. Some studies indicate an increased risk of 0.5 to 1 percent.

There is also a very slight risk of infection. Women who are RH(-ve) have a risk of antibody cross-over, but this can be easily prevented by giving the standard injection of Rh Immune globulin. It is still recommended following CVS that you consider having a blood test for Spina Bifida at sixteen weeks of pregnancy. This defect occurs in about one out of a thousand newborns and usually causes significant handicaps. The test will detect about eighty percent of cases of women carrying a child with this problem.

X-Ray

This can be used to assess pelvic size and shape, to assess the position of the baby and assess risk of obstruction during labour. Usually done at thirty six weeks and is not very conclusive as the movement of the pelvic bones in labour are not taken into account with the X-Ray result, so a caesarean section may be unnecessarily performed, putting mother and baby at further risk without first attempting a trial labour.

Regardless of the size of the pelvis there are very few reasons why a trial of labour cannot be given. Every woman and baby is different. There are many documented cases of small and even 'tiny' women giving birth vaginally to big babies. Birth advocate Vicki Chen is a petite size 8 and gave birth to a fourteen pound healthy baby naturally. Her birth video is amazing to watch.

Ultrasound in Pregnancy

Ultrasound is high-frequency sound waves that travel at ten to twenty million cycles per second. The pattern of these echo waves creates a picture of tissue and bone. Ultrasound is performed to confirm pregnancy, ascertain due dates, check for obvious abnormalities, the presence of twins, placenta praevia (low-lying placenta) and foetal growth retardation.

How many scans you should undergo in pregnancy is controversial. Some research indicates there may be a risk to the developing baby if there is an over exposure to full strength scans.

The jury is still out in relation to the research around regular ultrasound. Your obstetrician will assure you it is safe but I tend to err on the idea that less is best. A UK study followed 33,000 pregnancies between 1991 and 1996 and reported that a surprising number of parents were given false-positive ultrasound diagnoses, where an ultrasound image finds an abnormality that just isn't there (Steinhorn, 1998). In the five year period this study covered, forty three percent of the babies identified by ultrasound or other tests as having an abnormality were aborted. A further one hundred and seventy four babies whose ultrasounds suggested abnormalities were born healthy. It has been suggested that advances in ultrasound technology make them sensitive enough to pick up unusual features that can be temporary but may be interpreted as abnormalities.

You can reasonably expect an early scan around ten to twelve weeks and another at eighteen to twenty weeks. It is not necessary to be scanned at every antenatal visit, this is intrusive and can cause more concern rather than confidence that everything is okay.

Doppler and Nuchal Ultrasound

These are painless and non-invasive but are used to detect specific abnormalities. A Doppler can detect blood flow, especially as to how well the placenta is performing. A Nuchal Scan examines the baby's neck, looking for a thickening, which can indicate a risk of Down's Syndrome. Generally an amniocentesis will follow to confirm the diagnosis.

Doptone

This is a portable foetal heart monitor used to detect the presence and rate of the foetal heart. It can be carried out after twelve weeks and at any time during pregnancy with safety. It can be an extremely useful way of employing sound waves and is gentle and less invasive than other methods. It is an excellent tool used in labour as it provides freedom of movement for mum.

Vaginal Ultrasound

This involves the Doppler being covered with a lubricated condom like cover and inserted into the vagina. It has become popular with obstetricians because of its convenience, however it is often used unnecessarily and can be very invasive. Please make sure you understand why it is necessary before agreeing to this procedure.

Glucose Tolerance Test

There has been an increase in the diagnosis of Gestational Diabetes (diabetes in pregnancy) at around thirty weeks. As the pregnancy progresses the kidneys must cope with an increase in fluid filtration. This can result in a spilling over of small amounts of excess sugar into the urine. In the majority of cases this is inconsequential to the health of mother and baby. If however there is an increased level of sugar in the urine this may indicate a propensity to diabetes, especially when also associated with high blood sugar and a history of diabetes.

At around twenty eight weeks you will be given fifty millilitres of glucose to drink, not the most pleasant of tastes. Four blood samples are taken over the next two hours to assess blood sugar levels to check how well your body is able to produce insulin. If the blood sugar levels remain high this may indicate the presence of diabetes. Unfortunately there appear to be many false positives with this one and I have found that it is best to seek a second opinion. There are natural ways of reducing blood sugar levels which my clients have had success with as well. Many of these techniques are described ahead in this book.

Amniocentesis

The amniocentesis test is rarely done now, but when indicated may be done at sixteen to seventeen weeks to detect foetal abnormalities such as Spina Bifida or Down's syndrome. The sex of your child can be determined at this time as well.

Amniocentesis can be done at 24 weeks to assess the foetal well-being when there is Rhesus incompatibility. It also can be done at thirty to thirty nine weeks to assess the maturity of the baby's lungs if an induction or caesarean is necessary due to health of the mother. With the advent of skilled ultrasound technicians there is less need for amniocentesis.

Amniocentesis The Procedure

Amniocentesis involves inserting a needle into the womb to take a sample of the fluid surrounding the baby. An ultrasound is used at the same time to locate the placenta and the lie of the baby. Results may take two to three weeks to come back.

Amniocentesis Risk Factors

There is a one to two percent chance of spontaneous abortion following the procedure but it is unclear as the risk of miscarriage after sixteen weeks is about three percent anyway. The main drawback is that results can be slow sometimes, up to the twentieth week, which creates a huge amount of stress for the mother should she want to abort. By then the baby is very active in utero, making the decision very difficult. Counselling is recommended prior to the procedure.

Many factors need to be discussed prior to undertaking this procedure, especially what will you choose to do if the result is positive for Down's or Spina Bifida? If you would not choose to actively abort why take the risk? But then having the test can be reassuring and stop you feeling stressed by concern throughout your pregnancy. It is very important to discuss the options with your Maternity Carer as much as possible.

Although very rare, there is a very slight risk of infection with amniocentesis, and a slight risk that the baby could be damaged by the needle. There have only been a few reported cases of this out of thousands of cases every year.

Another risk of amniocentesis is the possible development of a Rhesus problem if the woman is Rh (-ve). If the mother is Rh-negative an injection of Rhesus immune globulin is given just after the amniocentesis to prevent this problem from developing. This is standard practice.

The chromosome test that will be performed on the amniotic fluid sample is ninety nine percent accurate to detect Down Syndrome and Spina Bifida (open spine deformity). These defects occur in about one out of every one thousand babies born and are usually very disabling.

There are many other birth defects and genetic diseases and disorders that cannot be detected accurately by amniocentesis or by ultrasound. Thus, having amniocentesis and/or ultrasound does not guarantee a normal child.

Nutrition in Pregnancy

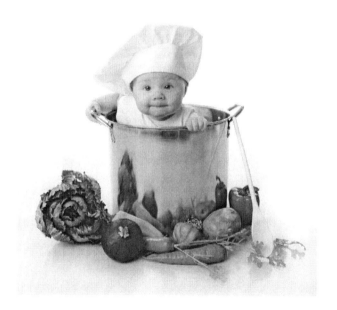

Our bodies produce millions of new cells every day, replacing those that are naturally completing their lifecycles. This process begins from the moment of conception, with cell replication at its premium during the first few weeks. Correct replication is essential to the health and wellbeing of your developing baby. What you consume each day provides the materials for your cells to uptake to complete their processes, resulting in healthier, more capable cells or cells with less ability to function.

So it stands to reason that a pregnant mum's cells are even more in need of good nutrition with two lives dependent on what is eaten. The Foresight Association has shown quite clearly that what we consume before and during pregnancy can affect the next two generations.

Most health providers would recommend pregnant women concentrate on a healthy diet as the main source of nutrients. However, research indicates that large segments of Western populations, even those well above the poverty line, are malnourished. Although the intake of food is high and obesity is prevalent, nutritional intake of micronutrients and minerals is inadequate.

Studies suggest that antenatal nutritional status affects the learning ability, behavioural and psychological status of the child (Smart et al., 1987). A more recent study investigated the relationship between low birth weight, diet, obesity and longevity (Barker, 2004). Results indicated that a baby exposed to low level nutrients grows less well and will develop a lower ability to produce insulin, the hormone needed to process sugars.

This baby, deficient in the ability to process sugars, may have a shorter life span if then fed by a mother who consumes a high carbohydrate or junk food diet. This is further compounded by a higher likelihood of the child being fed on junk food once weaned.

It can be a challenge to ensure good nutritional intake, as many of the most important trace elements are no longer readily attainable from the food available in shops. Most of the food has travelled great distances and has been stored in cold storage for many months, decreasing the nutritional value.

The Barker Theory

> "The quality of nutrition you received in the womb dictates the quality of your life outside the womb."
>
> From the documentary 'The Nine Months That Made You.'
> http://www.youtube.com/watch?v=51_E4hc2_JM

The Barker Theory is the result of over twenty years of research by Professor David Barker (Hertfordshire, UK), who concluded that lack of substantial phytonutrient intake during pregnancy resulted in low birth weight and the increase in chronic illness such as cardiac disease, high blood pressure, diabetes, stroke and arthritis. These are the sort of diseases usually attributed to Western lifestyles and expected later in life. Two important studies Professor Barker reasearched in detail were those by Dr Ranjan Rasheen and Tessa Roseboom.

Dr. Rasheen studied native people living in villages in India. Regardless of apparently excellent diets, little stress, fit and healthy lifestyles and lack of obesity, these people were filling Dr Rasheen's diabetic clinics. Dr Rasheen discovered that the majority had been low birth weight babies. Dr Rasheen and Professor Barker conducted a twenty year study, closely monitoring and following the lives of 200 low birth weight babies. When those babies reached twenty one years of age the following results were found:

> "Children born with low birth weight were found to be more insulin resistant at four years of age and then more insulin resistant at eight years and are even more insulin resistant now at twenty one years whilst already showing signs of cardiac disease. Over the passage of years the blood sugar levels are rising and is now much higher than their colleagues who were not low birth weight. Though these people present as thin and healthy they have the same diseases normally seen in obese people. Through the course of the study we realised that these babies were very thin but carried very high levels of fat, that would be seen in an obese

child not a thin child as these are. What your parents did has a bearing on what happens in your life, not only on the physical health but also on the personality of the child."

Dr. Ranjan Rasheen, 2011

Dr. Rasheen looked at every aspect of the pregnant diet and concluded the future health of the child was not dictated by getting the right balance of protein, carbohydrates and so on, or by the quantity of the food, but about getting the right micro-nutrients. Our life in the womb and not just our genes makes us more resilient later in life.

Tessa Roseboom (Academic Medical Centre, Amsterdam, 2009) followed the long term health of over 2000 babies born or conceived during the Dutch Famine that spanned five months following the end of the Second World War. Whatever genes they carried, all exposed to the famine whilst in the womb had diseases such as cardiac disease, high blood pressure, raised cholesterol, diabetes and breast cancer, yet siblings conceived after the famine didn't. Foetal exposure to the famine only had a detrimental effect if the exposure occurred during the first twelve weeks after conception, which is when the main blueprint for the human being is created.

"Early development sets up your constitution so therefore it also sets up how vulnerable you are to negative things you may encounter through your life. If you wanted a happy old age then the intake of phytonutrients during the nine months you spent in the womb is the most important time."

Dr. Barker, 2011

Particular nutrients have been researched to be very effective during pregnancy to help your body cope with the changes and extra stress of growing a baby. They also help to tone the uterus ready for birth and to produce an efficient uterus producing effective contraction for a quicker and easier birth.

Required Nutrients During Pregnancy

Recommended Daily Allowances (RDA) are based on the diet of a pregnant woman who is not experiencing stress, a rarity in our modern world. Research clearly indicates that the average woman is undernourished and requires considerably more nutrients than just the RDA. Thus I advise women to increase their intake of nutrients to have a better coverage.

(www.foodmatters.com)

Recommended Daily Allowances

Nutrients	Non-pregnant	Pregnant	Lactating
Calories	2100	2400	2600
Proteins (g)	46	76	66
Iron (mg)	18	36	18
Calcium (mg)	800	1200	1200
Iodine (mg)	100	125	150
Magnesium	300	450	450
Phosphorous (mg)	800	1200	1200
Zinc (mg)	15	20	25
Fat Soluble			
Vit. A (IU)	4000	5000	6000
Vit. D (IU)	400	400	400
Vit. E (IU)	12	15	15
Water Soluble			
Vit .B1 (mg)	1.1	1.4	1.4
Vit. B2 (mg)	1.4	1.7	1.9
Vit. B3 (mg)	1.4	1.7	1.9
Vit. B5 (mg)	14	16	18
Vit, B6 (mg)	2	2.5	2.5
Vit. B7 (mg)	?	?	?
Vit. B12 (mg)	3	8	6
Folic Acid (ug)	400	800	600
Vitamin C (mg)	45	60	60

It is essential to avoid ....

- all chemicals, especially alcohol, cigarettes and drugs
- fad dieting to lose weight. Weight gain is a normal healthy process and very important for successful breastfeeding.
- over indulgence in sugars or refined carbohydrates
- caffeine high foods such as coffee, tea, coke, chocolate. It takes your baby approximately thirty six hours to remove caffeine from its system.

There are certain foods that have been linked with Listeriosis, Toxoplasmosis and Salmonella. These foods are best avoided during your pregnancy, such as organ or offal and deli meats, salami, patés (especially liver) and soft cheeses brie, camembert, blue-veined cheeses, cold chicken and seafood.

Carbonated drinks, some fruit juices, canned foods and baked foods are best avoided as they often contain cornsyrup, which has been linked with autism. The Center for Disease Control and Prevention (2012) recently released a study in which it claims Autism is reaching epidemic proportions with one in eighty children in the United States being affected. A 2011 study by Stanford University School of Medicine reported that sixty two percent of autism risk can be attributed to environmental factors such as neurotoxic chemicals in our food which can be found in high fructose corn syrup. http://bodyecology.com/articles/autism-on-the-rise-what-mothers-and-expectant-mothers-need-to-know

Avoid Peanuts in Pregnancy

Peanut protein consumed by pregnant or lactating mothers may play a role in sensitising children at risk of developing peanut allergy. At risk children are those who have a parent or sibling with allergies, eczema, asthma or hay fever. After this sensitisation an allergic reaction occurs on subsequent exposures. A significant public health problem, peanut allergy often causes severe or life-threatening anaphylactic reactions and accounts for the majority of food-induced anaphylactic fatalities (News Edge Corp. 2001).

A study by St. Michael's Hospital/University of Toronto collected breast milk samples at hourly intervals from twenty three healthy, lactating women who had eaten fifty grams of dry, roasted peanuts (Vadas, Wai, Burks & Pererlman, 2001). Analysis detected sufficient amounts of peanut protein to be a potential allergen in eleven of the twenty three samples. The protein appeared in the breast milk within one hour of eating the peanuts in eight of the women, within two hours in two women and after six hours in one woman.

Nutrition - So What Can You Do?

I recommend sixty percent of the diet be raw, fresh vegetables and fruit, preferably organic. Many people rely on bank eating of vegetables, where they eat a huge amount once a week instead of small amounts every day. Bank eating does not work! Your body needs fruit and vegetables every day for optimum health and nutrition.

- refined foods might satisfy your hunger, but they starve your body of necessary nutrients. Aura photography taken of white bread and whole grain bread showed the absence of the energy field aura around the refined white bread whilst the whole grain's aura was bright and colourful.
- avoiding all added sugar is recommended, but a little salt can be added. Kelp salt is an excellent source of iodine.
- a high fibre diet with plenty of fluids will help prevent constipation, indigestion and heartburn
- eat when hungry, rather than from habit. Frequent and small nutritional meals are better than one large meal. Eat the whole spectrum of colour when choosing fruits and vegetables, the more variety the better.
- use dried fruits and nuts for snacks. Yoghurt, cottage cheese and rice, quinoa and nut milks are more readily absorbed and don't encourage mucous production.
- good sources of protein are beans, nuts, grains and seeds. Meat does not need to be your primary source of protein.

- make use of sprouts in daily meals. Sprouts are high in iron, Vitamin K and other essentials.
- drink at least two litres of purified water daily with a squeeze of lemon.

I find it interesting how often I hear people scoff at spending five dollars on a container of blueberries yet think nothing of spending that amount on a bag of crisps, a block of chocolate or a cappuccino. Somehow we have confused our priorities.

Watch 'Hungry for Change – Your Health is in Your Hands' http://www.hungryforchange.tv/

Eating Within the Zone

The average person's diet consists of food extraordinarily high in saturated fats, commercially produced food and refined sugars. The ratio of carbohydrates, proteins and fats is unbalanced and often the diet is low in protein.

Balance

It is important to eat a balanced ratio of carbohydrates, fats and proteins which are conducive to health and vitality, but particularly phytonutrients (from plants). When this ratio is balanced excessive levels of insulin in the body are avoided.

High carbohydrate food (cereal, bread, pasta, rice, and potatoes) may cause increased levels of insulin in the blood. Excessive insulin causes the body to store extra fat and stops the burning of fat that's already stored. Insulin also promotes the inflammatory reactions that are the cause of many common conditions. Excess insulin leads to heart disease, cancer, hormonal imbalance, diabetes and arthritis, lack of energy, weight gain, high blood pressure and high cholesterol, along with a myriad of pregnancy specific abnormalities.

The way our human predecessors consumed food was very different to what we know today. Animal protein was once sourced from wild game, carbohydrates were supplied from fruits, berries and roots in season. Wild game generally contains a far healthier type of fat than that of domesticated animals, which often contain high levels of saturated fat due to intense breeding campaigns.

You only have to look at how this fat solidifies on refrigeration to see the effect in the body. Fish oils are especially beneficial as they do not solidify. If they did, a fish would not be able to move in the cold water. If we all stopped eating red meat from domesticated animals we would be healthier and so would the earth, as much of the global destruction of our forests is a result of the creation of grazing land for domesticated animals.

A vegetarian diet is not necessarily lacking in protein. Consider that to gain twenty grams of protein from meat you need to eat one hundred grams. By comparison, the same twenty grams can be gained by eating twenty five grams of cheese or lentils or thirty four grams of soy beans. It has been proven that in terms of calories per acre a diet of grains, vegetables and beans will support twenty times as many people as a diet of meat. Growing evidence suggests the Australian diet is too high in unhealthy protein, processed carbohydrates, salt, and saturated fat and is too low in fruit and vegetables.

The Insulin Zone system aims to keep the glucose and insulin levels within a tight range by encouraging you to include forty percent low index carbohydrates, thirty percent healthy proteins and thirty percent healthy fats every time you eat. This is a way of eating everyday food in balanced ratio and does not deprive your body of any essential food item, nor does it take the fun and enjoyment out of eating. This is an easy to follow eating plan that incorporates everyday foods in a tighter ratio. It is best to master the zone system step by step under the guidance of a practitioner for more sustained benefits. It is important to realise that it is food eaten over a number of meals or days that has effect rather than individual meals or days.

Food Groups and Sources

Proteins

Provide all the essential amino acids, the building blocks of the body. Amino acids are essential for growth and repair of body cells and maintaining colloid osmotic pressure of blood.

Daily Protein Intake

A simple technique to help define your daily protein requirement is the palm method. The palm of your hand gives an approximate of the amount of protein required at any one meal. The protein should fit into the palm of your hand and be as fat as your hand.

Examples of healthy organic or free-range protein choices:

- soy
- legumes
- nuts (*Note that peanuts should be avoided during pregnancy.*)
- seeds
- sprouts (eaten within 18 hours of sprouting)
- eggs
- low fat cheese
- veal
- venison
- lean beef
- lean lamb
- duck
- chicken breast
- rabbit
- fish
- turkey breast
- quinoa

It is important to eat only healthy choices of protein that do not contain high levels of saturated fats. Some foods contain both protein and carbohydrates. The best choices of these are skim milk, low-fat yoghurt, tempeh and soy flour.

Carbohydrates

Carbohydrates are foods that require the pancreas to release insulin for glucose conversion so as to provide the body with energy. Unfortunately much of the media advertises the healthy benefits of eating high carbohydrate foods for providing energy. This is generally okay for someone who is exercising regularly and needs the extra energy, but for the average person it can be detrimental to maintaining healthy blood-sugar levels. Some carbohydrates require higher levels of insulin production than others and therefore need to be moderated (these tend to be high in complex sugars and starch).

Daily Carbohydrate Intake

The better choices are carbohydrates that slowly convert to glucose, commonly known as low GI carbohydrates. These tend to have a high fibre or water content and allow the pancreas time to rest and recover.

The optimal way to achieve the zone is to create a balance between the different carbohydrates. Examples: asparagus, bean sprouts, green vegetables, cauliflower, cucumber, radishes, watercress, spinach, eggplant, onions, parsley, pumpkin, turnips, peppers and fruits such as cantaloupe, rhubarb, strawberries, watermelon, melons, tomatoes, apricots, blackberries, cranberries, grapefruit, guava, lemons, limes, oranges, raspberries, peaches and kiwis.

Use the palm method to estimate the amount of carbohydrates necessary at each meal. For example fast metabolising carbohydrates need to be limited to one palm full per meal whereas you can have two palms full of the slower conversion carbohydrates. Therefore the ratio is one to two. Often a craving for bread or a carbohydrate fix can mean a need for protein.

Fats

Types of Fats/Oils

The modern diet contains large amounts of fat in contrast to what was traditionally available as food sources for humans. It is important to understand the different types of fat available.

Healthy fats help to slow the rate of entry of carbohydrates to the bloodstream, thus reducing their glycaemia effect. These good fats are generally mono-saturated and should be encouraged as a major source of fat in the diet. Found in olive oil, canola oil, grape seed oil, olives, macadamia nuts and avocados and have no effect on insulin levels. Monosaturated fats found in canola, olive and peanut oils may also help to lower cholesterol and decrease platelet aggregation. These are much less susceptible to oxidation.

Note that peanuts should be avoided during pregnancy.

Polyunsaturated fats are found in oils from plants such as safflower, sesame, sunflower and corn. Though these have been found to be beneficial in lowering cholesterol and decreasing platelet aggregation they are susceptible to oxidation. A high intake has been associated with an increased risk of cancer, so eat minimally.

The really unhealthy fats to avoid are those containing arachidonic acid such as organ meat, deli processed meats, fatty red meat and high fat dairy products. Saturated fats have their place in the diet, but some should be avoided, such as those found in high fat animal protein sources and dairy products that have been homogenised or pasteurised. Trans-fats are unsaturated fats which have undergone a chemical process called hydrogenation to turn them into saturated fats. These are found in packaged foods such as pastries, cookies, crackers and baked foods and are best avoided if possible.

Omega-3 and Omega-6 Fatty Acids

Linoleic acid is an Omega-6 fatty acid found in safflower, sunflower, corn oils, Evening Primrose oil (EPO), blackcurrant and borage oils. Omega-6 fatty acids can be manufactured in the body using Linoleic acid as a starting point.

Alpha Linoleic acid is an Omega-3 fatty acid found in cold-water fish, mackerel, herring, halibut and salmon. Lesser amounts might be found in shrimp and tuna. Flaxseed oil is also an excellent source but needs to be ground or taken as oil, it is not well metabolised during pregnancy.

A few Omega-3 fatty acids can be manufactured in the body using Alpha Linoleic acid as a starting point. These are the most essential oils required by the body. They are involved in energy production, the transfer of oxygen from the air to the blood stream and the manufacture of haemoglobin. They are also involved in growth, cell division and nerve function.

Essential fatty acids are vital for normal nerve impulse transmission and brain function. They are components of the cell membrane, involved in cell to cell communication, cell nutrient uptake and hormone regulation. Essential fatty acids are also involved in the manufacture of prostaglandins, substances which play a role in a number of body functions including hormone synthesis, immune function, regulation of the response to pain and inflammation, blood vessel constriction and other heart and lung functions.

Latest evidence suggests that the Australian diet lacks Omega-3 more so than Omega-6. Normal intake should be Omega-6 four times the amount of Omega-3. Due to our currently low intake of fish the average intake of Omega-6 is sixteen times that of Omega-3.

Eating cold-water fish three times a week or taking a daily supplement of Omega-3 can help rectify this imbalance. Be careful of the source of the supplement, make sure it is high quality and free of toxins. Unfortunately now due to farming of cold water fish, where the fish are fed on meat pellets, the Omega 3 levels are considerably lower than in free running fish. Also our seas are being fished out so a healthier and eco option is Hemp oil. Another option might be Barramundi as it lives on phytoplankton so is less likely to be affected by toxins and mercury, thus its flesh and oils are more pure.

Daily Fat/Oil Requirements

Fats and oils are essential as they slow down the insulin response at each meal when eating within the zone (30% fats/oils). Beneficial fats and oils aid weight loss, improve the taste of food and provide a sense of satiation.

Best choices include:

- almonds
- canola oil
- tahini
- avocado
- olives

- olive oil
- guacamole
- macadamia nut
- vinegar dressing (1 tspn olive oil and 2 tspn vinegar)

Vitamins and Minerals in Detail

The first three months after conception is a critical period for neuronal growth. If the mother's diet fails to supply enough fats, proteins, carbohydrates, vitamins, minerals and water for both her and the baby, some part of the baby's development may be affected. As with a building, different materials or building blocks are required at different times for optimal development. During this period of baby's development, large amounts of fats are deposited into the brain tissue from Omega-3, Omega-6 and other fatty acids (EFA's). The types and quantities of these fatty acids differ, depending on the period of development and the needs of the brain at that point in development. If you are reading this and feel that your diet may have been lacking in those first few weeks, don't panic, it is not too late. Research has shown that a diet high in nutritional superfoods, at any time during the pregnancy, can be of great benefit. An easy way to turn fruits and vegetables into superfoods is to blend them into a smoothie or juice. This increases the cell uptake of the nutrients and speeds up the digestive process, facilitating a higher absorbency rate. This chapter will help you locate the foods you require for specific nutrients.

Fat Soluble Vitamins

Vitamin A (Retinol)
Essential for normal growth of most body cells, particularly those making up the different epithelium, including the uterus. Helps in production of red and white blood cells and hormones concerned with reproduction and lactation. Vitamin A is essential for tooth formation, normal bone growth, vision and is involved in fat metabolism.

- large doses in pregnancy can cause cranial neural defects in the baby
- it is advised to avoid liver and vitamin supplements containing high levels of vitamin A, beta-carotene is a safe and more absorbable source.

    Sources: carrots, spinach, broccoli, eggs, dairy food, cod liver oil, tomatoes, fenugreek, sprouts, rockmelon, mango, capsicum, sweet potato, prunes, green peas, peaches, watercress.

Vitamin D
Essential for calcium absorption and bone formation, can be supplied by digestion or through sunlight on the skin.
> Sources: sunshine, salmon, sardines, herrings, milk, eggs, fish liver oils, corn tortillas. I recommend A.I.M.

Vitamin E
Prevents the oxidation of vitamin A and is needed for the utilisation of essential fatty acids, essential to fertility, reproduction, prevents miscarriage, aids in preventing pre-eclampsia, repairs and heals the body.
> Sources: sunflower seeds, pumpkin seeds, parsley, soy beans, vegetable oils, wheat germ, rolled oats, sunflower oil, beans and peas, milk, egg yolk, green leafy vegetables, lettuce, avocado, nuts.

Vitamin K

Vitamin K is manufactured by bacteria essentially in the gut and acts as a co-enzyme in the synthesis of prothrombin and other blood clotting factors in the liver. Prevents miscarriage, strengthens the uterine walls, prevents bleeding and aids in labour. Deficiency can result in haemorrhage.

> Sources: kale (possibly the highest ingestible source of vitamin K), kelp, alfalfa, milk, fish liver oils, cod liver oils, wheat germ, green leafy vegetables, carrots, soy beans.

Water Soluble Vitamins

These are readily excreted in urine, are easily destroyed and deficiencies can occur more readily, so must be replenished frequently.

B Group Vitamins

Involved in several metabolic processes, energy production and muscle and nerve tissue functioning, all of which are especially important in the increased metabolic activities of pregnancy. Individual B vitamin supplements should not be taken because a balance of all B vitamins is needed in the body.

B1 (Thiamine)

Essential in carbohydrate metabolism and normal brain growth, especially in the developing baby. Studies show that thirty to eighty percent of women are thiamine deficient by late pregnancy. Women with excessive nausea and vomiting are at most risk. Symptoms of a deficient mother include insomnia, stress, nervousness, jitters and paranoia. The growth of the infant may be affected by a deficiency, resulting in a smaller baby for gestational age.

> Sources: wheat germ, brewer's yeast, wholegrain bread, beans, cereals, rice.

B2 (Riboflavin)

Functions in tissue oxidation and respiration, is involved in protein and energy metabolism. Deficiencies are characterised by lesions on the lips, cracked lips and facial acne. Usually associated with other nutritional deficiencies. Not common in pregnancy.

> Sources: wheat germ, brewer's yeast, wholegrain bread, beans, cereals and rice.

B5 (Niacin)

Essential for glycolysis and tissue respiration, deficiencies are not notable in pregnancy.

> Sources: wheat germ, brewer's yeast, wholegrain bread, beans, cereals and rice.

B6 (Pyridoxine)

Essential to the development of the central nervous system. A deficient mother may display oral lesions, morning sickness, eclampsia and decreased protein metabolism. A deficient infant may result in excessive crying, jitters, fitting and irritability.

> Sources: wheat germ, yeast, soy beans, citrus fruit pith, rice ** needs to be supplemented if taking the contraceptive pill.

B12 (Cobalamin)

Essential for thyroid function, blood development and neural tube development in the baby, which occurs around the 24th -26th day following conception. Deficiencies are usually due to mal-absorption rather than a lack of. Deficiencies in the mother can result in infertility, anaemia, thyroid problems, neurological dysfunction, whilst in the baby can result in neural tube defects.

> Sources: animal protein, kidneys, mussels, fish, dairy foods, brewer's yeast, egg yolks, kelp, soy, wholegrain bread and seaweed.

Folic Acid

Essential for DNA synthesis, therefore is necessary for neural tube development in early conception. This must be taken pre-conceptually and in the early weeks following conception to prevent neural tube defects. Please ensure it is taken in combination with B12 as folic acid requires B12 to synthesise, if lacking will pull sources from the body to metabolise, this can lead to pernicious anaemia if sources of B12 are too low. The deficient mother may experience miscarriage and anaemia whilst may result in neural tube defects in the deficient infant.

> Sources: spinach, green leaves, broccoli, soy beans, strawberries, wheat germ, brewer's yeast, oysters, salmon and mushrooms.

Vitamin C (Ascorbic Acid) and other Antioxidants

Essential for providing an intercellular cementing substance necessary for supporting the vascular system, muscles, cartilage and connective tissue and assisting the uptake of calcium in bones. Essential to immunity and sperm growth. It assists the immune system by preventing the invasion of viruses and bacteria and aids in the healing process. Metabolic function of active tissues, iron metabolism and red blood cell formation relies on Vitamin C. Deficiencies are characterised by scurvy, which is almost non-existent in Western countries.

> Sources: capsicum, tomato, citrus fruit, rosehip, broccoli, kiwi, carrots, olive oil, yoghurt, soy bean, mango, potatoes, and sweet potato.
>
> ** Cooking and exposure to air destroys half of this vitamin.

Eating fresh fruit and vegetables frequently is the best source of vitamin C and antioxidants.

Minerals

Trace elements serve a variety of functions but act primarily as catalysts in enzyme systems in the cells. Deficiencies are uncommon, although in pregnancy the supply is often insufficient. Subsequent pregnancies can lead to long term deficiencies. Colloidal minerals are a very good source. I recommend ForeverGreen PURE as one of the best sources of minerals, as it contains 92 sea minerals in a bioavailable form. I have received excellent feedback from many pregnant mums on the benefits of PURE in assisting cramps and muscle fatigue.

http://73861142.myforevergreen.org/AUS_Pure.html

Hair Tissue Mineral Analysis

Hair analysis is a wonderfully straight forward way to test for levels of nutrients and toxic minerals. Minerals are essential to health and wellbeing, playing a vital role in many of your body's functions. Even if you maintain a highly nutritious food intake you may be lacking in some minerals or suffering from toxicity of others. This is due to many factors, perhaps most particularly to environmental pollutants and modern farming methods that deplete the mineral content of soil.

Hair Tissue Mineral Analysis (HTMA) is safe and non-invasive, all that is required is a few strands of hair. InterClinical Laboratories is the leading service provider of Hair Tissue Mineral Analysis in Australia. On their website InterClinical Laboratories list the benefits of HTMA as:

- safe, scientific, non-invasive pathology test
- reliable data on more than 35 nutrient and toxic minerals, and over 25 important mineral ratios
- valuable health information often not revealed in standard blood and urine tests
- discovery of nutrient mineral imbalances or toxic mineral excesses that may be affecting your health
- personalised patient and doctor interpretive test reports that assess your current mineral status, highlight areas of concern and recommend dietary changes and supplements for improved health and wellbeing.

http://www.interclinical.com.au/hairtissue.php

Boron

Required for calcium metabolism. An inadequate level of boron is also suspected in negatively influencing the body's uptake of magnesium and potassium, possibly resulting in bone density loss and elevated blood pressure.

Calcium

Critical for many biological functions including nerve transmission, fat and protein digestion, muscle contraction, healthy bones and teeth, blood clotting, nerve functions and oxygen transport. Occurs in large quantities in the body, with ninety nine percent being found in the skeletal system, bones and teeth. The remaining one percent is involved in important functions such as blood coagulation, neuro- muscular function, muscular contraction and relaxation and heart muscle function. Calcium with Vitamin D can aid in pain relief, and is especially beneficial when taken at the onset of labour. Calcium uptake relies on Vitamin C. An overdose in pregnancy can lead to muscle cramping. Deficiency may result in muscle weakness or cramps, brittle bones, rickets, osteoporosis, high blood pressure, insomnia and anxiety.

> Sources : sesame seeds, soy products, goats milk, nut milk, strawberries, raspberry leaf tea, dairy products, green leafy vegetables, fruit, shellfish, figs, molasses, broccoli, fish bone, legumes, beetroot, cress, alfalfa, seaweed, agar-agar, kombu, kelp and Irish moss.

Chloride

A component of stomach hydrochloric acid. It helps regulate the body's acid base pH. Essential for hydrochloric acid production, which usually decreases with age.

> Sources: sea salt, kelp and seaweed.

Chromium

Beer and wine can accumulate chromium during fermentation and are therefore considered to be dietary sources of the mineral. Chromium is effective in insulin action. Deficiencies may lead to glucose intolerance, diabetes, atherosclerosis and slow growth. Many people do not get enough chromium in their diet due to food processing methods that remove the naturally occurring chromium in commonly consumed foods.

> Sources: concentrated food sources include onions, tomatoes, brewer's yeast, oysters, whole grains, bran cereals, and potatoes.

Cobalt
Essential for formation of Vitamin B12, metabolism of fatty acids and synthesis of haemoglobin.

> Sources: raw milk, raw goat's milk, raw milk cheese, organic apricots, sea vegetables, apricot kernels, organic red meat.

Copper
Essential in ovary production and prevents constipation, morning sickness and afterbirth hysteria. Copper assists immune function, artery strength, helps form haemoglobin from iron, metabolizing vitamin C and the oxidation of fatty acids. Many women are found to be copper deficient after taking the contraceptive pill. Deficiencies may lead to osteoporosis, anaemia, inflammation, hypoestrogenism and premature ventricular contraction.

> Sources: leeks, garlic, parsley, broccoli, watercress.

Iodine
Important for thyroid hormone production. Some Australian states, especially Tasmania, tend to be low in iodine and supplementation is required. Iodine is needed by the thyroid hormone to support metabolism. Deficiencies may lead to thyroid enlargement and goitre.

> Sources: iodised fortified salt and foods. Kelp is an excellent source of iodine.

Iron
Essential constituent of haemoglobin for red blood cells to carry oxygen and for immune function. Iron is present in a variety of enzymes, essential for maintaining energy and preventing haemorrhage. Iron assists postnatal

healing, in meeting foetal development needs, and must be stored in the liver to supply the infant for the first three to four months of life.

Pregnant women who have good haematology reports in early pregnancy should not take iron supplements as this may lead to Heam-saturation which can create hypertension. Late in pregnancy if anaemic then iron needs to be taken. The more natural formulations are better absorbed.

I recommend liquid iron supplements, cell salts and bio-available pre-chelated iron sources such as Metagenics Hemagenics IC from Healthworld (follow this link for details on how to order).

A deficient mother may result in anaemia, excessive tiredness, pallor, shortness of breath, poor appetite, disorientation, haemorrhage, palpatations, pica, immunodeficiency, candida, low birth weight infants and emotional upheaval.

> Sources: prunes, brain, heart, wheat germ, kelp, bran, molasses, oatmeal, avocado, bananas, kiwi (combats iron deficiency), wholegrain food, green leafy vegetables, raspberry leaf tea, kelp, seaweed, eggs, caviar, lean red meat, parsley, pistachio nuts, pumpkin seeds, peaches, Milo, cocoa powder, yeast extract.
>
> ** Chelated Iron supplements are up to four times more readily absorbed than other forms.

Lithium

May play a protective role in treating sodium imbalances that contribute to atherosclerotic heart disease. Studies also show that lithium can prevent behavioural alterations related to social isolation and confinement.

> Sources: mustards, kelp, sardines and other fish and sea products, blue corn, raw or roasted pistachio nuts, mushrooms, summer squashes, okra and cucumbers.

Magnesium

Essential for all life forms, magnesium is needed for the production and transfer of energy, muscle contraction, nerve excitability and transmission, protein synthesis and assists in the function of enzymes. Magnesium activates over 300 enzymes. Magnesium deficiency is believed to occur commonly in pregnant women and regular supplementation can be valuable in preventing pre-eclampsia and hypertension (high blood pressure) as well as assisting a more efficient labour.

Deficiency may lead to eclampsia, bowel irritation, cramps, high blood pressure, muscular twitching, cardiac arrhythmia, apathy, weakness, cramps and muscle tremors which leads to convulsions, insomnia, headaches, depression, constipation and hyperactivity, excessive perspiration and diabetes. We tend to struggle to produce enough magnesium. People with chronic illness are likely to be particularly lacking.

> Sources: all fresh green vegetables, soy beans, wheat germ, figs, corn, apples, cashews, pistachio nuts, lettuce, walnuts, milk, eggs, seafood, dolomite.

Manganese

Development and growth, metabolism of fat and energy, reproductive system.

Deficiencies may lead to anaemia, glucose intolerance, fatigue, weight loss and adrenal insufficiency.

> Sources: cloves, saffron, wheatgerm, bran, hazelnuts, pine nuts, pecans, mussels, oysters, clams, cocoa and chocolate, roasted pumpkin and squash seeds, flax, tahini, chilli, roasted soybeans and sunflower seeds.

Molybdenum

Essential for enzyme action. Deficiencies can lead to bronchial asthma, dental cavities.

> Sources: leafy greens, liver, kidneys and water.

Nickel

Involved in a number of important biological functions, including production of hormones prolactin and aldosterone, maintaining the integrity of lipid and cell membranes and stabilizing DNA and RNA.

> Sources: plants supply about 900 mcg daily of nickel, dry beans, cocoa, baking soda and nuts (including hazel nuts, almonds and pistachios).

Phosphorus

Essential for foetal bone and teeth formation, assistance in the breakdown of fats, proteins and carbohydrates.

> Sources: dairy products, garlic, mushrooms, pumpkin seeds, sunflower seeds, whole grains, yeast, wheat germ, soy beans, Brazil nuts and almonds.

Potassium

Essential for blood Ph regulation, blood pressure, body fluid balance, acidity of urine, nerve and muscle contraction and nerve transmission. Deficiency may lead to dry skin, poor reflexes, apathy, weakness, confusion, extreme thirst, cardiac irregularity and poor digestion.

> Sources: bananas, potatoes, whole grains, wheat germ, soy flour, nuts, all fresh fruit and vegetables.

Selenium

This important nutrient is vital to immune system function and thought to help prevent cancer by affecting oxidative stress, inflammation and DNA repair. Selenium works in conjunction with vitamins E and C, glutathione and vitamin B3 as an antioxidant to prevent free radical damage in the body. Selenium has been found to be important to male fertility, as increasing selenium levels can lead to improved sperm motility. Preliminary research suggests that selenium supplementation may also help with asthma symptoms, but more studies are needed.

Deficiencies of selenium can occur in areas where soil content of this mineral is low. Diets high in refined foods may also lead to deficiency, as selenium can be destroyed by food processing. Taking anti-inflammatory drugs may reduce the body's supply of selenium. Low selenium levels can contribute to autoimmune problems such as psoriasis and thyroid disease. Low levels have also been tied to stomach, throat and prostate cancers, although more research is needed to determine if this is a cause or a result of the disease. Some studies suggest that selenium deficiency is linked to mood disorders. There are also indications that deficiencies in selenium may contribute to the progression of viral infections.

> Sources: brazil nuts, sunflower seeds, fish (tuna, halibut, sardines, flounder, salmon), shellfish (oysters, mussels, shrimp, clams, scallops), meat (beef, liver, lamb, pork), chicken, turkey, eggs, mushrooms (button, crimini, shiitake), grains (wheat germ, barley, brown rice, oats), onions.

Silicon

An essential trace mineral required for stronger bones, better glowing skin and more flexible and strong joints. Present in the body in the form of an ether derivative of silicic acid or silanate. It is important to include silicon in your daily diet as it may help boost the benefits of calcium, glucosomine and vitamin D.

Generally plant sources have a higher silicon content by comparison to animal sources, refined or processed foods. Refining and processing normally reduces the silicon content of foods. The silicon content in drinking water and beverages shows geographical disparity, and silicon is high in hard water and low in soft water areas.

> Sources: cereals, apples, oranges, cherries, raisins, almonds, raw cabbage, onions, carrots, eggplant, pumpkin, cucumber, fish, honey, oats, unrefined grains/cereals with high fibre content, nuts and seeds.

Sodium

Crucially important to many metabolic activities, one third of the body's sodium is for skeletal use, two thirds for the extracellular fluid, plasma, nerve and muscle tissue. Sodium functions metabolically for fluid balance, acid-base balance, cell permeability, cell life and potential and muscle contraction. An overdose results in fluid retention, muscle spasms and aching joints.

> Sources: natural sea salt, milk, meat, eggs, vegetables. Fast and refined foods often contain high levels of sodium but not in a healthy form.

Sulphate

Anti-inflammatory and anti-depressant, sulphate is needed for making stomach acid and digestive enzymes so that we can break down the food we eat into useful components. Sulphate keeps the gut wall healthy so that over large fragments of food cannot pass through. If they did, it would lead to the production of antibodies and to allergy. Sulphate protects us from cancer by detoxifying chemicals in food and drugs, chemicals made by the body and others from the environment. If we lived in the Garden of Eden we might make enough sulphate. In our industrialised society we do not tend to make enough, with people who are particularly bad at making it tending to have chronic illnesses.

The best way to increase your sulphate is by putting half a cup of Epsom salts in your bath about every third day, but don't stay in the bath longer than half an hour as the salts create a detox reaction which is not recommended in pregnancy (Epsom salts is the common name for magnesium sulphate). Sulphate passes through the skin into your bloodstream. Taking Epsom salts orally is not as effective, but if you have a sore throat I do suggest putting half a flat teaspoonful of Epsom salts from the chemist in a litre bottle of filtered water, and drinking in four sessions through the day.

Tin

Although there is not a tremendous amount of research available regarding the role of tin for our health, a study by the Clinical Research Resource for Cellular Nutrition and Trace Mineral Analysis suggests tin may provide some health benefits. The study involved 285 participants, some of whom were given tin supplementation for a few weeks, others for one or two years.

The study claimed side effects were equal to or less than other trace minerals and provided a number of "positive health effects including improvements with fatigue, some forms of depression, and a general increase in energy, well-being, and mood. There were also benefits with certain types of headaches, insomnia, asthma, or improvements with digestion, skin, or various aches and pains."

http://www.acu-cell.com/tin.html

You can take tin supplements if advised by your health professional, however tin is available in many foods, including most vegetables, seaweed, some toothpastes and herbs.

Zinc

Essential to every organ function, zinc helps to prevent morning sickness, stretch marks, stillbirths, premature births, placental abruption, difficult labours due to inefficient uterine contractions plus many other complications. Zinc is also of benefit to enzymatic reactions, reproductive health, growth and development and immune functions.

Deficiency may result in growth retardation, increased risk of pregnancy complications, suppressed immunity, diarrhoea, wasting of body tissue, poor healing and dermatitis, poor sense of taste and smell, excessive hair loss, memory loss, hyperactivity and white flecks on fingernails. Mild deficiencies are common in many societies with up to eighty percent of the population low in zinc.

The testes and prostate have the highest concentration of zinc in the male body. Deficiencies in males is one of the leading causes of infertility. Deficiencies in the female may lead to poor ovarian production, frequent abortion, prolonged gestation of pregnancy, postnatal depression, pre-eclampsia and low birth weight babies.

Sources: almonds, bananas, brewer's yeast, wheat germ, liver, red meat.

Zinc is the most easily destroyed of all the minerals through packaging or preparation. Daily intake through green leafy vegetables is essential. Best supplement sources are Zinc Drink rather than in tablet form. Supplementation of zinc and magnesium during pregnancy may assist with prevention of postnatal depression, as indicated by a study by Surrey University (click here to read their findings).

Metagenics Zinc Drink is available from Healthworld. Follow this link for details on how to order (found in the Appendix).

Optimal Super Foods ▨▨▨▨▨▨▨▨▨▨▨▨▨▨

Unless your diet is extremely high in organic, raw and freshly picked produce, you may not be eating a balanced diet and would be advised to include nutraceuticals into your everyday diet. When you give your body the quality nutrients you need and practice overall health supporting behaviours, you will optimise not only our own health but the future health of your growing child. The taking of vitamin supplements certainly assists but as Dr. Hugo Rodier (Nutrition Professor at University of Utah Medical School) states:

> "I'm not fond of Multi-vitamins I think they are poorly absorbed, very synthetic, too little of too many vitamins, so if you're going to supplement according to the medical journal of clinical nutrition then it better be whole food and this is what Phytoplankton is, microscopic whole food."

> Dr Hugo Rodier, 2006
> University of Utah Medical School

Superfoods

- Greek yoghurt
- quinoa
- blueberries
- kale
- chia
- oatmeal
- green tea
- broccoli
- strawberries

- salmon/ barramundi
- watermelon
- spinach
- pistachio
- eggs
- almonds
- ginger
- beetroot

- beans
- pumpkin
- apples
- cranberries
- garlic
- cauliflower
- leeks
- lentils

Marine Phytoplankton

Marine phytoplankton is a microscopic plant that grows in the ocean and is the basis for the rest of the food chain. It is a complete whole food that contains 400 times the energy of any known plant on the planet. It helps feed and detoxify the cells and is a powerful antioxidant. Invisible to the naked eye, marine phytoplankton are easily absorbed at a cellular level, making the nutrients instantly bio-available to your body. This is the first food on earth.

Marine phytoplankton has been named 'Mother Nature's Milk' as it supplies everything needed to sustain life. Many of the world's largest animals live on marine phytoplankton up to two hundred years. A study by the University of Utah (School of Medicine) states that marine phytoplankton also benefits the immune system by supporting the T-cells.

"It is one of the rare total foods"

Dr. Jerry Tennant, Tennant Institute of
Integrative Medicine in Dallas, 2006

FrequenSea

FrequenSea provides cellular nutrition for healthy cell replication, with marine phytoplankton in its most bio-available form, as well as Frankincense and Rose, which decrease stress by creating a calming effect on the body. Stress is one of the biggest challenges facing pregnant women and couples trying to conceive.

http://casadelsole.fgxpress.com/farmers-market/

PURE

Contains 1500mg of marine phytoplankton, is highly concentrated and is a potent mineral base. Pure is a nature balanced multi-mineral super concentrate extracted from nutrient-rich ocean water that has the salt removed. It contains 92 ionic minerals and trace elements essential to life. ForeverGreen has gone to great lengths to achieve the sourcing of this mineral base. It works because it is ionic and provides individual atoms for cellular metabolism. Powdered macro mineral molecules are too big to be used by the body. The beauty of Pure is that it provides readily available particles (ions) that can be metabolised.

http://casadelsole.fgxpress.com/farmers-market/

Hemp

Hemp is one of the most perfect foods for human consumption! Hemp is the only sustainable and pure vegetable source of EFAs. Hemp seeds contain up to thirty six percent protein, which is comprised of approximately sixty five percent Edestin. Edestin is important. Edestin is a globular legumin protein than can only be found in hemp seed protein and aids digestion, is low in phosphorus and is considered the backbone of human cellular DNA.

Hemp protein contains all twenty known amino acids, including the eight essential and two semi-essential amino acids (EAAs) our bodies cannot produce. Proteins are considered complete when they contain all essential amino acids in a sufficient quantity and ratio to meet the body's protein requirements. No other single food source has the essential amino acids in such an easily digestible form, nor has the essential fatty acids in as perfect a ratio to meet human nutritional needs.

Hemp seed is also an excellent source of calcium and iron. Whole hemp seeds are a good source of phosphorus, magnesium, zinc, copper and manganese. Hemp seed is gluten free and consequently will not trigger symptoms of celiac disease.

The ingredients in these optimal super foods are high in antioxidants and many other micronutrients, which is why they are so helpful in maintaining and restoring overall health.

Although as a society we may tend to rely on the prescription drugs of Western medicine, many health issues may in fact be assisted by the ingredients listed here since they work at the root of the problem, cell metabolism and communication. This is especially true when these ingredients are consumed together, maximizing their synergistic effect.

Transform Your Thinking

"The concept of primary prevention of complications of pregnancy, delivery and prevention of neonatal abnormalities through sound prenatal nutrition has been supplanted by secondary prevention, which consists of elaborate intensive-care nurseries which electronically monitor premature babies, many of whom would have been normal size at birth had nutrients been a priority before and during pregnancy."

Dr. Tom Brewer
www.drbrewerpregnancydiet.com/

Dietary Principles Based on Traditional Chinese Factors

Traditional Chinese Medicine (TCM) classifies food according to its energetic effects. Certain foods are viewed as warming and nourishing, others are seen as cooling and eliminating. Some foods are useful for building Qi (energy, life force) others have blood, yang or yin building proprieties.

A breakfast of a banana and yoghurt will generally have the same nutritional value in Western medicine no matter who is eating it. In Traditional Chinese Medicine it may be seen as beneficial for those with yin deficiency conditions but detrimental to those with yang deficiency or dampness.

Food in this context either assists or hinders our daily efforts to maintain health or recover from illness, depending on our constitution. It is not just a matter of eating nourishing healthy food but of eating nourishing healthy food that is right for your individual body type.

Thus your underlying constitution, including the strength of your digestive system, determines what foods are most suitable. Traditional Chinese Medicine also emphasises guidelines on how food should be prepared and eaten if it is to be utilised in the most efficient way.

The Five Flavours According to Traditional Chinese Medicine

Foods in traditional Chinese medicine are assigned according to the five flavours:

Sour, Bitter, Sweet, Pungent (spicy) and Salty

and the four natures:

Cool, Cold, Warm and Hot

The flavour of food can be used to predict its effects on your body.

- Sour calms and alkalises the body related to the liver
- Bitter creates heat in the body and is related to the heart
- Sweet acts as a tonic and balancer for the body and is related to the spleen and digestion
- Spicy removes wind and cold from the body and is related to the lung
- Salty removes stagnation and assists fluid balance and the kidneys.

Each of these flavours corresponds with one of the five phases, wood (liver, gallbladder), fire (heart, small intestine), earth (spleen, stomach), metal (lung, large intestine) and water (kidney, bladder).

If we follow good health practice, when our body is out of balance we may crave foods that can assist the body to rebalance. However when consumed excessively, the targeted organ will be weakened. For instance, overeating sweet flavours is detrimental to the spleen, excess consumption of salt affects our kidneys, overindulgence in sour food weakens the liver, an excess consumption of spicy foods impairs the function of lungs, while too many bitter flavours in the diet damages the heart.

Many foods belong to more than one of the five flavours. For example vinegar is seen as being both bitter and sour, cheese as being sour and sweet. Changing the way you prepare food can make it more suitable to your constitution. Raw food is the most cooling for the body, requiring more energy to digest than food that has been cooked. Examples of the same food prepared in a different manner are muesli compared with porridge, salads compared with stir-fries and roasted vegetables, or a piece of raw fruit compared with one that is stewed or baked.

Our eating habits have changed immensely since the invention of the refrigerator and freezer. What was once consumed occasionally is now readily available, leading to many health issues. I still recommend eating seasonally as best you can with food in freshest form.

The Five Flavours of Food With Examples

Bitter foods like rhubarb and dandelion leaf tend to drain heat and cool and may also have a purgative effect as they induce bowel movements. Sour foods (grapefruit and olives) are cooling and in small amounts aid digestion. Pungent or spicy foods (onion, cayenne pepper) have a warming action, promoting energy to move upwards and outwards to the body's surface. They also have useful properties in dispersing mucus from the lungs. Salty foods such as kelp and soya sauce are cooling and hold fluids in the body.

Sweet foods can be divided into two groups

1. sweet foods that are neutral and nourishing or warm and nourishing. These include meat, legumes, nuts, dairy products and starchy vegetables.
2. sweet foods that are cooling. These include fruits, sugar, honey and other sweeteners. Potatoes, rice and apples are all considered to belong to the sweet flavour.

Preparation of Food and its Influence on the Nature of Food.

Coldest: Raw, Steamed, Boiled, Stewed
Warmest: Stir fried, Baked, Deep fried, Roasted

Strengthening the Spleen

Traditional Chinese dietary therapy places emphasis on the efficient functioning of the spleen to extract maximum value from food. There are several simple but important factors that help to maximise Spleen Qi.

Eating a Suitable Breakfast

The most suitable time for eating breakfast according to the Chinese 24 hour energy clock is between seven and nine am. This is when the stomach's energy is at its peak as the body should be hungry and ready to start the day's digestive process. Lack of hunger in the morning implies a weakness in the digestive system, often resulting from faulty eating habits like eating large meals late at night or regularly skipping breakfast to save on calories or time.

Bread, fruit, yoghurt, muesli, bacon, eggs, pancakes, waffles or porridges form the mainstay of a Western approach to breakfast. However a sugary breakfast such as processed white toast and jam, or processed cereals with milk and sugar, is not a nutritionally balanced start to the day. There are a variety of breakfasts to suit all types. Soups, congees (rice porridge), stir fried vegetables and rice or noodles with meat or tofu are regularly eaten as breakfast in other cultures.

Breakfast does not have to be a huge meal, but should be eaten within an hour of waking. Depending on your underlying energic pattern and considering the season, cooler foods such as yogurt and fruit can be consumed in warmer weather, with warmer cooked foods such as porridges chosen in colder weather.

Some quick and easy suggestions to choose from include:

- fruit salad with nuts
- muesli and yoghurt
- muesli pre-soaked overnight and eaten with seasonal fruit
- fruit smoothies (a drink made by blending yoghurt, milk and fruit together)
- whole grain bread with hummus, tomato and avocado
- sushi
- oat porridges with stewed apple and cinnamon
- rice porridges with soya milk, apricots and almonds
- scrambled or poached eggs or omelettes with spinach and mushrooms
- miso soup with tofu
- noodle soup with vegetables.

Avoid Eating Large Meals Late at Night
A large meal late in the evening, before sleeping, strains your digestive system as the stomach Qi is near to its lowest ebb in the 24 hour cycle.

Eating late in this way can lead to food accumulation, creating digestive problems such as feeling bloated and full when you wake in the morning. Prolonged late eating can lead to chronic digestive problems.

Develop Regular Eating Patterns

Irregular eating times and irregular quantities of food are detrimental to an efficient digestive system. While meal times don't need to be rigid, eating regular meals will help develop a more efficient digestive system, unlike skipping meals, imposing self starvation or over eating. Eating regular meals every four hours is optimal.

Appropriate Fluid Intake

A small amount of warm liquid (such as green tea), with a meal can promote effective digestion. More than one to two cups, especially if chilled, has the potential to 'swamp' the stomach and impair digestion. Ideally the greater part of the fluids consumed in-between meals should be warm or at room temperature as chilled drinks cool and slow down the digestive process. Good quality organic red wine, in moderation, has warming properties when taken at mealtimes.

Enjoyment of Eating

Having a joyous approach to the food you eat is very important. It has been well documented that our attitude to food is very important, so whatever you put in your mouth really taste it. Eat with sheer joy and pleasure, not with a sense of guilt. Your body is designed to enjoy the food you eat. Your tongue is pre-programmed to recognise and enjoy different tastes and your sense of smell will stimulate the production of saliva. Sitting down to eat breakfast, having lunch away from the office desk and timing the evening meal so that it does not coincide with the TV news can all enhance your awareness and enjoyment of food. This will also aid healthy digestion.

Diet During Pregnancy

During pregnancy women can be prone to developing some dampness and heat. This can mean that foods you have previously thought of as healthy, for example dairy foods or orange juice, may contribute to problems by further increasing dampness. Pregnancy may also be characterised by food cravings. It would be pleasing to assume that these cravings were always directed toward beneficial foods and they sometimes are, but not always.

Even apparently unhealthy cravings, such as a desire for fried take away foods, can indicate a real dietary need, in this case for more high quality fat in the diet. If the craving is for very unusual substances such as clay or ashes it is termed 'pica' and thought to be due to nutritional deficiency.

Food effects individuals differently. If you have an underlying yang deficiency you might find it unpleasant to drink a glass of iced water, while your friend with an excess internal heat condition will crave drinks straight from the fridge. A person prone to phlegm disharmonies may immediately notice phlegm forming in the back of their throat following an ice cream, while others notice no such effects. A person with a yang deficiency will enjoy a warm curry, while those with a yin deficiency find that hot spicy foods can trigger feelings of hot flushes.

It is important in traditional Chinese medicine to help people find healthy foods that suit their body type, rather than following set dietary guidelines that ignore individual constitutional differences.

Water in Pregnancy

According to Susan Perri (The Birthkit, Issue 35) "in traditional Chinese medicine the water element embodies the virtue of knowledge, most importantly knowledge of the self. Balanced water relishes quiet and isolation to tune into the quiet inner knowing. Balanced water moves slowly and with clarity. It is described as 'sitting in the lap of God' or the essence of finding comfort and strength in knowing one's life purpose."

The water element can be encouraged with foods that are naturally salty and represent some connection to water, for example, seaweed, miso, tamarin, kidney beans, millet and root vegetables. Keeping water in the diet and in the body can help the kidneys do their job of flushing the toxins out of your system and maintaining electrolyte balance.

Dandelion (Taraxacum official, commonly known as Dandelion Tea), uses the leaves and flowers as kidney aids. They are high in potassium and will help maintain the essential balance of electrolytes while flushing out the system. The root is an excellent liver tonic.

Nettle (Urtica dioica) is another natural diuretic. Nettle is extremely nourishing to the kidneys and adrenals. Nettle is especially good for stress. Recommended use is infusion. Nettle is a popular herb in midwifery practice.

Diet and Postnatal Recovery

There is a long documented history in traditional Chinese medicine of women taking dietary remedies to encourage lactation and to promote their recovery from childbirth or a miscarriage. Specific foods are seen to be especially valuable, for example:

Foods that tonify Qi (energy) include;

Oats, rice, potato, sweet potato, pumpkin, mushroom (button and shitake), yam, date, grape, kidney beans, tofu, beef, chicken, tuna, egg, jasmine tea and spices such as basil, cinnamon, clove, dill, fennel, fenugreek, ginger, nutmeg, rosemary, thyme.

Examples of every day Western foods that can be used to build Qi:

Oat porridge with dates; roast sweet potatoes, pumpkin and yams with rosemary; chicken stir fry with shiitake mushrooms and rice; Shepherds pie with beef mince, mushrooms, carrots and mashed potato as a topping; tuna fish pie made with hard boiled eggs and served with mashed potatoes and peas; stir fired tofu, eggplant and mushrooms with sesame seeds on rice; home made muesli slice with honey and dates.

Complimentary Therapies & Remedies

Psychosomatic Therapy

My journey is to experience
'the discovery that body, mind and soul are all one'.
This is Psychosomatic Therapy.

Hermann Müller (2011)
Psychosomatic Breakthrough, Cert III PSYCHO1A

The shape your body is in right now provides many clues to your current state of balance. This state of balance has a profound effect on the baby you are growing. We are all the result of our own experiences in the womb. By developing awareness you are able to create a happy, peaceful experience for your baby, and in turn a happy, healthy child.

You are probably familiar with the term 'Emotional Baggage', which describes the negative effects of past traumas that most of us carry around in our hearts. But what about 'Body Baggage'? What is 'Body Baggage' and how does it affect you? The song lyrics 'Pack up your troubles in your old kit bag and smile, smile, smile' explains in simple terms how most of us deal with emotional issues and traumas in our lives. Rather than deal with issues and resolve them at the time they occur, we tuck unresolved negative experiences away to be dealt with at a later date.

This creates a false sense of security and an emotional safety net of sorts, but nets are full of holes. The holes being that the 'kit bag' you have packed your troubles into is your body, creating 'issues in the tissues'. The day for dealing with the troubles eventually will come, often due to a trigger of some sort, most likely ill health or another form of physical or emotional discomfort. Sometimes, unfortunately, we are forced to look at the 'issues in our tissues' from a hospital bed.

Your body is your vehicle to carry you through this life and it requires free-flowing energy to function at its best. You have created this body from the moment of your conception, it is the only one you have so why not love it? When your body is overloaded with unresolved negative experiences it becomes blocked, creating stagnation and lethargy. What happens inside your body manifests on the outside, this is the outer sheath's response to the inner core's condition ('This is the shape I am in'). Blocked energy in your spirit may become excess or insufficient tissue in your body. You see this where bodies may become fragile, thin and weak, or the opposite where they appear hard or armoured with flabby, insensitive tissue. Your baby is creating its vehicle (body) as it grows inside you. The thoughts and emotions you experience directly effect your baby and its vehicle.

We are vibrating energy. Every cell in your body has an electro-magnetic field measured at four watts of energy, and it is understood that we emit one hundred watts of heat most of the time. This electrical field acts like a transmission system, allowing nerve signals to travel at immense speed throughout the network of the body. Messages are received and emitted constantly throughout the day. Neurons retain these messages and accumulate them into programs and beliefs in preparation for a ready response when the emotions are triggered by a situation e.g. 'this always happens to me...' The more entrenched they become the more likely they are to eventuate.

Our emotional response to an event or situation is based upon these programs. Peptides are released in response to our emotional reactions, with each person responding to a situation according to their own programming. The more our behaviour repeats these programs the more entrenched they become. Most people have little understanding of the programs they are running subconsciously, going about their daily lives reacting rather than creating. It is a bit like hitting a ball into the pack on a snooker table. As the ball hits the other balls they respond randomly. When there is focus however, the ball is hit purposefully and directed to the pocket. The ball's response is deliberate and created, not random, so the ball goes where you want it to go.

You have the same ability to direct the thoughts of your mind to create happy, harmonious thoughts which in turn create a happy, harmonic body. Every cell in the body has the capacity to hold emotional memory. These emotions, positive or negative, are used as the blueprint for building tissues and structures in the body. The structural outcome is the result of the perception of what is required for the body to survive or protect itself - these are the 'issues in the tissues'.

The memories that caused you pain have also caused you to form protective habits. For example children who are frequently subjected to verbal, emotional or physical violence or conflict may grow up to avoid these situations at all costs. The outcome of this habitual behaviour can include inability to resolve conflict within personal relationships, difficulty feeling safe, and frequent triggering of the fight or flight response, becoming passively aggressive. Frequent responses of this nature place a tremendous pressure on the physical body and can result in illness such as Chronic Fatigue Syndrome, lethargy and depression. Every person has issues in their tissues and the experienced practitioner understands how to read a person's face and body to gain understanding and acceptance of the person and their life's journey.

The Chakra System

Chakra is Sanskrit for 'Wheel of Light'. The seven main energy centres or chakras receive and radiate energy at seven central points from the base charka in your pelvis, up your torso to the top of your head. Each chakra is situated in a particular part of the body for the specific purpose of the function and expression of the emotions of that area of the body. The caduceus cord (medical symbol) has some base in this concept. Two snakes intertwine up the body. One represents the female aspect, the other the male. Each point where they meet forms a chakra. In a person who is deeply spiritual the chakras can become radiant light and energy. This is why holy paintings of saints depict a white orb around the person.

Clairvoyant psychics and energy healers see the seven chakras as wheel like vortices of energy. Each chakra relates to a colour and is connected to specific organs and glands in that area of the body. The chakra itself lies in the etheric body, its vibrations flow through a stem that enters the physical body and connects into the spinal column at specific points where there are nerve plexus or ganglia. These nerve centres translate the vibrations received in the area into physically felt nerve responses, creating actions and reactions that we experience as feelings.

The benefits of chakra balancing for health and wellbeing have been written about by many intuitive healers. Though I do not have psychic sight I do have a sense of feeling the energy of the chakras on the body. I use this intuition to assess the balance of the chakras and then use sensitive healing techniques to balance the chakras. Using a pendulum is an excellent way of contacting the higher subconscious. When a pendulum is worked over the body it will swing in the direction the chakra is rotating. Depending on the state of the chakra at the time the pendulum will swing vigorously or sluggishly. This gives insight into the overall health of the body in that area.

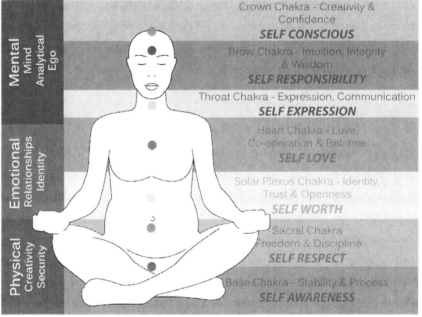

Crown Chakra - Creativity & Confidence
SELF CONSCIOUS

Brow Chakra - Intuition, Integrity & Wisdom
SELF RESPONSIBILITY

Throat Chakra - Expression, Communication
SELF EXPRESSION

Heart Chakra - Love, Co-operation & Balance
SELF LOVE

Solar Plexus Chakra - Identity, Trust & Openness
SELF WORTH

Sacral Chakra - Freedom & Discipline
SELF RESPECT

Base Chakra - Stability & Process
SELF AWARENESS

Mental — Mind, Analytical, Ego

Emotional — Relationships, Identity

Physical — Creativity, Security

The chakra points are also picked up on the feet, face and hands and correspond to the same areas on the body. Psychosomatic Therapy assesses the physical response in the body to the activity of the chakra in that area.

Every part of the body is important and essential to the overall wellbeing and productivity of the body. Self-awareness brings understanding to this principle. The mind trains every cell, neuron, muscle, tissue, bone and joint to coordinate thought, emotions and movement. When we lack this understanding we judge, talk negatively to ourselves and others, responding to our body in a negative way. The body in turn creates a body that fulfills your beliefs about yourself. For example, if you push yourself hard following the high expectations of the mind, the ego wanting to be first and the best so pushing the body beyond what it can handle, the body responds by becoming rigid to give itself strength against the strength of the mind. Eventually, when pushed far enough, the body will break either physically or emotionally. However, when there is balanced communication between the mind and body there is time for self, a sense of peace and harmony. The body can relax and trust itself and remains soft, flexible and toned, thus far less likely to wear out.

> "From the tips of my fingers to the tip of my toe I am one with my Soul in that instant of stillness and perfect balance!"
>
> Hermann Müller
> Face to Face With Facts, Personality Potential

Issues in the Tissues

> "Most psychologists treat the mind as disembodied, a phenomenon with little or no connection to the physical body. Conversely physicians treat the body with no regard to the mind or the emotions. But the body and mind are not separate, and we cannot treat one without the other."
>
> Dr Candace Pert
> http://candacepert.com/

It is understood that every thought, emotion, idea, notion and belief has a neurochemical reaction. Dr Candace Pert is widely known for her research into understanding the neuropeptides in the body. These peptides, the messengers for the body, are found on the cell wall throughout your body. They provide information and feedback so your body can react to a situation.

Research has shown that our emotions are inexplicably linked to these messengers and particularly to our immune and endocrine systems through the central nervous system. When strong emotions are felt but not expressed appropriately they become stored, creating an excess production of epinephrine, better known as adrenaline. This excess results in chemical breakdown and a weakening of the immune system.

Thus your thoughts, words and emotions are intricately linked with the health of your physical body. Your body is attuned to react to your held belief system, good or bad. So the key is to change the messages that are being sent around your body by changing the original emotional charge creating the belief.

Your body shape, the amount of excess tissue or lack of tissue, the way you stand, your posture, your face, hands, feet - every part of your physical body provides clues as to your life experiences and the emotional baggage you carry with you. Geometry is an important indicator. The first thing I notice when looking at another being is the shape of their face and body and the way their energy flows throughout, for example is it uplifting or draining?

These issues in the tissues are a result of the fears that you hold, the way you react to situations, your ability to cope with stressful situations and how positively you approach your life. The brain thinks - it cannot feel. It is your body that senses and feels and has the ability to hold onto pain and hurt until it is given permission to let it go. The Body-Mind protects us from being hurt by desensitising itself from painful experiences so that we can survive until we learn to overcome them. Imagine for a moment the joy of living without your emotional baggage.

Psychosomatic therapy can help you do this by guiding and teaching you to remove the emotional barb from past memory and experience. These emotional barbs (neuro emotional charges or NECs) can be likened to beach balls that keep popping up out of the water regardless of how many times we push them under. They float under the surface until something creates a charge, for example a smell, a sound, music or an emotional situation. This charge then results in a reaction that is either pleasant or unpleasant. We feel at the mercy of the forces within us until we learn how these NECs can be removed with simple psychosomatic techniques such as breathing and moving.

You will find over time that you are more able to focus and live in the here, in the now, rather than clinging to the past or worrying about the future.

How Does Psychosomatic Therapy Work?

Psychosomatic Therapy involves a thorough assessment of your 'tree of life' (your body) from the tips of your toes to the top of your head. Your feet and legs indicate the roots of your tree, how you ground in life, your ability to stand up for yourself and hold your ground now and in the past. Your torso is likened to the trunk of the tree. Does your tree stand tall and straight, or does it droop, sag, bend and curve? Is your tree rigid or flexible? Assessment is made through your posture, body shape and the way you stand, walk and move. Your chest and arms indicate how you extend your heart to the world. Do you protect or over nurture and forget to nurture you?

Your face is the fruit, telling the reader where you are right now. Are you comfortable in your body or looking and searching for the answers outside of yourself? Through this wonderful process you are able to acknowledge who you truly are and learn more about yourself than you probably ever have done before. Psychosomatic Therapy gives you the opportunity to come home and be comfortable in your own skin.

Your body has many emotional trigger points. Once the trigger points (emotional release points) within your body have been identified your therapist can begin the process of releasing that unwanted energy. This doesn't happen in one single visit, after all you have spent a life time gathering your emotional baggage. However over time, as your emotional baggage is released, you can expect to feel a greater sense of calm and a greater sense of knowing within yourself as you begin to live in the here and now rather than focusing on the past or worrying so much about the future. If you are considering pregnancy, or are already pregnant, psychosomatic therapy can help you to become more balanced and positive and help you to become more attuned with your body, which is so important when you are preparing to give birth.

Psychosomatic Therapy is Based in Three Principles: Focus, Balance and Structure

Focus

Most people are at the mercy of what they think. With focus you can learn to train your mind to think positive, loving thoughts, focusing only on those thoughts that are beneficial to you. When the mind becomes so busy worrying over another person or past event, then the body becomes stressed in response. The event is over but you are choosing to hold onto the pain, by doing so punishing your body over and over again. You cannot change another person, you can only change yourself. When we allow ourselves to react to another we give our power to them and dismantle ourselves one building block at a time. Like a pile of bricks on the ground, we then have to rebuild and put our self back together ('pull yourself together'). If we learn to accept that it is what it is without any expectation then we can just be in the flow. When your focus is in the present you listen to your body's messages and respond to the signals, thus fulfilling your body's needs and reducing stress. So the trick is to remain present, keep yourself in the here and now. Let go of the issues from the past, you cannot go back and change what has already been.

Happy, peaceful pregnancies and birth come from within. A successful birth relies on a relaxed mind, being able to let go and trust in the process that your body has been programmed to do. Your mind is not required and the majority of complicated births occur when the mind gets in the way. Distracting the mind is probably one of the most important jobs a good midwife will do, allowing your body to get on with what it needs to do. You can make a big difference to your birth outcome by practicing throughout your pregnancy so it becomes a natural way to be. As you get to know your body you will listen to what it is saying.

Balance

There are two intertwining aspects to your being, your heart and your mind. The challenge is to give balanced attention to both. In Psychosomatic Therapy we see these two aspects as the two sides of the body. The right is the mind, external, the ego, the analytical, male yang energy. The left is the heart, the inner aspect, intuition, the soul, the emotional, female yin energy.

The right side, the ego, pushes us hard to find the answer that cannot be found outside of self. The left side, the soul, already has the answer and awaits your acknowledgement that ultimately the answers lie within you. Just being you is the joy you are looking for. When you come home, trusting your soul, following your path and doing what feels right for you, the peace of being at home will be a natural way of being. When you are focused and tuned into both aspects of your being you listen to and trust your intuition (inner tutor) and will make decisions that are right for you and your baby. You will tune into your body, trusting your baby's souls journey as you work together as one, ultimately trusting your body to birth confidently.

Structure

The blue-print of your life is carried within the stem-cells and DNA of your body. It is your body that understands how to be pregnant and to birth. When you experience tension it is your body telling you that something is out of alignment. It is the body's natural state to create balance and to heal itself. Your body will perform miracles when it is supported and given the tools to heal. The tension you feel is to bring attention to the tension so that you can pay attention to it, change your posture, move and exercise or massage the area that is tense. By doing so you acknowledge the tension and allow the issues in your tissues to be released.

Attention to your structure brings attention to your body. When you are focused on your body you are not focused in the mind, thinking about the future, the past, or in another person's story - the focus is on you, right here, right now. Your body can relax and re-structure. Your body knows what to do, it just needs to be given permission to let it go. Women who follow these three principles have easy healthy pregnancies and births.

Exercises

Postural Integration

1. Stand with your feet facing forward directly under the hip bones. Your feet are like the wheels of a car, they must face forward in order to follow your path directly. Have a look at your stance. Do your feet face forward or do they head off in opposite directions? As I spoke about in the balance section, if you are balanced then both male and female sides will be even. If you notice that your right foot goes off in a different direction then your mind is taking you away from the centre. If it is your left then you are a wandering soul looking for emotional support.

    Practice walking straight, both feet pointing ahead. This may take some time as you have developed a lifetime of habits. An excellent way to check this is on the sand of the beach, checking to see if your footprints are straight or are they twisted in the wrong direction?

2. If your head is forward of your body, this compresses your neck and chest, making it difficult to breathe. Psychosomatically the head forward posture indicates that mentally you are ahead of your body, your thoughts are creating stress. It may be helpful to have a friend or your partner take a photo of you standing side on so that you can see how far ahead you are holding your head. Stand by the edge of an open door and notice if your ankle, hip, shoulder and ear are in alignment with the door edge. Make sure your feet are hip distance apart and facing forward.

    If your body is straight your ankle, hip and shoulder are all in alignment. The best way to check your alignment is to stand with your back against the wall, feet directly under your hips and facing forward, heels touching the wall or skirting board. Your shoulders and the back of your head should touch the wall. Pull in your navel, relax your knees and relax your body back into correct alignment. You can gently press your solar plexus point, located in the centre front below the bottom of your rib cage (below the sternum), and breathe deeply, feeling how it feels to relax and come home to your centre.

3. Learn to walk on the balls of your feet. When we are light and mobile we walk on the balls of the feet, hence the saying 'she is on the ball'. Dance around the room, you will see you cannot dance on your heels. Watch how children run and play, it is on the balls of the feet. We do not naturally walk on our heels. Another way to learn this is to walk backwards, moon walk. You cannot walk backwards on your heels, it is on the ball. Once you feel confident with this then reverse the action and walk forward.

4. Whilst standing walk up and down on the spot, one ball of the foot then the other, keeping knees soft. This also softens the ankles and assists with correct posture.

The whole time you are focused here you will be present in your body, not in your mind.

Breathe

When you breathe with full lung expansion your whole being benefits from oxygen being circulated through the body. Your lungs act as a container, whilst the diaphragm pumps air in and out of the body but also activates the lymphatic system, one of our detoxification processes. Seventy percent of your body's waste products are removed via your breath, twenty percent via your skin, seven percent via urine and the remaining three percent via faeces.

Deep breathing is the fastest way to trigger your parasympathetic nervous system, through what some practitioners call the relaxation response. The parasympathetic nervous system, which is stimulated in times of stress and anxiety, controls your fight or flight response, including spikes in cortisol and adrenaline that can be damaging when they persist too long. It is also responsible for increasing the 'feel good' hormoncs or endorphins which are welcome when you are stressed.

Many adults have lost the ability to deep core breathe, that is the ability to expand the lungs to their full capacity whilst activating the centre core muscles of the abdominal area (the whole of your abdomen from the rib cage to the pubic area). Lack of activation results in shallow, stifled breathing and is one of the reasons many people feel so tired. Emotional responses early in life result in us holding our breath. The more we hold our breath when emotionally upset, the less we use the full capacity of our lungs, eventually becoming shallow breathers with restricted musculature.

By connecting with your core as you breathe you create a centre for where you exist in your body, your home. When you are able to come home you find confidence, peace and great potential. Practising the deep breathing exercise below enables you to activate your core, bringing attention to your body and helping you to be inside your body. As your mind is focused on breathing and core activation it cannot take you away to your thoughts or stories.

The Exercise:
This activation is the same as that used in Pilates to engage the abdominals before beginning an exercise.

1. Sit straight or stand comfortably in good alignment. If you need assistance stand up against a wall with your feet in correct position. Soften your knees and ensure your shoulders are back against the wall. Rest your head against the wall and look straight ahead. This may be uncomfortable to begin with if you have created unsupporting postural behaviours.
2. Imagine you are pulling your navel button towards your back. At first this may feel like you are doing little, if anything, until you reactivate this area. Every time you bring attention to this area you will feel it soften and react more.
3. Once you have engaged your abdominals take a breath in. Relax the shoulders and fill your lungs to the very bottom of the rib

cage. Imagine your lungs are like a balloon that you are filling from the bottom to the top. At first you may feel like you are breathing quite shallowly and your lungs may feel stiff. Again, the more you practice the more the elasticity will return and your muscles will regain their tone.

4. Once you have taken the breath in hold it for a few seconds whilst maintaining activation of the navel. If possible pull the navel in further then gently and slowly breathe out.

5. Once the last of the breath has been expelled remain quiet in this space (known as the gap). It is here that you find the deepest of peace. Then begin the exercise again.

6. Practice this breath as often as possible and certainly use it for relaxation and meditation. The more you practice this the more you will be able to let go of unwanted issues in the tissues and find your inner peace. If whilst doing this exercise you feel emotion come up do your best to continue to breathe through the feeling. Allow the emotions to just flow like a river without attaching memory or stories to them. This is your body's way of releasing old unwanted baggage. I have used this practice consistently for the past three years with amazing results. It is easy and incredibly effective.

Practising this breath throughout pregnancy will create a way of being. When it comes time to birth you will work naturally with this breath, allowing yourself to let go and let your body do what it is programmed to do without your mind getting in the way.

Psychosomatic Therapy Personal Development Training

There is a way to identify and release your body baggage and you can learn to do it yourself without the added financial discomfort of paying someone else to 'fix you'. It is your very own experience that has created the 'issues in your tissues', and you know your body better than anyone else, so who is better qualified than you to heal you? Psychosomatic Therapy is how you can learn to do this. By learning to use your own powers of observation, touch and desire to find your own inner light, you can identify and release the pain from your own body. Correct breathing techniques and balanced posture helps your body to regain boundless reserves of energy.

Psychosomatic Therapy also works by teaching you how to balance your often unbalanced masculine and feminine selves, allowing you to unleash your soul's potential to be all that you can be. Life is about balance. Psychosomatic Therapy can help you achieve this, bringing you home to live comfortably in your own body.

http://www.casadelsole.com.au/index.php/therapies/
pychosomatic-therapy/psychosomatic-therapy

Fiona's Story

Birth outcome is the result of the ability to ignore the mind and listen to the body. The more a woman is able to drop into her body and ignore outside stimulation the better she will work with what her body is communicating to her through sensation and emotion. In order for your body to perform at its best your mind and body must work in unison. The high obstetric intervention rates are testimony to this as women lean toward trusting the external world for guidance rather than what their body is telling them.

Fiona, at 39 weeks, burst into tears during one of her last visits to me. Although Fiona had experienced a totally healthy, uneventful pregnancy, her obstetrician had suggested inducing early as she was going on holidays. Because Fiona had faith and trust in her carer she believed they knew what they were doing and so felt pressured to agree. I on the other hand have a different approach. I asked Fiona 'How does this feel to you? Does this feel right?' I asked her to check in on her gut feeling, her intuition (inner tutor) by breathing deep and sitting quietly, allowing her to gain access to her inner knowing and connect with her baby.

It took very little time before she stated 'No, this is wrong, there is no valid reason to do this'. So I asked her 'what do you want to do about it?' Fiona replied 'I want to be left alone to have my baby when it is ready to come, not when someone dictates'. We discussed strategies that she could employ when next discussing her progress with her obstetrician.

What is most important here is that there is no medical reason for induction and mother and baby were both very healthy and without risk.

Because of the stress induced somatic response in her body, Fiona's back was aching and for the first time there was a little swelling (oedema) in her feet. Oedema can be a psychosomatic response to fear. Through some gentle manipulation I released the tension in her body, whilst massaging her feet quickly reduced the oedema and Fiona was able to release the pent up fear emotion. Once this happened she relaxed, the backache disappeared and the swelling in her feet visibly reduced. By ensuring the connection between the mind, body and emotions, balance was restored very quickly.

In this situation **Focus** is created by focusing the mind on what is important and the present situation. **Balance** is restored by connecting the heart and the mind, whilst **Structure** is attended to by releasing the body's stored tension. Fiona refused induction and continued her pregnancy for another three weeks before she went into labour naturally and delivered a beautiful bouncing boy four hours later. Her birth story most likely would have been very different had she been induced three weeks early.

Neuro-Emotional Technique

As explained in Psychosomatic Therapy, the cells of our body hold memory. When we have a strong emotional reaction to an event our body produces hormones and peptides in response. These peptides lock onto the cell surface like a key and lock, resulting in a cellular reaction. Each time the same neural pathway is triggered by an emotional response this pathway becomes more embedded. Over time this pathway becomes dominant, resulting in habitual reactive behaviour.

You may feel the physical and emotional effects of unresolved stress exhibited as unexplained pain, anxiety, behaviours that do not serve you. An emotional response is generated by neuropeptides and their receptors and these travel quickly around the body. Future triggers that spark the memory of the event may initiate the same reaction as you originally had to the event.

These physical responses to emotions may in fact be conditioned responses triggered by a neurological or meridian deficit. For example if you find yourself reacting in the same way to a similar event frequently and find yourself saying such things as 'here we go again' or 'this always happens to me' then you have created a neural emotional charge (NEC).

These charges tend to be stored in the organs of the body and can be located by your therapist using muscle testing. Once located there are words that can be used to trigger the response and techniques used to explore the source of the charge, when it first occurred and what was the original memory. Once triggered specific points are used to distract the brain as explained in Psychosomatic Therapy and EFT. Once this happens the neural branch is broken and the brain can no longer connect the emotion to the memory. The memory is still present but without the emotional charge.

Eventually the memory of the event will diminish too. NET is an incredibly simple yet effective technique that clears the NEC, by doing so breaking your conditioned response. It is a non-intrusive technique that uses muscle testing to identify the physical location of stuck, negatively charged emotion in your body, then by accessing acupressure points of the spine releases the meridian or neurological blockage.

NET breaks health into four main areas, of which any or all of the four may be impacting on health:

- emotional or stress factors
- the effects of toxins on your body
- nutritional needs or deficits
- structural needs

NET practitioners test all four areas (the Home Run Formula) as it is essential that all are addressed in order for the conditioned response to be fully cleared. NET is a highly respected therapy with over 1000 practitioners across Australia & NZ and many more in the USA. For more info go to the NET therapy website site or my website. http://www.casadelsole.com.au

Ka Huna Massage

Ka Huna is no ordinary massage! Imagine a massage where your practitioner dances and glides around the table, using mainly their arms and forearms to provide deep, effective muscle relaxation that takes you to a truly blissful state.

What makes Ka Huna massage so beautiful to receive is the intention, focus and deep caring nature of the practitioner. Rhythmic and heart centred, it can only be explained as a deep state of unconditional love and compassion, designed to encourage a holistic natural healing state of the body, the 'aloha' spirit that is sacred to the people of Hawaii.

Through the balance of body, mind and spirit you are able to let go of withheld pain in a gentle, loving way.

A therapeutic massage technique, Ka Huna Massage is based on the teachings and practices of the ancient Hawaiian Ka Hunas. In the language of native Hawaiians, 'huna' means 'secret knowledge' and a master practitioner of any of the huna arts is known as a 'Ka Huna'. Traditionally, massage ('lomi lomi') was practiced in the Hawaiian Islands both for relaxation and as one of the Ka Huna healing arts.

Benefits of Ka Huna Massage:

- stimulates the lymphatic, circulatory, respiratory and digestive systems
- creates a sense of deep connection between you and your baby
- gives great relief to pregnancy backache
- stimulates natural endorphins, reducing stress, depression and tiredness
- is stimulating and uplifting to the soul.

The link below provides a video demonstration of Ka Huna massage and a directory of Australian practitioners:

http://www.massagetreatment.com.au/

Reflexology

The feet, hands and ears are micro-systems correlating to the whole body. Reflexology is more than a foot massage, it is the stimulation of thousands of nerve endings (approximately 7200 in each foot), that correlate to organs and glands in the body. By stimulating specific points on the feet balance can be created, enhancing healing and assisting the body to let go of emotional baggage. The trained therapist is able to skilfully hone in and discover areas of imbalance and sluggishness that could lead to disease if unattended.

> "Chemicals cannot cure emotional pain and surgery is not able to remove emotional hurts since dis-ease arises from within the self, resentment, anger, frustration and fear buried deep within the sub-conscious mind creates internal, physical, emotional and spiritual imbalance"
>
> Stormer, C., 1996

My Reflexology Journey

I was first introduced to reflexology when I was pregnant with my third child (Vanessa) in 1989. I met a wonderful local reflexologist, Elizabeth Bowden, who understood the magic of the feet long before there was a reflexology association. I asked her to be one of our presenters at our ten week childbirth class and teach pregnant couples how to massage their feet for improved health and to assist with an easier labour. Elizabeth was asked to attend many births and it was through this that I first understood how wonderful this modality is. Whilst I was pregnant with Vanessa I received regular sessions which felt wonderful and I am sure contributed to my uneventful pregnancy. When I was due Elizabeth massaged my feet during one of our childbirth classes as a demonstration and that night I went into labour. This story is at the end of the book.

After Vanessa was born it was difficult to go back to work with three children so I became a direct selling natural skin care consultant as it gave me income with flexibility. During this time I became very interested in the feet and with the help of Elizabeth's charts began teaching foot massage techniques to my consultants and customers. My business was very successful because of it. In 1995 whilst working as the Midwife Coordinator for the Childbirth Information Service I received a flier promoting Maternity Reflexology for midwives, conducted by UK midwife Sue Enzer, the pioneer of the maternity reflexology course taught to midwives and reflexologists today. I attended this training and was in awe of what seemed like an incredibly simplistic but incredibly effective tool. Reflexology has become one of my main modalities over the past eighteen years. When in doubt, look to the feet.

Though the modality of reflexology has been transformed over many centuries, what remains at its base is the understanding that reflexology aligns the energy zones that channel through the body. Most of us have been educated about the skeletal, nervous, cardiovascular, lymphatic, viscera, muscle and skin systems. Few have been taught about the central core energy that exists within the body - referred to as the intuitive or psychic, spiritual energy system, including the aura and meridians. Alex Gray in his book 'Sacred Mirrors' has created excellent examples in his artwork for all the systems of the body. The Meridians, recognised by traditional medicine and Eastern philosophy, are effectively rebalanced through the art of Reflexology. The flow of energy around and within the body has been discussed and documented throughout ancient texts for thousands of years, especially the Indian known as Prana and Chinese known as Qi. Western science is only beginning to grasp the concept of this energy field through the work of Quantum physicists, known as bio-energy, quantum energy or the matrix.

"Bio-energy paradigms conceptualise disease as a 'disruption' of energy exchange, and 'intoxication' of the body, especially through stress. Healing is based on the principle of conducting cosmic energy through the healer, in particular the hands, eyes, thoughts and words. Qi creates order out of chaos as it flows toward the 'higher concentration' (unlike entropy, where energy flow is toward dissolution)."

EFT and the Role of Energy in Therapy - Dr David Lake and Steve Wells 2009 http://www.eftdownunder.com/about.html

Using the meridian and spiritual energy systems reflexology goes deeper, complimenting and assisting the body to become:

"a permeable channel for the circulation of the subtle and fine energies of spiritual consciousness that are ever present and interpenetrate the self and surroundings. Parallel lines of force stream through the body extending out of the crown of the head and curling back around to the feet creating a toroidal flow."

Wilber, K. & McCormick, C. 1990

The Soles of the Feet Mirror the Body

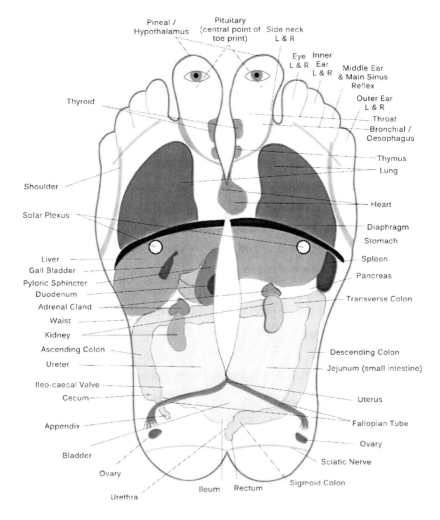

Spinal reflex runs up both inner aspects of feet.

Scientists have clearly shown this invisible energy passes through all matter, affecting every living system on the planet. Magnetic fields surrounding the earth influence behaviour, mental function, physical energy and biological welfare of man and are affected by the moon and solar cycles.

Emotional Anatomy of the Feet

The feet are the sole of the body and carry you through life, they imprint our character, telling us so much about what is going on with the body, mind and spirit. An experienced reader of feet, I am able to understand much about the people I meet when I look to their feet. I love summer as I get to see people's feet, which gives me so much insight into the person, even more than from face reading.

Reflexology concentrates not just on the physical body but on the total wholeness and soul of your being. 'There is more to the feet than meets the eye.' The foot is made up of twenty six small bones and over thirty ligaments that cushion the full impact of your body weight as you jump, run or walk, every day of your life. They depict male/mental and female/emotional balance, indicating how balanced left/right brain integration is. The soles of the Soul sense and inform every organ and muscle of your body about what you are stepping into.

Every organ and body system is reflected in the feet. The big toes reflect the head. Below the little toes reflect the shoulders, lower foot the backside and the spine is the same shape as the inside of the foot. There are 26 bones in the foot and 26 bones in the spine.

The toes are individual sensors that reach out like antennae to seek collective knowledge and explore life to the full. Being on the balls of your feet and on your toes conveys an eagerness and enthusiasm for life, which can be enhanced through reflexology. By massaging the toe pads and necks of the toes we can stimulate the head, brain, face and sensory reflexes. Each toe symbolises a specific aspect of the mind, with significant consciousness being immediately mirrored onto the toe pads. For this reason the toes should be studied in their entirety as well as separately.

The right foot and toes represent past thoughts and perceptions, as well as the mental, male logical thinking and how much influence this has on your life. The left foot and toes represent present ideas and perceptions, creative female thinking, the inner personal world and how much this has influence on your life. It is not unusual to see one foot larger than the other, indicating a priority for either male or female energy or a need to support oneself more on one side compared to the other in the past.

Length and shape is important, indicating to the experienced reader the degree of balance shown and the individual potential of the person being read.

Big Toe - the Thinking Toe

Indicates the strength of the mind and reflects the intuitive, intellectual thoughts that expand beyond the body to the greater world. It also represents the meridian energy of the spleen and liver.

The direction, size and proportion of the right toe indicates how much the mind is directing your life and how much past thoughts or male influence has had upon you in the past.

The direction, size and proportion of the left toe indicates how much you are able to stay centred in the present with your thoughts connected to your heart and intuition. It can also represent how much influence females have on your thoughts.

Second Toe - the Feeling Toe

Represents the feelings of self and to relationships in general, overall feelings, emotions and interrelationships within the environment. When longer than the big toe can indicate a demanding nature and need to control others. This meridian energy is related to the stomach and we understand how our stomach is tied up with feelings.

The right feeling toe indicates how your mind directs your feelings, how you experience your feelings in the external world or the past, and possibly the males in your life as well as accepting people for who they are with compassion and empathy.

The left feeling toe indicates your feelings towards yourself, your relationship with you and the female creative energies in your life and how you are feeling about yourself in the present. Accepting yourself with compassion and empathy.

Third Toe - the Doing Toe

Projects the thoughts regarding activity, personal achievements, self actualisation and inner control, how we actively take part in the world. Also connects with the bladder meridian.

The right doing toe indicates how much you do in the world. Do you walk your talk with compassion and empathy, is it a priority? Does your mind push you to be very active? Do you express your feelings through your actions in relationships?

The left doing toe indicates how much time do you have for yourself, the influence of significant females in your life and do you walk your talk? Are you able to actively express your feelings and intuition? Do you do what you want to do or do you pull back at the detriment of yourself in the perception of pleasing the external world or significant others in your life?

Fourth Toe - the Communication / Relationship Toe

Shows the impacts of ability to communicate the inner world to the outer world in relationships and pleasure as well as the gallbladder meridian.

The right communication/relationship toe expresses how you relate in your external relationships, particularly with the men in your life. Do you express and communicate with compassion, acceptance and understanding or do you hold back and hide your true inner self from the world?

The left communication/relationship toe expresses how well you communicate your needs to yourself. Do you listen to your inner tutor and act on this regardless of people's expectations? Are you open and loving to you and those around you?

Little Toe - the Social Toe

Displays the degree of self security. Influenced by family, upbringing and social systems that effect the expansiveness and freedom of thought as well as the kidney meridian.

The right social toe indicates how secure you feel in the external world and within your family of origin. The longer and straighter the toe the better your ability to be at peace within the harmony of your family. Are you truly comfortable being with yourself around your family and peers?

The left social toe indicates how secure you are with yourself and how much you trust your own guidance and are able to accept and understand your present family for who they are and who you are with them.

Emotional Anatomy of the Foot

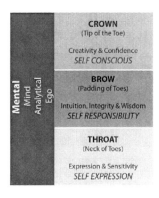

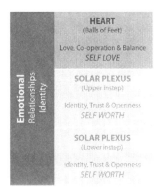

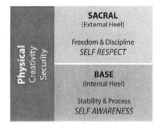

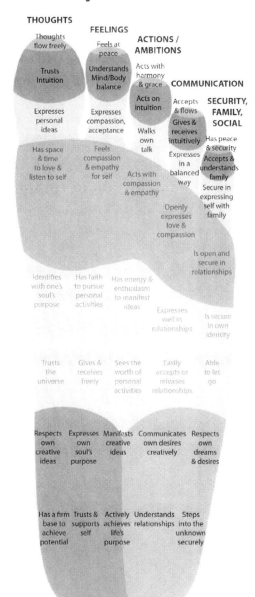

Feet

Let's take a closer look at what your feet may be saying to you.

Toes reflect - antennae, new thoughts and ideas
Toe pads - provide space to think and play
Neck of toe - indicator of expression of true self
Balls of feet – feelings, love, acceptance
Instep (upper half) - activities, energy and enthusiasm
Instep (lower half) – communication, relationships, creativity
Heels – mobility and security, move ahead with ease and confidence

Right foot – past thoughts and perceptions, masculine, relationships and reactions to the external world and other people
Left foot – present thoughts and perceptions, female, reactions to the internal world, emotions and who you are with people
Right toes represent the mind, the past and the external world.
Left toes represent the feelings, the present and the internal world.
Toe length and shape indicates individual potential.
Heavy Right foot - weighed down by unresolved emotions of the past
Heavy Left foot - currently carrying a heavier load and more burdens

SKIN

Pertains to the meaning of that area on the foot affected.
Soft and pliable - spontaneous and balanced
Excessively soft - lacking substance, lazy, lacking inner strength
Flaccid – no energy, gives in
Oedema - overburdened
Hardened - defensive, protective, stubborn
Sensitive – vulnerable, self-conscious, easily hurt
Shiny – emotional friction, worn away
Rough – going through a rough or harsh time, strained
Peeling – layers shredding for the new
Flaking - irritated, 'getting under skin'
Athlete's Foot (Tinea) - ideas rejected, irritation and frustration

Fragile - delicate and easily hurt

Smooth and dry - exposed feelings

Blistered - friction, inner burning, inner irritation

Wrinkled - drained and sapped, over-worrying

Calluses - emotional barriers, mind controlling the heart, protection, need to go with the flow

Cracked - divided and torn between head and heart

Plantar Warts - dislike of self

Itching - heel - itching to move on; instep - itching to resolve the issue

Burning feet - inflamed and angry

Cold Feet - fear, lack of enthusiasm

TOE NAILS (Protection of Outer Forces)

Big Toe - defends personal ideas and thoughts

Second Toe - concepts of self, feelings and emotions

Third Toe - activity and control

Fourth Toe - looks after communication, relationships and pleasures

Little Toe - covers concepts of expansion, mobility, security in relationships and family

CHARACTERISTICS OF TOE NAILS

Ridged - opposing thoughts to others

Horizontal ridges - disease and vulnerability

Vertical ridges - fiercely protecting one's perceptions

Very ridged - insecure and uncertain

Split - divided and undecided between self and others, wanting to break away

Spoon shaped - depressed in centre, feeling vulnerable and less protected

Hang nails - extra support

Curled over - a need for protection and for a greater sense of security

Ingrown nails - deep need to protect, threatened and vulnerable

No nail - unprotected, vulnerable and exposed

Nail tearing - pulling strips off self

Broken - feeling the need to break free

Thickened – extra protection

Fungal – inflamed, vulnerable, being taken advantage of

Yellowed – fed up and tired

TOES

Flexible – secure, alert, relaxed

Rigid – insecure, definite ideas, control, unbending, consuming ambition

Well spaced – open-minded, actively search universal truth, plenty of space for thoughts and ideas

Wide apart – feels separate and alone

Well proportioned, flexible toes – think clearly

Upstanding - unable to stand up to own ideas and face the world with confidence

Toes in a line – solid, consistent

Uneven toes – inconsistent, up and down

Overlapping – no room for ideas, lack of freedom of thought

Crushed – dominated, smothered, stifled

Squashed and cramped – feeling hemmed in, smothered

Sunken into their socket – nowhere to go, held back, over controlled by others' concepts

Twisted – turned away from the truth

Sloping – off track, insecure, standing alone and separate, needs space to think

Concealed – shy, withdrawn and hiding, hoping not to be noticed

Bent – fears responsibility or failure, frightened to face up to having own ideas, bending to others' beliefs

Hammer toes – ideas hammered and knocked back

Crooked – modifies and adapts thinking to please

Webbed – interdependent on one another for extra back up

Daily massaging and stretching of your toes is a good way to release emotional issues and help to create a greater sense of balance.

Reproductive Reflexology

Regular massage of the feet assists detoxification and balancing of the body's functions. Pre-pregnant and pregnant women especially need to be nurtured, listened to and respected for their individuality. We must first look after the mother if a happy, healthy baby is to be created. Every woman is different and her concerns and fears are completely individual. Women find all too often they are caught in an impersonal maternity system as just another pregnant woman. Reflexology enables you to stop, be pampered and listened to.

When beginning to work on someone's feet I totally open myself to them, giving them the trust and confidence they need to open up. Women receiving regular reflexology are healthier with far less intervention and a better ability to cope with social stress. However most important is the effect that reflexology has on labour, with women reporting over and over again labour times of three to four hours without the need for drugs or interventions.

Ongoing studies continue to reveal that reflexology can truly be of great benefit to all pregnant women regardless of age or social situation. Studies conducted in the UK regarding reflexology in maternity care gathered outstanding results. Women who received regular reflexology sessions throughout their pregnancy had shorter and more effective labours, less intervention and better birth outcomes.

Reflexology gives me the ability to analyse feet and to receive insight as to when a woman is ready to birth. When it's 'All Systems Go' the pituitary point on the big toe enlarges significantly (see photo), the base area under the inner ankle becomes warm, enlarged and sometimes reddened. The feet have a strong zingy energy.

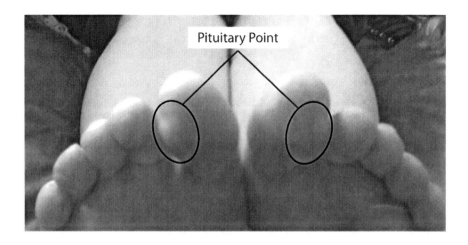

Pituitary Point

Jenny's Experience of Reflexology During Pregnancy

Jenny was referred to me by her obstetrician who thought that a course of reflexology may have a positive effect on Jenny's condition. Jenny was in great distress with a painful burning sensation in her thigh region, to the point where she was almost unable to walk.

Almost immediately on reflexology assessment I found a very tender zone on the reproductive area of the foot of the affected side. I did a midwifery assessment by gently palpating Jenny's uterus to ascertain in what position the baby was lying. The baby was lying in an awkward position, which would have accounted for the mother's pain. In the midwife role I used gentle movements and talking gently to the baby to move baby off the mother's lumbar region. I also encouraged Jenny to take up pilates as movement is very important (see the pilates section), stretching and working with the body allows the body to let go and assist the baby into the right position for birth.

Jenny expressed quite a few fears at this time. As psychosomatically the hips are about 'moving forward with ease', I picked up that Jenny's pain was related to her fears of being a single mum. I continued to work the specific areas on the feet whilst allowing Jenny to express her emotions. As we did this the pain subsided and with encouragement her baby moved into the correct position.

I gave Jenny several exercises to go home with and practice that could help keep the baby in the right position (these are explained in the Breech Section). Jenny expressed relief at being able to express how she really felt and then letting it go. The redness in her thigh began to dissipate quite markedly throughout the session. When she left she was able to happily walk with ease.

Over the next few sessions I built a trusting relationship between her and the baby. In time Jenny began to express some of the emotional turmoil happening in her life. She was experiencing loneliness and isolation at being a single mum, lack of financial and family support, deep seated fears about parenting and an overall sense of being out of control throughout the pregnancy.

As I was able to provide her with pregnancy and birth support her fear subsided. We then began to look at what support mechanisms Jenny required to create a happy, stress free life. Using psychosomatic principles we were able to work through her fears and Jenny learned how she is master of her own life. Once she began to give herself recognition and support for being strong and brave she was able to create a new reality that provides support and love.

Psychosomatically, we can see that Jenny's subconscious thoughts of lack of support had affected the cellular structure within her spine, resulting in imbalances along the spinal column. The physical body is created in response to these negative or positive patterns, thus Jenny's body created the issues in her tissues. The spine is the support system for the body, so if there is a feeling of not being supported the spine is one of the first places to reflect this.

After explaining this philosophy to Jenny I gave her techniques to boost her self-esteem and sense of self-worth. Over the final weeks of the pregnancy Jenny began to gain confidence in her own ability to birth her baby well and be a good parent. By the time Jenny was ready to birth she had developed personal survival skills and was feeling far more nurtured, stronger and ready to give birth and take on the challenge of parenting. As a consequence Jenny's spine was no longer imbalanced and she went on to birth easily.

Reflexology at Home

This is a suggested home foot massage session that can be done between visits with your practitioner. You can do this before bed, whilst relaxing in front of the television, or if you have a supportive partner they can treat you to this massage every day, reducing the risk of pregnancy complications.

I teach this technique to my pregnant client's partners and they become so skilled that they are a great asset in labour. With mother and partner working as a great team, the sense of achievement they feel at birthing their own baby is palpable, creating greater confidence to parent well. After all it is their baby not the maternity provider's. It is not necessary to have a thorough understanding of the reflexology points to gain benefit, however if you find a point that is particularly tender you can refer to the charts provided here for more insight.

Massage gently and firmly using a relaxing crème, and be particularly careful to massage gently those points specifically related to the reproductive system as shown on the Reproductive Points Chart.

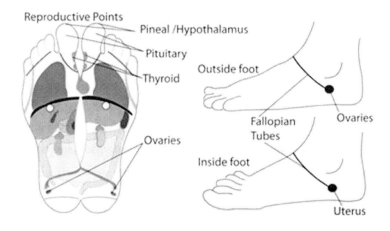

You can massage them more vigorously if you are overdue and want to encourage labour (discussed in more detail under Induction in the labour and birth section).

1. Relaxing the foot - take the foot in both hands and roll the ankle back and forward between the palms of the hand. This loosens up the ankle and warms the foot. Bring your hands to either side of the foot just below the toes, around the heart chakra area, and do the same.

2. Waking the spine - hold one foot in the palm of one hand. With your other hand use the thumb to walk up the bony structure on the inside of the foot. Walk from the base of the ankle to the top of the big toe. Do this several times to relax the spine. Note where any areas are tense or uncomfortable and spend more time on these areas to relax and release any tensions in the back. The side view picture gives you an idea of the correlation between reflex points and the spine. Gently work the sacral and pelvic reflex points on the feet to break up any toxins or blocked energy in this area.

3. Massage up and down the plantar (underneath) aspect of the foot. This massages all the internal organs and is very relaxing. Again note if any areas feel tense or have discomfort. Spend more time gently massaging these points to relax and release.

4. The adrenal point is a very important reflex point in pregnancy. It is found just on the inside of the ligament that runs down the foot, almost in line with the second toe about half way down the arch of the foot. Most women will feel some discomfort when this is massaged. The more stressed you are the more sensitive this point will be. It is very important to relax and massage this point regularly to help reduce the amount of adrenalin being released in the body. One drop of lavender oil massaged here is excellent for relaxing the adrenal zones. Be careful not to use any more as lavender is a strong oil.

5. Massage along under the toes, just at the top of the padding on the ball of the foot and into the neck of the toes. This may be sensitive, especially if there are allergies or sinus issues, but gives excellent relief.

6. Massage each toe individually, in fact give the toes lots of attention. Stretch them out to encourage them to be long and straight. Toes are meant to reach out and receive the messages of the world. If yours are cramped and turned under then pay particular attention and encourage them to become straighter. Regular massage can correct a bunion development especially if the emotional issue is dealt with. Check out the 'Emotional Anatomy of The Feet' chart in this section for more detail about what your toes are saying to you.

7. Shoulders - massage along the top of the foot especially around the sides under the little toes to release the shoulders.

8. Heart and neck - massage around the other side of the foot at the base of the big toe around the side onto the padding. This may be tender if there are emotional issues and often just massaging this area will release pent up emotions. Allow your tears to fall, breathe and let it go.

9. The mother's chest is often constricted as the baby grows and the organs and glands are pushed up into the diaphragm. A nice relaxing movement is to knead using the knuckles across the ball of the foot. Pressing the sole of the foot over a small ball works well too.

10. Gently press your thumb across the diaphragm reflex under the ball of the foot and back again in the other direction to assist with breathing. Then press into the centre of the foot to relax and release the solar plexus point.

11. Gut massage - begin on the left foot. Massage across the lower arch of the foot backwards and forwards to massage the intestine and ileocecal valve. Then track up the side of the foot (ascending colon) and move across to the right foot to massage the small intestine and descending colon (see 'The Soles of the Feet Mirror the Body' chart).

12. Massage the heel of the foot towards the arch in an upward movement.

13. Lymphatic Drainage - very important in pregnancy. Massage to simply open the meridians and facilitate the elimination of fluids. Working on the topside of the foot, place all four fingers over the tips of the toes. Lightly massage from the toes towards the ankle with very light little finger movements. Once at the ankle direct the massage towards the inside of the ankle to the bladder reflex. Massage around the ankle in the same way and direct the flow towards the bladder as well. Imagine you are directing fluid down the foot and then into the bladder for elimination. Do this several times until you feel the foot soften and the fluid reduce.

14. Hips, legs and pelvic area - massage around the base of the external ankle and up the leg, particularly on the bony section. This will generally be quite tender, especially if there is tension in this area in the body. Massage along the edge of the foot below the ankle. You can use your knuckle to massage around the heel to release any sciatica pain. This can be quite tender but a wonderful release if persisted with. Avoid massaging in the inner aspect of the heel where the uterus lies.

15. A pregnant foot often has quite a protrusion around the uterine area. Gently massage this area to relax and release. Do not work this area vigorously unless you are overdue and wanting to start labour.

*For specific points to massage for issues in pregnancy see the 'Complimentary Therapies For Discomforts of Pregnancy' section.

As you have read already, reflexology assists detoxification. Pre-pregnant and pregnant women especially benefit from regular reflexology sessions. My aim is to assist a woman to be relaxed, ready and attuned to give birth by releasing the issues in her tissues.

Muscles are designed for one action, to contract or grow shorter. The contraction occurs when the muscle receives an electro-chemical signal from the central nervous system to do so. When the signal stops the contraction stops and the muscle relaxes back to its former length.

It takes no energy to relax and lengthen a muscle, only to contract and shorten. When we voluntarily contract a muscle, then relax it, the muscle should almost completely soften. The relaxed muscle holds almost no electrical activity. Full voluntary control of a muscle is the ability to contract the entire span of the muscle and then to relax it fully to its length. Reflexology facilitates this.

Complete the session with a Brazilian Toe Massage.

Brazilian Toe Massage

This simple massage creates a very relaxing healing environment and can be done easily by your partner or a friend. Many people feel this as a soft fuzzy glowing sensation throughout their body and often remark how incredibly relaxed they feel afterwards. Some people experience profound emotional release and visions.

Remember we are all individuals so each person will experience it differently. The technique is very simple. It is important not to break the circuit at any time.

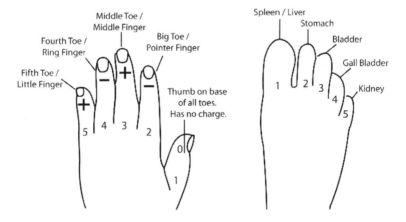

The corresponding hand to each foot carries a positive or negative charge on each finger in relation to the same toe:

- Thumb is neutral / earth - Big toe
- Second finger is negative – 2nd toe
- Third finger is positive – 3rd toe
- Fourth finger is negative – 4th toe
- Fifth finger is positive – 5th toe

1. With the feet facing you place the thumb lightly at the base tip of the big toe and place the pointing finger lightly on the top at the tip of the nail.
   ** Pressure is not required. It is an energy exchange.
2. Visualisation is an excellent tool to use with this technique, even visualising something as simple as a colour then imagine placing this colour somewhere within your body that you feel needs extra energy or healing.
3. You will feel a pulsation under your fingers. When this settles it is time to move to the next toe.
4. Without losing contact, move the top finger onto the second toe then follow with the thumb underneath and hold until you feel the energy like a pulse begin to move whilst repeating the visualisation, possibly using a different colour if you are inclined to do so.
5. Again without losing contact move the to finger to the third toe then follow with the thumb underneath. Continue in this way with the fourth and fifth toe respectively.
6. Finish the technique by placing the fingers on top of the feet with the thumbs gently holding the solar plexus reflex point under the ball of the foot (see the chart).
7. Take three deep breaths, imagine clearing all negative energy and renewing with new energy.

When you are ready open your eyes and smile at each other.

Vertical Reflexology Therapy

Vertical Reflexology Therapy (VRT) is a powerful modality developed by Lynne Booth (UK), based on reflex points on the feet observed when the person is standing. Because the body is in an upright vital state the energy exchange between the zones massaged and the body part targeted is rapid, bringing effective relief quickly. As you are encouraged to remain upright and mobile as much as possible during labour, this is an ideal time for your support person to provide VRT. With VRT the stimulation is short, only a few minutes at a time, meaning the labouring mother on the move is able to receive effective relief quickly without needing to remain in one position for long. I have undertaken the advanced training in Vertical Reflexology Therapy and have outlined here a few of the techniques I have found of most help for pregnancy and labour as self-help techniques. Working the hands and feet at the same time can be far more effective than only working one point at a time.

For best results I advise employing a reflexology practitioner with VRT training, but for the sake of simplicity the following can be of benefit.

1. Massage around the ankle until you find a point that is the most sensitive. This is the point to be activated and released. At the same time massage down the spinal reflex on the inside edge of the foot until you find the corresponding tender point. Activate (press) these two points together for relief. Continue to work your way around the ankle a few times to release and relax these zones.
2. Massage each toe on top and around the sides. This is very relaxing and releases endorphins that clear toxins and re-balance.
3. Massage up and around the calves, especially about half way up. Place both hands around the calf and massage towards the front

with the fingers meeting in the front. Do this several times. This is a great release for the thoracic and chest area.

4. Lymphatic Stimulation - Massage on top of the feet, from the toes towards the ankle. Once at the ankle direct the massage towards the inside area of the side of the foot where the bladder reflex is situated. As you massage have an intent that you are sweeping fluids down the foot to be excreted by the bladder. Very soon the person you are massaging will need to pee to release the excess fluid. I have done this on one foot with

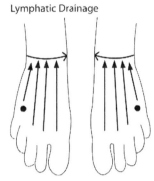

Lymphatic Drainage

the mother going to the toilet before I did the second foot and the difference was remarkable. Fluid retention on the foot I had worked was gone whilst the foot I hadn't worked was still quite swollen and visibly bigger.

5. To energise the feet use the knuckles. Roll your hand into a fist and massage the knuckle joints into the foot in a rolling, grinding style across the metatarsals. Be gentle as the top of the feet can be quite tender. The effect is very stimulating and can be used when mum is feeling tired or needing a boost of energy. Particularly good in labour.

6. To stimulate contractions stimulate the reproductive areas on the feet, the uterine point on the internal side of the foot and around the ankles.

7. The nails are also a micro-system and you can massage the nail area with good effect.

For more information and to find a practitioner click on
http://www.boothvrt.com/view/2/what-is-vrt

Facial Massage

The face is an easy area for you or your support person to access. It is wonderful to lean back into the chest of your partner while they massage your face. Facial massage can be deeply relaxing and healing especially when combined with an ear massage at the same time, and is particularly useful in labour and for relieving tension and aches in pregnancy.

Using one finger or the thumb massage in a circular motion onto the point you are focused upon. Do this for about thirty seconds, then gently massage over the point to shift any blockages of energy in the area. Generally stimulate one point at a time unless they are replicated on both sides of the face then both sides can be massaged. If a point is tender focus here until it relaxes.

Chakra Facial Massage

The chakras can also be identified in the face, hands and feet. The following diagram depicts the chakras in the face, plus the three zones (mental, emotional and physical). Your face is the fruit of life and indicates how you are at this point in time. The more it is massaged and relaxed the better the effect - plus what a wonderful anti-aging tool!

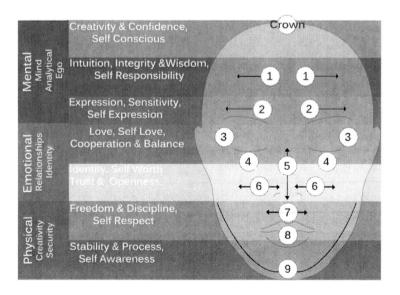

The Chakra Facial Massage diagram (above) will help give you a map to follow for specific complaints you wish to treat, which are listed in the 'Complimentary Therapies For Discomforts of Pregnancy' section.

Massage Technique

Begin at the top of the head and connect with the crown chakra. Place your thumbs lightly on the crown and gently spread your fingers either side of the forehead at the hairline.

1. Massage the fingers across the forehead from the centre to the hairline using both hands together. Massage the temple area particularly if there is mental tension.

2. Massage firmly with the thumbs across the eyebrows. The eyebrows are the boundary between the head and the heart (the eyes are the window to the soul). When there is a lot of mental activity the eyebrow area can become very tense with trying to hold back all that heavy mind energy from the heart ('the thoughts weigh heavy on the heart').

3. Tension often builds at the edge of the eyes, so this is a great place to massage away the tension of the day and to relax the eyes. After massaging this area rub your hands vigorously until they are very hot. Now place your lovely hot palms over the eyes. Totally relax into this and feel the wonderful release.

4. Bags under the eyes represent all those uncried tears. Now is the time to let the emotional pain go. Massage in circles working outwards towards the ears.

5. Massage down the nose and then in an upward motion, softening and moulding the centre of identity.

6. Emotional tension can be gathered around the nose as this is the area of identity. Your identity is changing as you become a mother.

7. Some people have strong tension in the sacral area, across the lower cheek and just above the mouth, especially if nostrils are pinched in and the mouth is quite small. These people have

difficulty expressing their true self and this area can be quite tight and painful.

This area also correlates to the sacral, naval and reproductive area of the body. In pregnancy and birth this is best relaxed and open. The more this is massaged the more relaxed the sacral area in the body can become.

8. The mouth represents the pelvic area, vagina and birth passage. The mouth tells us how you taste life, is it sweet, bitter or sour? Massage the lips, open the mouth, do lots of funny mouth exercises to stretch the lips and muscles around the mouth. Practice lots of sensual kissing. I encourage lots of kissing and caressing in labour to assist the opening of the cervix. It is well known amongst natural birth advocates that the mouth is akin to the birth canal. 'Soft lips soft cervix'.

9. Massage along the jaw line. Use the thumbs firmly to press into acupoints to release any tensions here.

Massage the throat, neck and shoulders. We all carry tension in these areas and we can never have too many massages to release this.

Giving facial massage is a wonderful opportunity to do a face reading. Face reading is a powerful tool that allows you to gain greater depth of understanding of the person, their challenges, their strengths and where they are at right now.

You can learn to face read by contacting a Psychosomatic Therapy Trainer. For more insight into face reading please follow the link to my website:

http://www.casadelsole.com.au/index.php/therapies/
pychosomatic-therapy/psychosomatic-therapy

"It is so nurturing to look into the eyes of a person you have never met before with a warm smile of recognition. Sometimes being noticed comes like a shock to them to be worthy of being seen. The Art of Reading Faces creates an atmosphere of comfort, acceptance and understanding at a subconscious level between the observed and the observer, an attitude of 'I know you so well, it is so good to meet again".

Hermann Müller
Face to Face With Facts, Personality Potential

Auricular Therapy

The first documented use of auricular therapy, by traditional Chinese medicine practitioners, was recorded around 500 B.C. Not only do the feet and hands reflect the whole being but so do the ears. The twelve major meridians which circulate blood, energy and life force (Chi) throughout the body converge either directly or indirectly on the ears.

Stimulating specific points on the ears will affect the rest of the body, especially corresponding areas that reflect imbalance. Dr. P. Nogier (1957) wrote in a German acupuncture periodical about the significance between specific sites on the ear and other parts of the body, charting the inverted foetus theory.

The diagram here shows the visual analogy of the ear in the shape of a baby. You will see that the reflex points on the ear correspond to the organs and glands of the baby. W. Flocco and Dr. T. Oleson published research in an Obstetrics and Gynaecology article (1993) suggesting that ear, hand and foot reflexology reduced pre-menstrual symptoms by forty-six percent. When the feet and hands are unavailable the ears provide the perfect alternative.

The ears are an excellent massage tool for many ailments. There are thousands of energy points on the ears and the therapy itself is quite extensive. I have only focused on a few beneficial points for specific conditions. Try massaging the large outer section of the lobe when you have back ache and feel the soothing results.

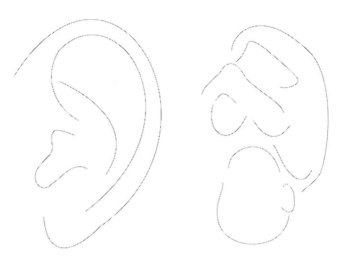

Auricular Therapy Points

Massage on the outer ear from top to the bottom several times when tired and feel how invigorating it is.

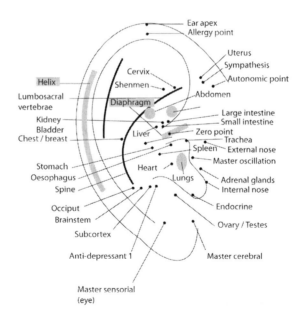

Eastern Techniques

Eastern Philosophy - Yin and Yang

Eastern health philosophy is based on the fundamental principle of yin and yang, the balance of opposites, the polar cycle, positive and negative. Yin is the accumulation, organising and storing of energy. Yang is the expansion and use of energy. As described in the Psychosomatic Therapy section, we function from these two components. Yin energy is the feminine, gentle, relaxing and meditative heart energy whilst Yang energy is the male doer, active mind, driver. Each is equal and one cannot exist without the other.

Regardless of gender, some people are more yang energy and others are stronger in yin energy. Health is dependent upon the maintenance of both yin and yang aspects. People born with a stronger yang constitution will be seen as strong energetic types who tend to suffer from more acute, dramatic yang imbalances, often as a result of pushing beyond capacity and exhausting the body. Those with a stronger yin constitution will have the opposite, tending toward chronic long term illnesses, taking longer to recover and may be seen as more sensitive people. This is why in pregnancy some women appear to take it in their stride while others can be quite fatigued and find balance more difficult. The following table can help you understand your constitution, making it easier to make choices that better suit your body-type.

The following table can help you understand your constitution.

Yang	Yin
• large, strong and sturdy bone structure	• smaller, slighter bone structure
• energetic, more aggressive nature	• more passive, gentler energy
• healthy, rosy glowing complexion	• paler, softer, lighter complexion
• fiery, somewhat angry disposition, tend to strongly debate	• somewhat timid, anxious, fearful, will look for more passive and agreeable approach

- testosterone dominant
- acute illnesses
- high libido and sexually active
- rigid body type

- oestrogen dominant
- low libido and sexually submissive
- chronic illnesses
- collapsed body type

The Five Elemental Energies

Yin and *yang* describe the basic principles of the flow of energy. The seasons with their four phases are a good example of this cyclic flow.

- Wood - early yang phase – the months during which the daylight is longer and warmer (spring)
- Fire - late yang phase - full active energy (summer)
- Metal - early yin phase - when the days withdraw and become shorter and colder (autumn)
- Water – late yin phase - little activity (winter)

These phases can be seen through all cycles of life, even throughout the cycle of a day. The morning is Wood, afternoon is Fire, evening is Metal and the late night is Water. The fifth element, Earth, is the essential aspect that brings the elements together and that is balance. Without balance the system would fall apart. Earth is the centre and must be present at all times. The five elements govern the flow of energy throughout the body.

Metal - Conception & early pregnancy. The transitional early yin energy from summer to autumn, the withdrawing inwards of energy and governs the lungs. A cleansing and letting go of the external world to come within. It is experienced as the contemplative quietening and releasing of energy.

Metal is associated with the harvest, the collecting and dispersing of what has been gained through the previous season.

Water - The fullness of pregnancy. The concentrated yin, the depth of winter, governs the kidneys. It is the energy of the seed, the fundamental energy of life, the 'pregnant pause', the will to sustain and have courage.

Wood - Labour. New yang and fresh energy associated with spring and its flow, oversees the liver. It is the motivating force within us, the need to create and express ourselves, our will to open up and expand. When wood is abundant we develop, procreate and create.

Fire - Birth. Yang energy of growth and fullness, expansion, warmth, loving and compassion, the summer element associated with the heart. When abundant life is joyous, exuberant, full of wisdom and strength. Fire energy when in balance brings harmony, acceptance and peace.

Earth - Balance, the center, and must always be present. Earth dominates change and rules the spleen and digestive system. Experienced as nourishing, balanced, centered and understanding energy. An energy of maturity, the ripened soul, Earth nourishes the flesh and the bone structure. It is the ability to see the whole picture with a broad and open heart and mind.

Ailments have a yang or yin dominance. The therapies described in this section can have both yin and yang effects depending on how they are applied and what outcome you are hoping for. If you tend toward the more yang constitution then the therapies that relax and reduce stress will have beneficial effects. If you are more yin then you will require plenty of rest, relaxation and high energy foods and formulas that boost up your constitution. Yin constitutions require gentle understanding and a space to express your fears and concerns. Yin constitutions may be more prone to postnatal depression, therefore boosting your system with the nutrients suggested will assist with preventing this condition.

Creating a balanced life through reducing stress and maintaining a healthy diet, good elimination, daily movement, emotional balance and meditation is imperative.

Balance is the key to longevity and health and it begins in pregnancy. Balance will assist in preventing the ailments of pregnancy and encourage an easier pregnancy and birth. Doing anything to extreme damages the body. Extreme highs are followed by extreme lows. For example being a gym junkie does not increase your health but taxes the body and burns precious muscles stores. Not exercising at all creates many health issues.

Every person is different, so what is balanced and moderate to one person will be very different to another. I see these differences in my children. One son has strong yang energy and tends to have boundless energy, diving, surfing, kite boarding and doesn't like to sit around reading, preferring to be active. His brother on the other hand has more yin energy and therefore a different constitution. Though he thoroughly enjoys the same pursuits he tends to tire more easily and likes to take things a little more gently and slowly, as well as enjoying a good book and relaxing games and music.

Three Treasures – Jing, Qi and Shen

Some liken the Three Treasures to a candle. Jing is the wax and wick, the essence of life, without which there would be no light (life). Qi is the flame, energy, the life-force, and dictates how long the candle will last. The glow of the flame is likened to shen, the strength of the light. The stronger, larger and better quality the candle the steadier the flame and the longer the candle will last, creating greater shen.

Jing

Jing is the essence of who you are genetically and determines your life span. A strong, concentrated energy, jing is said to be the root of our vitality, stored in all five primary organs as a back up. Jing is stored in the kidneys, which in Chinese medicine include the reproductive organs, brain, skeleton and adrenal cortex and is concentrated in the sperm and ova. Strong jing energy in the 'kidneys' will lead to a long and vigorous life.

Jing begins at conception as the refined essence (jing) of the mother and father merge and become one within the new embryo cell, creating the new jing (the constitution). Original jing (prenatal jing) given by the parents sustains the growing baby growing who, via the umbilical cord, is totally reliant upon the mother for sustenance and oxygen. Immediately after birth the baby is independent, activating its own jing and assimilating nutrients from food and the creation of its own energy source (this is known as postnatal jing).

Left over original jing is deeply concentrated and stored as a back up reserve, only to be used when life is threatened. The more relaxed and non-stressed the mother is the more original jing is available to the baby, creating a good store and a strong constitution. As the baby develops, postnatal jing is also stored and continues to be released and recreated in small amounts within the individual for the rest of their life. Old Chinese wisdom states that if a person cares for the cavity of jing (located in the lower abdomen) and does not waste it recklessly it is very easy to enjoy a life of great longevity. Psychosomatic breathing, yoga and pilates activate this energy centre by focusing on the core, the house of jing.

It is so important to listen to your body and rest when it dictates. Whilst it is okay to feel fatigue, you must not become exhausted as jing is burned up by stress & fatigue. If qi energy runs low we are forced to tap into original jing reserves, severely diminishing our life force. Eventually we will use up all the reserves and our body physically dies. We innately understand this. You have probably heard people say after a traumatic event or great shock 'it took years off my life'.

Qi

Qi is the invisible life force that flows through all life and can be seen in the movement of our universe, from the circulation of the planets to the air we breathe. Qi energy flows through your body via the twelve meridian channels, nourishing the inner organs with life force. Just by looking at someone you can see how well this energy is flowing. Those who are vital and active have strong qi energy compared to those who are frail, weak or sensitive, move slowly and tire easily.

Qi has two components, nutritive qi which nourishes us and protective qi which protects us. Both are gained from food and air. The more fresh and full of life force the food and breath is the more qi you will have. Your blood system is governed by qi. Red blood cells are yin and nourishing, whilst white blood cells are yang, aggressive and protective. Qi is understood to be produced by the spleen and lungs.

Shen

Shen is the heart and the spirit (higher consciousness). Governed by the primary organ system of the heart, shen is expressed as love, compassion, kindness, generosity, acceptance, forgiveness and tolerance. Shen is the divinity within all of us that we attain to and is driven by the combination of jing and qi. When we are relaxed we create jing, which then allows for a large amount of qi which gives us strong shen. When jing and qi are strong the mind and spirit are strong and emotions are balanced with an acceptance of the cycle of life. All activities are governed by shen. When the emotions are not in balance they strive for dominance, creating discord and eventually illness. Moderation in all things is the supreme way to health.

To attain true happiness you must first attain balance in life. The ancient philosophies emphasise the need to live in balance and harmony with nature and the cycles of life. When there is balance in the body there is balance in the mind. You will find this philosophy flows through all the complementary therapy practices, and is the basis of psychosomatic therapy which teaches that through focus, balance and structure we can achieve this.

Heartfelt giving without expectation or reward is the easiest way to build shen. By seeing the divine beauty in all things we become a channel for divine love. It does not matter whether you are paid for your service, the exchange happens in the heart. When the heart is pure and gives freely then the reward of shen is far greater than any financial reward. Some herbs help to open up the flow of shen and to stabilize the emotions.

Specific herbs can also assist jing and qi, which are necessary for the body to be strong so that shen may radiate.

Traditional Chinese Medicine (TCM) is based upon the principles explained simply above and follows the philosophy that medicine and food are of the same origin. Commonly used tonic foods are ginseng, dang gui and lycium. Herbs are used in the majority of cooking and are deemed an important food group. Specific herbs are described in the herbal section.

Wild foods were once a stable part of the diet but due to westernised agricultural practices they are rarely eaten now, thus an extremely valuable part of the diet has been forgotten. It is only recently that science has turned its attention to a new category of nutrition, the bionutrients and phytonutrients. These healthful, nutritious plants contain much more than vitamins and minerals. They are anti-aging, immunity building and cancer preventative. Superfoods such as phytoplankton and hemp (recommended throughout this book) contain dozens of phytonutrients that perform truly remarkable tasks in our bodies.

The best and simplest way to attain these phytonutrients is FrequenSea http://casadelsole.fgxpress.com/farmers-market/

Meridians

Meridians are energy channels that flow throughout your body, connecting all the organs and glands. It is understood meridians are formed within the first few weeks after conception as the anchor for the internal systems. To be in good health your meridian lines need to be clear of blockages that prevent the free flow of energy. A demonstration of the flow of meridian energy can be seen in the extraordinary art work of Alex Gray.

http://alexgrey.com/art/paintings/soul/painting/

There are twelve main meridians points:

- lung - grief
- large intestine - stubborness
- spleen - frustration
- stomach - seat of emotion

- heart – self love
- small intestine – abandonment
- kidney - fear
- bladder – pissed off
- heart constrictor – blocking emotions
- triple warmer – enthusiasm for life
- liver - anger
- gall bladder - resentment

Acupressure

Acupressure works on the principle of boosting the natural energy system found within the meridian system of the body. All pressure point therapy has its base in the meridians. Facilitating the flow of energy along these meridians assists health during pregnancy and the easier birth of the baby. Acupressure employs a firm but somewhat gentle pressure to specific points on the body, in the birthing situation focusing on points on the arms and legs as these tend to be easier for the therapist to access. This therapy is based on an energy exchange, so the more relaxed both giver and receiver are the greater the exchange.

Acupressure works effectively for reproductive issues in women from fertility to pregnancy and birth as it is effective in both yin and yang conditions. Acupressure is particularly good for women who have gone over their due dates or when things slow down and the labour needs to be sped up. It will not work if you are not ripe and ready. Natural therapies and remedies are only effective when all systems are ready as the very nature of natural remedies is to work in unison with nature. Patience is a virtue at the end of pregnancy.

Relaxation is very important for a woman in pregnancy and labour. Endorphins which have a direct relaxation effect are released by the power of touch through these techniques. I have included a few points that can be of benefit to the novice but recommend that you visit a trained therapist for more intensive treatment.

If you are a novice begin slowly and gently and do not apply pressure longer than three minutes. If the point is sore relax the pressure until you find a comfortable state, reduce the pressure gradually until very light touch at the end of the three minutes. Afterward close you eyes, relax and allow the effects to take place.

Acupressure points to work for specific conditions are listed in the 'Complimentary Therapies for Discomforts of Pregnancy' section.

See diagrams that follow for detail.

Most Effective Treatment Points

Stimulating Labour - Spleen-6 (SP-6) Inner Ankle
* Only to be applied from 37 weeks, after which can be stimulated twice daily.

Assists ripening and preparation of the birth canal, cervix and uterus. Also helps get baby into the correct position. To induce labour it is recommended the pressure is applied three times a day.

Find this point by placing your hand around your ankle (inside leg), little finger over the bony prominence of the ankle. It is

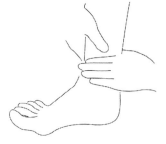

Stimulating Labour - Spleen SP-6
(Inner Ankle)

in line with the centre of the index finger on the side of the leg just under the leg bone. Use the opposite thumb to press on this point. Generally you will feel a sensation, a buzz or tenderness.

Apply firm pressure to both ankles during a contraction. Hold between contractions as an effective point to stimulate more effective contractions, or to help deliver the placenta. In a single blind controlled trial, acupressure for 30 minutes on SP-6 with a woman in her first pregnancy who was 3-4 cm dilated reduced labour times, reduced the caesarean rate and decreased labour pain (Kashanian & Shahali, 2009). The results were statistically significant when compared with the control group who received a light touch at this point for 30 minutes.

Large Intenstine-4 (LI-4)

* Only to be applied from 37 weeks. Fleshy thumb point, also known as the Gateway Point. Place your left thumb on the top of the fleshy mound of webbing between the thumb and index finger with the other index finger under (palm side). Gently but firmly press your two fingers together. This gateway point can also be found on the foot between the big toe and second toe. This is an excellent relaxation point.

Use firm pressure while pressing between the two fingers to produce an intense sensation, sometimes it can be quite tender.

Acupressure here can provide general pain relief in labour, whilst enabling regular, strong and efficient contractions, assisting the progression of labour. Also useful in pre-labour to try and get things moving, if contractions are mild or irregular, or if labour slows down at any stage. Apply pressure for a few minutes or 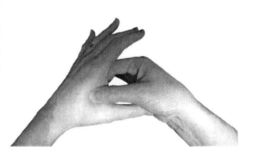 stimulate on and off on each side of the body. Having two people do this at the same time can be really effective and quite calming for mum.

Back Pain & Fear

* Only to be applied from 37 weeks.

K3, also known as Bigger Stream or Kidney 3, is on the inside of the foot, halfway between the Achilles-tendon and the side of the ankle-bone. Pressing here may have a calming effect whilst assisting lower back pain. Recent studies have found acupressure can significantly assist in decreasing pain, especially for later stages of pregnancy (Ekdahl & Petersson, 2010).

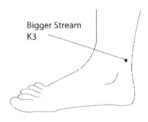

Bigger Stream
K3

Increasing Stamina and Energy

ST-36, also known as Three Mile or Stomach 36, is on the front of the leg, one hand width (four fingers) below the kneecap, on the outside, in the dip between the shinbone and the leg muscle. A good point to work to reduce oedema, diarrhoea and constipation. Also strengthens the overall constitution, relieving anxiety and depression.

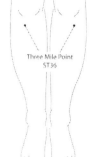

Three Mile Point
ST36

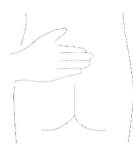

Yu Points (also known as Shu points) are found on both sides of the lower spine. Massaging these points can benefit all the internal organs and is very relaxing to do throughout pregnancy. An easy way to relax these points is to stand against a wall and roll a medium size ball up and down the wall with your back, or use two smaller balls on either side of the spine. Roll on the floor or on a wall. It is a great way to massage the spine and relax these points.

Directions for Floor Exercise: Place two tennis balls in a sock and tie the end with a string, rubber band or twisty so the balls stay together. Place them on a carpeted floor and lie down gradually on the balls, with your spine between the two balls. If it hurts because the balls are hard, double a thick towel over them for padding. After lying on the balls for five to ten minutes, deeply relax, lying flat on your back with your knees bent, eyes closed and take slow, deep breaths for another ten minutes to discover the benefits.

Above Tears GB41

On the top of the foot, in the indentation between the bones about two fingers width from the webbing between the fourth and fifth toes. Massage this point for relief of shoulder tension, hip pain, water retention, headaches and sciatica.

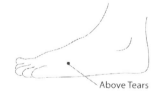

Above Tears

Acupressure Points – Front

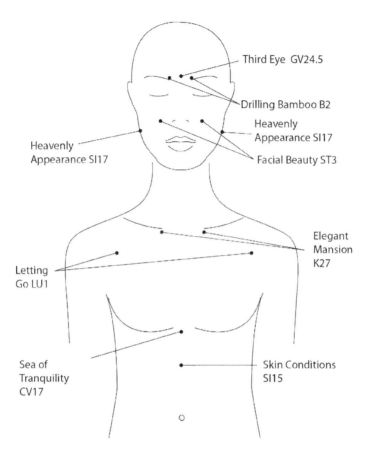

Third Eye GV24.5 (Governing Vessel) between the eyebrows in the groove where the bridge of your nose meets the forehead. Balances the pituitary gland, relieves hay fever, headaches, indigestion, ulcer pain and eyestrain. Also relaxes the central nervous system for relieving anxiety and insomnia.

Drilling Bamboo B2 (Bladder) the indent either side where the bridge of your nose meets the ridge of your eyebrows. Relieves eye pain, headaches, hay fever, eye fatigue and sinus pain.

Heavenly Appearance SI17 in the dip between the bottom of the earlobe and the top of the jawbone. For relief of nausea, ear pain and itchy throat.

Facial Beauty ST3 below the cheekbone, in line with the pupil. To relieve eye strain and pressure, congestion of head and nasal passages and toothaches.

Elegant Mansion K27 (Kidney) in the hollow below your collarbone, next to the breastbone. Relieves allergies associated with chest congestion, breathing difficulties, asthma, coughing and sore throats.

Letting Go LU1 approximately four finger widths up from the armpit, about an inch inward. Deep breathing while holding these two points opens the respiratory system, calms and releases repressed emotions such as grief, frustration, and anger. Try crossing your arms whilst holding these points so that the opposite hand is on each point. For relief of confusion, emotional repression, asthma, fatigue and breathing difficulties.

CV 17, also known as the **Sea of Tranquility,** can be found four finger widths up from the base of your breastbone, in the centre of your chest. Massage gently, keeping your spine straight whilst focusing on breathing slowly and deeply. This is a wonderful emotional balancing point.

Acupressure Points - Back (see diagram next page)
The following three points are the emotional release points for assisting in the letting go of past memories and hurts. You can massage all these points to relieve head tension, insomnia, eye strain, fatigue and neck stiffness.

- **Gates of Consciousness GB20 (Gallbladder)** below the base of your skull, in the hollow between the two vertical neck muscles.
- **Heavenly Pillar B10 (Bladder)** back of your head, half an inch below the base of the skull, on the muscles half an inch outwards from your spine.
- **Wind Mansion GV16 (Governing Vessel)** press on and off into the hollow at the centre of the back of your head, at the large hollow below the base of your skull.

Bearing Support/Skin Conditions close to the spine, just off the top of the shoulder blade. Assists strengthening of immune system, especially for resistance to colds and flu infections.

Heavenly Rejuvenation GB21 a fingers width below the top of the shoulder, halfway between the neck and the outer edge of the shoulder. Massage this point to relieve shoulder and neck tension.

Acupressure Points - Back

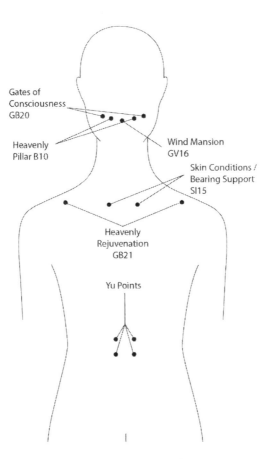

Acupressure Points - Front Leg

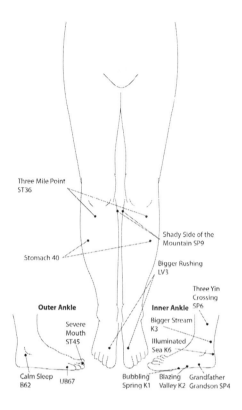

Acupressure Points - Front Leg

Three Mile Point ST36 (Stomach) four finger widths below the kneecap on the outside of your leg. Supports and improves circulation and digestion and gradually improves the absorption of nutrients. Good for anxiety, depression, low energy, leg pain and low immunity.

Shady Side of the Mountain SP9 inside of the leg (side), just below the knee, in the flesh not on bone. For relief of swelling, varicose veins, water retention, oedema and cramps.

Stomach 40 once daily for three minutes on each shin. Apply mild pressure in slow, clockwise movements. On the front of the lower leg, about eight fingers width above the external malleolus. Assists in cleansing and detoxing your body. Also known as the Phlegm Point.

Calm Sleep B62 (Bladder) gently massage in a circular motion in the first indentation directly below the outer anklebone. Can be very relaxing and assist with insomnia.

UB67 *Caution - only work this point or warm with moxa after 35 weeks to assist a baby to move into the correct position.

Severe Mouth ST45 (Stomach) on the outside of the base of the nail of the second toe. Relieves nausea, indigestion, toothaches and abdominal pain.

Bigger Rushing LV3 (Liver) apply gentle pressure in circular, anti-clockwise movements at the point between the second toe and big toe, three fingers' width from the edge (repeat three times a day). Can assist in unblocking withheld or suppressed emotions, particularly anger and depression, can relieve nausea and cramps and has a relaxing and stress reducing effect. (Stress is one of the factors that causes an increase in blood sugar levels in the body).

Bubbling Spring K1 (Kidney) on the sole of your foot, between the bones of the second and third toes, just below the ball of your foot (about two thirds the distance from the heel to the base of the second toe). May be quite tender. Apply firm pressure for about one minute. Stimulate by pressing on a small ball or massage with your thumb to assist with fatigue, insomnia and relaxation.

Blazing Valley K2 (Kidney) on the arch of the foot, halfway between the big toe and the heel. Massaging this point can relieve oedema and fluid retention.

Illuminated Sea K6 (Kidney) gently massage in circular motion on the point directly below the inside of the anklebone in a slight indentation. Relieves insomnia, heel and ankle pain, hypertension and anxiety.

Bigger Stream K3 (Kidney) * Only to be applied from 37 weeks. Use circular movements in clockwise direction on this point on the inner side of the foot, between the side of your ankle bone and Achilles tendon. Apply this pressure for three minutes. Assists with strengthening the immune system.

Three Yin Crossing SP6 (Spleen) * Only to be applied from 37 weeks, after which can be stimulated twice daily.

Grandfather Grandson SP4 inner side of foot, about two centimetres from the ball of the foot. For relief of indigestion, abdominal cramps and stomach ache.

Acupressure Points – Back Leg (see diagram next page)
CAUTION - It is best to avoid pressing any points around the sacral (lower back) and lower abdomen until after 37 weeks pregnancy. You can use these points as a guide and use gentle palm pressure to relieve symptoms rather than direct acupressure.

Sea of Vitality B23 (Bladder) - CAUTION - if there are disintegrating discs or fractured bones do not press or apply any pressure. This point may also be very tender if you have a weakness here. In either case, do not apply pressure, instead the light touch of a stationary hand may provide gentle healing.

Sea of Vitality is at waist level in the lower back, between the second and third lumbar vertebrae, not on the spine itself. You will find the spot about two to four finger widths away from your spine. This point can relieve lower sciatica and lower back ache and fatigue that may result from back pain.

Womb and Vitals B48 (Bladder) one to two finger widths outside the sacrum (the large bony area at the base of your spine) and midway between the top of the hipbone and the base of the buttocks. Massage in gentle circles plus apply full hand gentle pressure to relieve lower back ache, sciatica, pelvic tension, hip pain and tension.

Commanding Middle B54 (Bladder) in the centre of the back of your knee crease. A great pressure point to gently massage to relieve back pain, sciatica, knee pain and back stiffness.

Beautiful Baby K9 (Zhubin) is located above the inner ankle bone, directly below the calf muscle. The name 'Zhubin', means 'Guest Building'. It is thought this 'guest' refers to the growing baby. This pressure point is traditionally used to calm the mind and to build blood in the body. It can be used to treat hypertension, fear, anxiety, nightmares, and mental disorders.

Acupressure Points - Back Leg

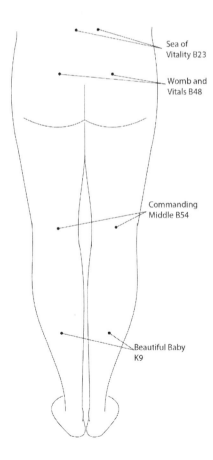

Sea of
Vitality B23

Womb and
Vitals B48

Commanding
Middle B54

Beautiful Baby
K9

Acupressure Points – Inside Arm

Crooked Marsh P3 found at the centre of the elbow crease, an excellent point to press or massage to relieve nervous stomach, anxiety, arm and elbow pain.

The following four points, P4-P7, are found up the middle of the underside of the arm, can all be pressed or massaged to relieve and settle the stomach and calm the mind.

Cleft Gate P4 is five finger widths above the centre of the inner wrist crease, between the tendons. A good point for calming grief or depression.

Intermediary P5 four finger widths above the centre of the inner wrist crease, between the tendons.

Inner Gate P6 (Pericardium) on both sides of arm. Morning sickness and motion sickness point. Found two finger widths above the inner wrist.

Big Mound P7 (Pericardium) bend wrist upward and you will find the point in the middle of the crease, between the two tendons that run from the hand up the arm. Allow the wrist to relax back in a laid out position while applying pressure. Do not press so hard as to cause pain or soreness and do not use it if doing so results in tingling fingers. Emotional balancing point.

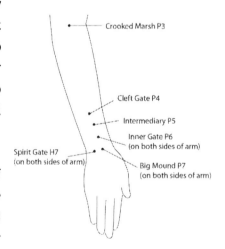

Spirit Gate H7 (Heart) inside of the wrist crease, in line with the little finger. Relieves anxiety, cold sweats, and insomnia due to over excitement.

156

Acupressure Points - Outside Arm

Crooked Pond LI 11 (Liver) can be found at the outer end of the elbow crease. Gently massage this point to trigger the colon to relieve constipation and to help boost the immune system.

Outer Gate TW5 (Triple Warmer) is found when the arm is slightly bent. Feel for two pressure points on either side of the large tendon, they should feel slightly harder than the tissue either side of the tendon. Apply steady pressure first on one side of the tendon and then on the other with the arm relaxed.

Active Pond TW4 (Triple Warmer) with the back of the hand facing upwards, apply pressure to the back of the wrist. Be sure to keep the wrist straight as bending of the wrist can lead to pinching of the nerves, resulting in loss of nerve sensation and inflammation of the joint. Stimulating the nerves causes nerve impulses to flow through the joint, releasing natural anti-inflammatory chemicals into the body. Both these points are excellent for conditions such as carpal tunnel and oedema

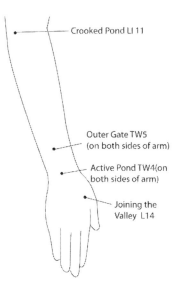

Crooked Pond LI 11

Outer Gate TW5
(on both sides of arm)

Active Pond TW4(on
both sides of arm)

Joining the
Valley L14

Joining the Valley LI4 (Large Intestine) * Only to be applied from 37 weeks. This is on the back of the hand on the webbing between the thumb and index finger. Press and release for about nine counts. Improves the immune system.

Su-Jok Hand Therapy

Reflexology is excellent on the hands as well as the feet, but I particularly like to use the Su-Jok therapy on hands. Korean Professor Park Jae Woo developed the theory of Su (hand) Jok (foot) in the late 1980's about the same time Reflexology was being developed as a therapy in the Western world. Su-Jok is a popular modality practiced throughout Asian and European countries. I was first introduced to the concept two years ago in New Zealand where I met Dr. Vesna, who had moved to New Zealand from Russia. Dr. Vesna is extremely experienced with many years of practice in Acupuncture, Acupressure and Su-Jok.

The Su-Jok modality is based on finite acupressure points derived from the practice of Acupuncture on the hands and feet. The diagrams and maps are different from those used in hand and feet reflexology where each hand and foot represents that side of the body. In Su-Jok one foot and one hand represent the whole body. I have been very impressed with the great results I have seen using this modality. What I have found as the main difference is that in Reflexology we are often massaging using the thumb and fingers with a deep firm massage. Su-Jok uses a more finite approach similar to acupressure, using a probe to run over the area to pinpoint the area of discomfort. Seeds, magnets, colour and heat using Moxa are then applied to the area as frequently as you can.

In Su-Jok the hand and foot are depicted with the map of the body flowing down from the wrist/ankle to the fingers/toes.

- the head and neck are at the wrist/ankle
- organs and glands of the torso correspond with the palm of the hand/foot
- second and fifth finger/toe are the arms and hands
- third and fourth inner fingers/toes are the legs and feet
- reproductive system sits at the joint of the third and fourth finger/toe

- thumb and big toe become their own micro-system, with the top of the thumb/big toe being the head and neck, the venus mound on the hand and ball of the foot the lungs
- knuckles and toe joints correspond to the joints of the limbs
- back of the hand and top of the foot represent the skeletal structure of the body.

Su-Jok Hand Therapy Diagram

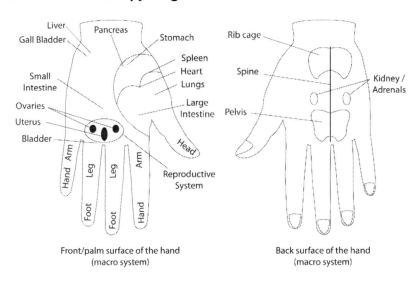

Front/palm surface of the hand
(macro system)

Back surface of the hand
(macro system)

The Insect Correspondence System

(see diagram following page)

The Insect Correspondence System is an even smaller microsystem, similar to the ears. Each finger and toe corresponds to the whole body. Finite pain points can be located on the hands/feet fingers and toes and released with direct contact. It is called the insect system as an insect has three sections, similar to the three sections of our digits.

The insect bodies consist of three parts - head, chest and abdomen. The head is the third digit, the chest the second and the abdomen the first digit closest to the hand. The side view of the finger or toe represents the side of the face/body, arms and legs folded at the joints.

Front/Palm Surface of the Hand
(micro system)

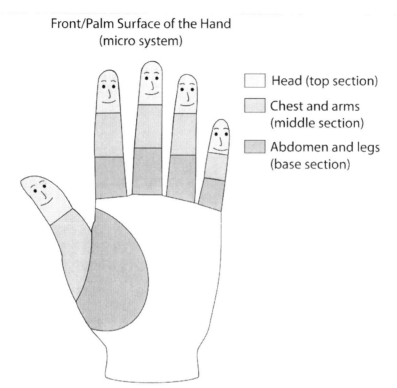

☐ Head (top section)

☐ Chest and arms
(middle section)

▨ Abdomen and legs
(base section)

The front of your hand represents the front of your body, the back of your hand represents the back of the body and the bone structure (spine).

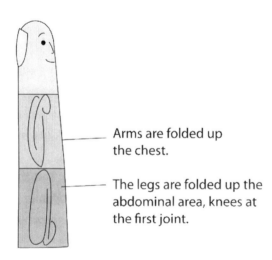

Arms are folded up
the chest.

The legs are folded up the abdominal area, knees at the first joint.

The Five Theory Elements

Each finger or toe represents the whole body and one of the five elements described in Eastern philosophies.

- Thumb – Wind (green)
- 2nd Finger – Heat (red)
- 3rd Finger – Humidity (yellow)
- 4th Finger - Dryness (orange)
- 5th finger - Cold (blue)

I use the 5th (little) finger often as many of the reproductive issues stem from a cold condition. We want to warm up the organs in those areas by stimulating the uterine point on the little finger with moxa, red elastic band, red texta or the warm red side of a magnet. This has a warming effect on the uterus.

Su-Jok therapy brings about balance, enhancing medical treatment. However I would warn to be careful not to stimulate the uterine points during pregnancy. Definitely stimulate the uterine point if wanting to stimulate labour.

Su-Jok can be used to reduce many everyday ailments and discomforts. For instance Su-Jok is wonderful for reducing back ache. Locate the areas of discomfort on the hand and foot corresponding to the spine and then begin to massage this area or place a seed on it and press frequently until the pain subsides.

Su-Jok doesn't treat the symptom but the focus of the disease or discomfort. For instance it will not treat a high temperature but if you understand where the high temperature is coming from then the affected organ can be treated with Su-Jok.

Systems of Correspondence

Each organ or part of the body has numerous corresponding zones on the hands and feet. The following diagrams give an idea of the zones that can be stimulated for the uterus and vagina. I find treating the hand easier, simply because it is easy to get to and the person being treated can self-treat throughout the day. Active points on the feet are also very effective but can be too uncomfortable when walking on the seeds. Anyone can find points on the hands and feet guided by the diagrams because the hands and feet have similar structures.

Stimulating Points with Su-Jok

Here is a simple exercise to try this therapy. Using the following diagrams as a guide, take a pencil or some other pointed object and start pressing around the parts of the hand that correspond to the parts of the body that you have a problem with. Don't stop at the point of sharp pain, continue probing until you find the point of the most intense discomfort.

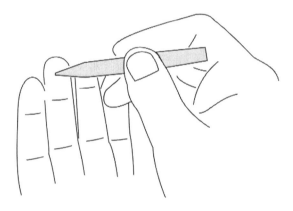

Whilst applying pressure, you will be able to feel a small sphere around which the worst pain lies. The very act of pressing on the painful point is healing as it is shifting the blockage, which then travels through the meridian channel to the affected organ or gland. If the pain doesn't subside after a few minutes of gentle pressure then tape a small seed over the point, which can be stimulated on and off throughout the day. Use any seed you like, however, be guided by a possible similarity between the seed and the organ treated.

For example:

- use kidney beans for kidney or reproductive issues, they are also red which is warming
- for brain, use parts of small walnuts
- for stimulating heat use pepper corns, these are readily available and very 'active'.

If you are not sure where the point of strongest pain is, put several seeds together. Fix them over the entire correspondent region and stimulate by rubbing throughout the day. Replace the seeds regularly as you will note that after one or two sessions, the seeds lose their power and become dry. Taping seeds to the points on the feet can be a great way to stimulate a point whilst walking.

Su-Jok for Fertility

Being a midwife and natural fertility specialist I was particularly drawn to Su-Jok because it is so effective in assisting conception. I have witnessed first-hand how effective it is with two clients with long term fertility issues now pregnant since instigating intense therapy. Reproductive organs have many corresponding points on the hands and feet. By stimulating these it is possible to increase fertility, reduce the ailments of pregnancy, to stimulate labour if overdue or if needing to increase the intensity of labour.

Basic Fertility Stimulation

Often conception is not happening because there are imbalances in other organs and glands besides the reproductive system, such as the thyroid, pancreas, adrenals or pituitary gland. Thus by searching for the point of discomfort you can stimulate other areas that may be involved. All these can be stimulated with Su-Jok therapy. By stimulating, using the appropriate colour, warming up or cooling down these points and meridians, balance can be restored quickly. For women it is important to stimulate the uterus and ovaries. For men it is important to stimulate the male genitals corresponding points and prostate.

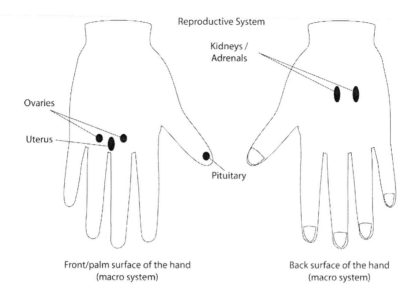

Front/palm surface of the hand
(macro system)

Back surface of the hand
(macro system)

Points corresponding to the male and female reproductive systems are the same. The pituitary gland, ovaries, uterus and adrenal glands are best warmed up with moxa.

Seed Therapy

Whatever the acute problem, apply three seeds on the reproductive point and wear them as long as you can. If this is not appropriate during the day then be sure to wear them through the night - heal yourself while sleeping! The prolonged wearing of seeds, for several months in a row, has been documented to have assisted severe cases of endometriosis.

All of the above are only basic ways of stimulation according to Su-Jok therapy. You can explore Su-Jok therapy with workshops conducted across Australia and New Zealand. I have had the great pleasure of being trained under the guidance of Dr. Vesna Zdravkovio, Su-Jok Therapist, and have been given permission to teach the basic Su-Jok training to other therapists as a post-graduate training. The advanced training will be conducted by Dr.Vesna.

Emotional Freedom Technique (Tapping)

Emotional Freedom Technique (EFT) is an emotional, needle free version of acupressure based on new discoveries regarding the connection between your body's subtle energies, your emotions and your health.

Another way of removing the Neuro Emotional Charge described in Neuro Emotional Technique and Psychosomatic Therapy, EFT allows insight into what really limits our physical and emotional health and wellbeing.

EFT works on the principle of tapping on a specific acupressure point while focusing the mind on what it is you wish to deal with. It is healing that is changing the way we perceive emotional and physical dysfunction and disease. The tapping interrupts the thought and memory process in the way that breath, movement and massage of the emotional release points do in Psychosomatic Therapy and the tapping points on the spine relate to specific meridians in Neuro Emotional Technique.

The theory is that by interrupting the emotional process attached to the memory the old emotions are released. I can personally vouch for these processes. I am focused far more in the present now and even if I do find myself thinking about a distant memory it feels like a story without any emotional response. It is so wonderful to feel free of emotional baggage.

EFT has reportedly been successful in thousands of cases covering a substantial range of emotional, health and performance issues. There are testimonials online if you wish to explore this further.

Using Tapping in Pregnancy

Sit in a relaxed position and explore how you feel about your pregnancy, labour or birth. Find a fear or emotion that you wish to clear. Note where you feel tense in your body when you state the fear or emotion. For example 'I feel so scared when I think about birthing my baby'.

Set up your statement and begin tapping on the Karate point shown in the diagram below :

1. State 'Even though I have this feeling about (state the problem) I accept myself.' Repeat three times.

2. Then Sequence: Tap 6-8 times on each point while staying focused on the problem. State the problem out loud or in your mind. Take a deep breath and check your emotional level.

3. Repeat the sequence if any intensity remains or if other issues come to mind.

4. Now begin tapping with the positive outcome you would like to achieve, for example 'Even though I feel scared about giving birth to my baby, I choose to feel calm and relaxed.' (Use the words that have meaning for you).

    You can continue doing rounds of the sequence as you move through and change the wording. For example, you might say 'I am confident about giving birth, experiencing labour and birth is an easy process. I am looking forward to my body birthing easily.' Be prepared to persist with the procedure until all aspects of the problem have been addressed.

This is a wonderful technique to overcome pregnancy anxiety, fear around the birth or being able to cope as a parent.

EFT Tapping Points

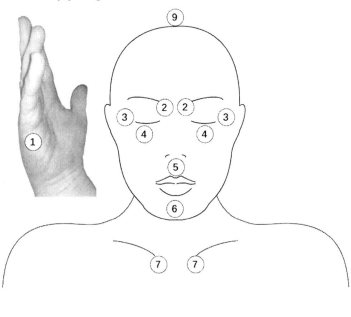

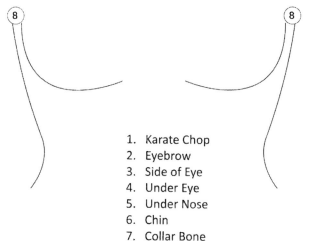

1. Karate Chop
2. Eyebrow
3. Side of Eye
4. Under Eye
5. Under Nose
6. Chin
7. Collar Bone
8. Under Arm
9. Top of Head

Herbal Remedies

Herbs and homeopathic remedies can provide you with welcome relief from the minor discomforts of pregnancy.

* These are not to be used as a medical substitute and should be taken under the guidance of a trained practitioner. If symptoms increase please seek further advice from your midwife or doctor.

Traditional use and knowledge of the plant based on observation and experience is valid. The herbs that I recommend here are well known amongst traditional midwives and natural therapists, having been used for centuries with great efficacy.

The good news is that the majority of readily available herbal teas are safe to drink during pregnancy. A couple of daily cups of chamomile, peppermint, rosehip, raspberry leaf tea, nettle and valerian tea are very safe and very relaxing. Raspberry leaf is a wonderful uterine tonic, relieves nausea and vomiting and assists in milk production. High in vitamins, minerals and anti-oxidants, raspberry leaf helps regulate the action of the uterine muscles and seems to assist in shortening labour.

As noted by R. F. Weiss (1999), a leading German physician,

> "Where there is a long tradition of use by a population, the herb's action has to be considered established, even without double blind trials. For example, there is general knowledge regarding the use of prune juice for constipation. We know what prune juice does and that it is safe. It is not necessary to study its safety and efficacy".
>
> 'Herbal Preparations and Dosage Guidelines'.
> Midwifery Today E-News 1(44).

Similarly, widespread use of a herb over time for a particular effect suggests there is validity to that knowledge. The World Health Organization recommends that in a rational approach to evaluating the safety and efficacy of herbal products, historical and cultural usage should be combined with modern scientific research (2006). The herbs recommended here have established research to support their use.

Herbal Preparations and Dosage Guidelines

Storage - Store dried herbs away from light and heat.
Quality and freshness of a herb is a direct result of the care taken in harvesting, drying and processing. These are the most important factors in the effectiveness of the herb. Water-based preparations must be made from dried, not fresh plants. In the fresh plant the cell wall is still intact, so most of the constituents cannot be extracted. Drying is necessary to rupture the cell wall and allow release of the constituents. A larger quantity and broader range of the nourishing properties of the plant are available in water preparations.

Infusion
Made by adding one cup of boiling water to 1-2 teaspoons of dried herbs (leaves, flowers and stems), steep for 10-15 minutes. Drink lukewarm sweetened with honey if desired. DO NOT BOIL.

Infusions are used to prepare the leafy portion of plants. Leaves have tougher cell walls so it takes longer for the constituents to come out of the plant into solution. Cold infusions are used for a few plants which contain valuable constituents that would be damaged by heat. Simple teas are appropriate for flowers and seeds which open and release their contents easily, or for herbs where the volatile oils are a major constituent.

Decoction
Prepared with seeds, root or bark by boiling 60-125gms of the herb in approximately 2 cups of water for 15-20 minutes. Let steep for another 15 minutes and drink lukewarm. Decoctions are used to extract the more dense parts of plants such as roots or barks.

Tincture

Can be made by several methods but this one is probably the simplest. Take 60-125gms of the powdered herb and add 600mls of brandy. Shake well. Place in a dark cupboard and shake every 12 hours for 3 to 4 weeks. Strain into a tinted glass bottle with a tight cap and store.

Tinctures are alcohol based preparations. Some herbs work better in tincture form as some plant constituents are more soluble in alcohol than in water. Some plants are more effective medicinally if the fresh plant is made into tincture, in other cases dried plant is more beneficial, and with some herbs it doesn't matter.

Fomentation

Prepared by making an infusion or a decoction with the prescribed herb(s), and soaking a clean towel or nappy in the preparation. Wring out the cloth and place on the affected area. Can be used as a hot pack, or iced for a cold pack.

Infused Oils

The fresh plant is packed into a jar, covered with olive oil and allowed to sit for two weeks. Salves can be made by simply adding beeswax.

Glycerites

The sweet fraction of oil (oil minus the fatty acids) does not have the same extractive properties of alcohol. Most herbs are not effective in this preparation.

Powdered, pre-packaged herbs

Have been extensively exposed to air, causing oxidation and rapid loss of potency. Grinding and encapsulating the herbs oneself is the best way to maintain high quality if capsules are preferred.

Dosage

The usual dose for infusions or decoctions is one cup three to four times daily:

- external preparations or fomentations should be used as often as possible, at least four times daily
- tinctures are administered by placing a few drops under the tongue, or mixed with a glass of water and sipped three to four times daily
- external applications of herbs, such as poultices, compresses and fomentations are used to accelerate healing and prevent or draw out infection
- essential oils are very strong and are rarely used internally.

Best to buy herb teas in their whole form stored in brown paper bags or containers resisting light.

Herbal Remedies for Normal Childbirth

The following list offers information about natural, safe and effective herbal remedies that are tried and true and long valued by women worldwide as allies for the transformative process of childbirth (recommended reading Wise Woman Herbal, Susan Weed, Ashwood Publishing, 1989).

Black cohosh (Caulophyllum thalictroides) may help labour progress with less intensity, taking the edge off powerful contractions and allowing the mother to remain more relaxed and open. Take 15 drops of the tincture in a cup of warm water every half hour until a good rhythm is established.

Blue Cohosh (Cimicifuga racemosa) carries a significant amount of oxytocin-like properties, which may assist the initiation and maintenance of the process of labour.

Blue/Black Cohosh Roots Combination assists to establish and regulate labour.

Comfrey Leaf (Symphytum officinale) for use after birth, *** For External Use Only - do not drink.**

The herb in infusion form can be used topically for any perineal tears, stitches or general soreness in the pelvic floor. Soak in a comfrey sitz bath several times a day. The bath can be prepared by adding a litre of comfrey leaf infusion to a litre of warm water and mixing these in the sitz bowl before use. Soak for up to twenty minutes each time.

Dong Quai (Angelica sinensi) may encourage the expulsion of a reluctant placenta. This herb usually yields good results within one or two doses. Take 15 drops of dong quai tincture every 15 minutes for a maximum of three doses.

Ginseng/Ginger Roots (Panax, Zingiber officinale) assists energy during labour and birth. Ginseng is renowned as a strengthening tonic overall and is useful in difficult or prolonged labour in which the mother feels exhausted and unable to go on. Ginger root is a warming, stimulating tonic that will give a boost while easing contracting muscles. Use 20 drops of tincture hourly as needed. As labour moves into the pushing stage, a one-time dose of 30-40 drops can be used to boost energy.

Nettles (Urtica dioica) are a favourite preventative herb used by midwives the world over. The leaves and stalks are safe enough to be consumed as a tea every day. If you find you just cannot drink this tea, or in the quantities recommended, you can take it in capsule form (2 capsules 3 times a day). Nettle tea is a superior natural thirst quencher, high in vitamin K, iron and important anti-oxidants. Mixed with other woman-friendly herbs such as oat straw, red raspberry leaf and red clover, these herbs support the expanding blood volume and tone the uterus. It is a wonderful and refreshing drink hot or cold.

Taken during labour, it provides all important blood clotting vitamin K for mother and baby and has an anti-haemorrhagic effect. After the baby comes it continues to refresh the mother by boosting the adrenals, hormonal and circulatory systems and helps increase milk production. Leaves are a source of:

- histamine, which helps to reduce the symptoms in an allergic response, including hay fever, asthma and sinus
- serotonin, which acts as a neuro-transmitter to the central nervous system and is helpful for relieving stress, fear, nervousness, depression and insomnia
- melatonin, an antioxidant sometimes referred to as an anti-ageing hormone, that may give relief from chronic fatigue syndrome, seasonal effect disorder, depression and sleeplessness.

Nettle is valuable for strengthening the adrenals. Eating nettles or drinking the tea has been a folk custom to make hair brighter, thicker and shinier and the skin clearer and healthier. It is a mild diuretic to relieve fluid retention and stimulate the lymphatic system and is known to eliminate bad breath. Nettles increase excretion of uric acid through the kidneys, making them an excellent remedy for assisting pre-eclamptic symptoms. The herb is used to balance blood sugar, and a tincture of the seed has been found to raise thyroid function and reduce goitre. A healing ointment is prepared by steeping cut nettle leaves in oil.

Partridge Berry or Squaw Vine (Mitchella repens) is a great uterine tonic. Use as a tincture, take as directed. If you are experiencing pelvic congestion (signalled by constipation, bloating, haemorrhoids, varicose veins, and/or menses with clots) add 5 millilitres of ginger root and 5 millilitres of cinnamon per 30 millilitres of partridge berry.

Raspberry Leaf Tea (Rubas idaeus) is probably the most popular herb for pregnancy. It acts by toning the uterus, increasing its efficiency during labour and birth and reducing the chances of post-partum haemorrhage.

Raspberry leaf is a wonderful uterine tonic, relieves nausea and vomiting and assists in milk production as well as being very high in vitamins, minerals and anti-oxidants. Raspberry leaf also helps regulate the action of the uterine muscles, seeming to shorten labour.

Dose: one cup daily as an infusion, building up to several cups by late pregnancy. Try adding Lemon Grass (Andropogon Citratus) or one of the mint teas to improve the taste, and chamomile tea which has the added benefit of helping insomnia. Most herbal teas act to alkalise the body, whereas caffeine drinks cause acidity.

Skullcap/Passionflower Combination (Scutellaria laterifolia, Passiflora incarnata) specific for pain relief and nerve nourishment. Helps settle the nervous system and adrenals. Helps reduce fears and anxiety, particularly when the fear of pain becomes greater than the pain itself. This formula may help to normalise blood pressure if there is a tendency to rise above an acceptable normal range. Can be taken following the delivery to help settle and relax the mother. Use 10-20 drops of tincture hourly, or every half hour if necessary as labour deepens.

St. John's Wort (Hypericum perforatum) massaging the oil into the lower back seems to take the edge off painful labour contractions felt in that area for about twenty minutes. Reapply as needed while the woman's back is massaged. St John's Wort is so named because the plant opens its yellow flowers in the northern hemisphere around the feast day of St John the Baptist in late June. Wort is an old English word for plant. St John's Wort has been used to treat nervous conditions since ancient Greek times and was also used for its sedative and anti malarial properties. In the 19th and 20th centuries, St John's Wort was used to treat hysteria and nervous diseases with depression. It has also been used to treat wounds, bruises and sprains.

Today, St John's Wort is officially listed in the national pharmacopoeias of Czechoslovakia, France, Poland, Romania and Russia. In September 2000, the British Medical Journal published a study by German researcher Hermut Woelk, comparing St John's Wort with the antidepressant imipramine as a treatment for mild to moderate depression, which concluded that the herbal treatment was 'therapeutically equivalent' to imipramine. It has been noted though, in some of the correspondence regarding the trial, that imipramine is an older antidepressant and may have more side effects than some modern antidepressants in conventional use.

Yarrow/Shepherd's Purse (Achillea millefolium, Capsella bursa-pastoris) wonderful to have on hand in case of unchecked postpartum bleeding. Yarrow is well documented for its haemostatic properties that help reduce excessive blood flow. This tincture must be prepared with fresh flowering shepherd's purse. The dried herb is not as effective. Use 10-15 drops of this formula, only after the placenta has been delivered, every 15 minutes until bleeding is under control.

Aromatherapy for Childbearing

Of the five senses, smell has the most direct link to the brain. Many people find that an aroma can have surprising effects, reaching past our conscious thoughts to trigger emotions and memories. It is precisely this ability to gently reach past our mental armour that gives aromatherapy its power as a system of healing.

Essential oils have been used throughout the world for thousands of years, as far back as 3000 B.C. Extracted from the plant, herb or flower by a lengthy process of distillation, essential oils are highly fragrant and concentrated. In some cases when oil is undiluted it can be a skin irritant so the best way to use an essential an oil is in a balm or oil.

Oils to Avoid Early in Pregnancy

Oils that must be avoided during the first three or four months of pregnancy include those that are described as:

- 'emmenagogue' meaning that they induce menstrual flow
- those that are recommended for use during labour to strengthen contractions.

The following oils should be avoided in their concentrated form:

- aniseed, armoise, arnica
- basil, birch, camphor, myrrh
- origanum, pennyroyal, peppermint (perfectly safe as a herbal tea)
- rose, rosemary, sage, clary sage
- cypress, fennel, hyssop, jasmine, juniper
- marjoram, saviour, thyme, wintergreen
- and any other oil described as toxic.

Chamomile and lavender are best avoided in early pregnancy but are wonderful in late pregnancy for relieving back ache and as a calming effect on the adrenal points on the feet. Massaging the feet with crème containing a few drops of lavender is excellent in labour.

Methods of Application

Any touch therapy helps relax the mother by releasing endorphins, and the scent of the oils helps calm breathing. The oils are absorbed through the skin and have medicinal properties. I regularly use the oils during a reflexology foot massage.

Immersion

Oils added to salt then added to water are better absorbed. A few drops in a bowl of hot water or atomiser will help scent the room and calm the breathing. Four drops of the oil of choice to 2 teaspoons of base/carrier oil such as sweet almond can be massaged into the feet and legs during labour. Be careful not to put onto the mother's hands as may be too strong.

Compress

Add four drops of essential oil into a bowl of hot water, swish to disperse. Drop a washcloth on top of the hot water and wring out.

Apply:

- clary sage with lavender to the lower abdomen for pain relief (excellent during labour)
- jasmine and rose to the lower abdomen to help with placenta delivery
- rose to the perineum to help prevent tears.

When the cloth is cold, repeat. After every three repeats, add a few more drops to the water.

TRUessence Aromatherapy

Choose the oils you use carefully. I recommend TRUessence. TRUessence has taken the use of medicinal plants to a totally new level. TRUessence has carefully screened growers all over the world to find essential oils that are not only 100% pure but are also grown, harvested and distilled correctly to create intensely active essential oils. All TRUessence products are distilled and extracted for therapeutic use, but with the addition of the HYDressence Plant Life Concentrate, they go beyond traditional aromatherapy. These oils are water-soluble, able to be ingested safely, making them more bio-available. Mixing a few drops in a glass of water or pure juice creates healing synergy that accelerates and accentuates the body's natural healing influences.

- Red Dragon – five different herbs to enhance circulation and stimulate the central nervous system
- White Dragon – a blend of eight different whole herbs that boost the immune system

- Green Dragon - a blend of eight different whole herbs that promote detoxification
- Rainmaker - a blend of seven different whole herb and flower extracts formulated to sweeten the other Dragon Plant Life Concentrates or to be used by itself as a hydrating floral experience.

Essential Oil Properties

Bergamot (Monardia fistulosa) extracted from the rind of a specific type of orange. Helps relieve urinary tract anomalies, is uplifting and has an anti-depressant effect.

Clary Sage (Salvia sclarea) **Not to be used during pregnancy** but excellent in labour. Strengthens and tones contractions, relaxes and reduces tension. Antiseptic, antidepressant, antispasmodic, emmenagogue, aphrodisiac, uterine tonic. Lowers blood pressure. Use on a compress for pain and relaxation, or as an antidepressant and euphoric. Put some on a tissue and breathe in during each contraction, it will assist the effectiveness of contractions.

Chamomile (M. chamomilla) extracted from the blooms of one of two types of chamomile plants, German chamomile (the most common) or Roman chamomile. The oils are closely related and have pain relieving anti-inflammatory properties, good for muscle aches, best used after sixteen weeks of pregnancy.

Geranium (Pelargonium graveolens) distilled from small glandular formations in the flowers and foliage of the geranium plant is used as an antiseptic, antidepressant, astringent, diuretic, fortifying, healing, refreshing, toning, uplifting. Balances the body, relieves depression and fatigue. Is wonderful postnatally as it stimulates the lymphatic system, relieves fluid retention and helps engorged breasts. Helps heal wounds and sores.

Jasmine (Jasminum officinal) antidepressant, antiseptic, antispasmodic, aphrodisiac, helpful during labour, increases milk flow, general tonic. Expensive, but strong, so a little goes a long way. Uplifting, calming, boosting effect on emotions. Boosts confidence, relieves pain and helps expel the placenta. Can be used after sixteen weeks of pregnancy.

Lavender (Lavandula officinali) **Best not used in early pregnancy.** With its sweet and unforgettable fragrance is one of my favourites, especially as I live on the wonderful island of Tasmania where some of the purest lavender in the world is grown. Antiseptic, antibiotic, analgesic, antidepressant, diuretic, antiviral, antifungal, antispasmodic, healing, sedating, toning. So gentle one drop can be used without dilution on the skin, but you can blend it to make it go further. Just putting a couple of drops on a pillow can be just as beneficial. It is physically and mentally relaxing during labour and offsets pain.

Lemon Citrus (Limonum) antiseptic, antibacterial, antifungal, astringent, diuretic, stimulant, tonic. I use a few drops of lemon on a tissue for mother to inhale if she needs to clear her head or if she feels nauseous during transition. Don't use directly on the skin.

Mandarin (Citrus nobilis) antiseptic, refreshing, tonic, digestive stimulant, mild relaxant. Inhale on a tissue to help an upset stomach. Add to massage oil and massage the legs in upward strokes toward the heart to alleviate swollen feet and legs.

Neroli (Citrus aurantium) sedates the nervous system, relaxes and regenerates the skin, when combined with coconut oil can be especially good for preventing stretch marks.

Peppermint (Mentha x piperita) relieves digestive ailments, nausea, headaches, assists breast engorgement and improves circulation, excellent as a foot balm, uplifting and energising.

Rose maroc or Rosa damascena - *not to be used until after 37 weeks pregnancy.** Antiseptic, antibiotic, anti-inflammatory, aphrodisiac, menstrual stimulant. Especially good for grief, sadness, shyness and uncertainty. Tonic to the digestive system, especially the liver. I suggest a mix of 40 drops of rose in 15 mls of carrier oil, apply to the perineum twice a day for two weeks before the birth to help prevent tears (see Perineal Massage).

Rosemary (Rosmarinus officinalis) *not to be used until after 37 weeks.** Excellent in labour. Antiseptic, analgesic, general stimulant, menstrual stimulant, astringent, diuretic, tonic. I use a few drops on a tissue if mother needs to become more alert. Stimulating, increases breast milk production.

Sandalwood oil distilled from the roots and inner wood of the sandalwood tree. Has an antiseptic and relaxing effect, extremely uplifting and balancing when applied to the back of the neck. Use in moderation as the scent can be overwhelming.

Tea Tree Oil one of the most well known oils used as an antibacterial and antifungal. Especially good when used on the feet or as a local antiseptic.

Ylang Ylang (Cananga odorata) is one of the most beautiful essential oils, extracted from the fragrant blooms of the ylang ylang tree. This intoxicating, sweet smelling oil can be used as an antiseptic. Also has mood lifting, aphrodisiac and sedative properties. May assist in lowering blood pressure. Helps anxiety, nervous tension, fear, shock, anger and emotional problems. Place a couple of drops on a tissue and breathe deeply to normalizes a racing heartbeat and rapid breathing, wonderful during an anxiety attack and during transition in labour.

Labour and Birth

Prepare the oils to be used at birth ahead of time so that you have the correct measurement, avoiding the risk of over use and a counterproductive heavy aroma.

One drop of lavender or jasmine can be gently massaged onto the tummy and/or lower back as well as onto the adrenal points on the feet from the beginning of labour. Jasmine is effective at strengthening contractions, but some women find the scent too cloying in the warm birth environment. Lavender may be more acceptable. A few drops mixed in cool water will make a refreshing mixture with which to sponge your face and body. I find the feet the most effective way to administer oils.

Early First Stage

To calm and relax: to a 10ml bottle, add four drops lavender and two drops neroli essential oils, add organic vegetable oil to fill. Massage temples, forehead, chest and solar plexus. Massage solar plexus points on the feet also. Remember to breathe deeply.

Active First Stage

To a 10ml bottle add six drops lavender, one drop each neroli and rose essential oils and add organic vegetable oil to fill. Massage the solar plexus, heart chakra, chest and neck. Inhale the blend deeply while resting.

Use lavender essential oil in a base of pure light olive oil for massage during labour. Place small drops of pure lavender onto the adrenal points on the feet to calm. Be careful not to get onto your hands and or near your face as the perfume could be too strong.

Add a few drops of clary sage to a tissue and breathe the aroma during contractions to calm and enhance the effectiveness of the contraction.

Transition

For shaking, shivering, nausea, fear or exhaustion brought on by hard and fast contractions, inhale the following blend between contractions to help you endure this phase and give you an added boost of strength for delivery.

To a 10ml bottle add four drops lavender, four drops each sage or clary sage and peppermint, add organic vegetable oil to fill. Massage the lower back, with emphasis on the sacrum, and add to a tissue and breathe in the vapours.

Make up a spray bottle with water or hand lotion that is strongly ginger scented. If you are experiencing nausea, spray a little of the lotion on to your hand to sniff when needed. This helps about seventy five percent of the time, as well as putting one or two drops of ginger oil onto the wrists. The nausea usually subsides, although sometimes it comes on too strongly to be arrested. Vomiting is to be expected during transition.

Wintergreen may assist urine retention during labour or postpartum to help avoid having to be catheterized.

Second Stage
To a 10ml bottle add four drops each peppermint and rosemary, add organic vegetable oil to fill. Inhale before you begin pushing to help you gain the needed courage and emotional strength for this stage.

Postpartum
Jasmine is best used immediately after baby's birth to help expel the placenta quickly and cleanly. It will also help tone the uterine muscles and help them return faster to their pre-pregnant condition. Jasmine is also a very good antidepressant and promotes the flow of breast milk. Oil of fennel is well known for promoting breast milk flow. (Recommended reading ' An A-Z Aromatherapy' by Patricia Davis).

Homeopathics in Pregnancy & Birth

Dr. Samuel Hahnemann discovered homeopathy in the late 1700's and it was well used in main stream medicine right up to the 1950's when many Homeopathic Hospitals were actively in practice. This healing modality assists the body's natural healing mechanisms.

Homoeopathic remedies work on the principle of like meets like. Substances that cause symptoms in overdose amounts cure those same symptoms when given in minuscule amounts. For instance peeling an onion brings tears to your eyes and makes your nose run, but a small amount of onion juice in homoeopathic form cures those symptoms during a cold or hay fever. Homeopathics are available through homoeopathic practitioners.

For best results I advise you to consult a trained homeopath. I have provided some simple suggestions for you to try. Generally the 6c potency is adequate. Give 2-3 doses within an hour or two whilst symptoms are strong then reduce to 2-3 times a day until symptoms abate.

Homeopathy Dosage Directions

Select the remedy that most closely matches your symptoms. In conditions where self-treatment is appropriate, unless otherwise directed by a physician, a lower potency (6X, 6C, 12X, 12C, 30X, or 30C) should be used. You will find instructions for use are usually printed on the label.

Many homeopathic physicians suggest that remedies be used as follows:

- take one dose and wait for a response
- if improvement is seen, continue to wait and let the remedy work
- if improvement lags significantly or has clearly stopped, another dose may be taken

The frequency of dosage varies with the condition and the individual. Sometimes a dose may be required several times an hour, other times a dose may be indicated several times a day. In some situations, one dose per day (or less) can be sufficient.

- if no response is seen within a reasonable amount of time, select a different remedy.

Aconite for distressing labour pain, fear and anxiety.

Arsenicum for vomiting in labour.

Arnica used at the beginning of labour and repeated as needed during and after labour (provided no other remedy is indicated at these times) will help prevent troublesome after pains. Give Arnica 200c as soon as labour starts, if no other remedy is indicated and the mother is progressing normally. Repeat as needed, every half hour if the labour is progressing rapidly and/or very difficult pushing occurs. Arnica will lessen the need for other painkillers and may prevent haemorrhage. Repeat immediately after birth to prevent postpartum haemorrhage. Homeopathic Arnica 200c, either 4 tablets or 6-10 drops taken under the tongue immediately after birth and then every four hours will assist an aching body.

Caulophyllum to increase contractions, soften and relax the cervix and lubricate the birth canal.

Belladonna assists high blood pressure.

Arnica Montana for excessive pain, bruising and sore feelings. This is a good one to take throughout labour to help with recovery.

Chamomile helps with extreme back pain, but only if the contraction feels as though it begins in the back and radiates down the inner thighs or if it feels as though it draws forward from the sacral region and grips and pinches in the uterus. The extreme pain is often associated with extreme restlessness and irritability.

Kali Carb assists when you want your back pressed and you are finding it hard to move because of pain.

Kali Phos is excellent for tiredness and exhaustion, also great for birth attendants and support people.

Gelsenium gives a spurt of energy, assisting in second stage of labour when the cervix is open but you may be feeling too sleepy to push.

Carbo Veg is excellent for birth trauma or foetal distress, it is the great reviver. Take it to boost energy and give it to a listless baby or one who has breathing difficulties.

Pulsatilla is excellent for turning breech or posterior presenting babys, give one dose, wait three days and give one more dose if required, maximum three doses. Refer to 'Breech Babies" section for more tips. During labour pulsatilla can be given to allay panic and fear, the 'I can't do this anymore' moment during transition, give one dose, wait thirty minutes, a maximum of three doses should be given.

Also good for overdue labours and for increasing effectiveness of contractions, particularly if labour is slowing down.

For slow labour give one dose, wait one hour before giving another, maximum three doses.

Cell Salts

Dr. Wilhelm Schuessler, the originator of this approach to healing, theorised that the human body contains certain vital inorganic elements which are essential for normal cell function. These elements must be present if good health is to prevail. Disease results when one or more of these elements is deficient. Taking these elements in tissue salt form creates a ready supply through the blood stream.

Cell Salt Solutions

Instead of dissolving the cell salt directly under the tongue solutions can be made by combining cell salts in purified water. Under each condition outlined in the 'Complimentary Therapies For Discomforts of Pregnancy' section I have added cell salt suggestions. You can combine these salts by placing 2-10 tablets of the cell salt together in a 200-250ml bottle of purified water and sip throughout the day.

Calcarea Fluor beneficial for muscular and elastin tissue, loose teeth, haemorrhoids, varicose veins, ulcers, decaying, abscesses, goitre, prolapsed uterus, hiccoughing, excellent for blurred vision and cataract.

Calcarea Phos excellent for bones, teeth, blood, connective tissue, anaemia, leg cramps, assists aches and pains, gastric juices and saliva. Known as the great tissue restorer.

Calcarea Sulph recommended for skin, liver, bile, mucous membranes, blood and for any pus discharge from wounds and pimples, excellent for tonsillitis, croup, diarrhoea and constipation.

Ferrum Phosphate particularly good for any blood condition, fever, inflammation, congestive disease, bronchitis, sore throat, coughs, colds, rheumatism, bladder and kidney irritations, congestive headaches. May help in anaemia and the healing of contusions and sprains.

Kali Mur unites with albumin to form filarin, present in every organ and tissue, essential for brain formation. Good for thick white discharges from mucous surfaces and grey coated tongue. Excellent for croup, dysentery, catarrh of nose, throat and other organs, rheumatism, mumps and whooping cough, dissolves blood clots and excellent for stroke victims.

Kali Phos recommended for brain, nerves, muscles and blood, mental or nervous disorders, loss of memory, prostration, brain fatigue, nervous headaches, neuralgia pain, sleeplessness, nervous indigestion, hysteria, heart palpitations and depression. Excellent for the weepy, suspicious patient. Gives people drive. Exceptional in asthma and other respiratory illnesses, also urine retention, muscle spasm and stomach ulcers.

Kali Sulph useful for the outer skin layer, acts as an oxygen carrier, vital to normal functioning of the glands and water balance. Symptoms are chilly, dizzy, toothache, headaches, pain in hands and feet. Use for catarrh of nose, throat, stomach and urinary organs, coughs, bronchitis, eye diseases, delayed menses, measles, rash and chicken pox.

Magnesia Phos excellent for brain, nerves, muscles, good for cramps, aches and pains, neuralgia of face, head, earache, toothache, stomach cramps, asthma, menstrual cramp, diarrhoea, angina and great for reducing blood pressure. Works more efficiently if taken with hot water.

Natrum Mur excellent for all aches and pains.

Natrum Phos helps regulate digestion and waste activity, use for stomach acid attack, sour vomiting, colic spasm, rheumatism, arthritis, gout, heartburn, urinary tract infections.

Natrum Sulph regulates the intercellular fluid water quantity and bile consistency. Use for diarrhoea, gallstones, dizziness, vomiting during pregnancy, influenza headache, jaundice, congestion of the liver, gut hepatitis, reduces blood pressure.

Silica helps connective tissue, skin, hair, nails, helps combat infections, excellent for any skin problem, use for chronic nasal catarrh, bone problems, gout and arthritic pain, acts as a muscle relaxant.

Colour Therapy

Colour triggers an emotional reaction at the subconscious level, often connected to a past experience. It has been used for healing by many cultures throughout history. It is widely understood that colour creates mood and ambience. Colour can have a strong influence on the body physically and emotionally and can be used in many ways such as:

- by wearing the colour
- through visualisation, directing the colour to specific areas of the body
- placing a coloured card or paper under a glass of water enhances the water's healing affect in the body with the properties of that colour.

Each colour has its own properties and effects. Black and white tend to be neutral as they both contain all the colours of the spectrum. Black absorbs whereas white reflects.

Cultural belief has shaped the use of colour. For instance in western societies, white is associated with daylight, purity, spirituality and cleanliness whereas black is seen as dark, mystical and often associated with evil. Other cultures hold the opposite regard, such as China, where red and black are seen as the higher vibration and spiritual colours. The colour of vegetables and fruits also affects their health benefits.

Colour is vibrational, therefore sitting with a colour without word or sound is often the best way to gain the insight and healing colour can bring. All colours are equal, it is your personal experience that creates the like or dislike of particular colours.

If you particularly dislike a colour this is the one you most need to sit with to discover the emotional trigger and allow its healing properties to clear the attached emotion. It is a good time to ask 'why am I reacting or feeling this way to this colour?'

The Primary Colours

Red
Physical, action, related to the Base Chakra, Self Awareness.

Positive properties: courage, vivaciousness, strength, passion, grounded, warmth, energy, survival, masculinity, excitement, uplifting, power.

Negative properties: anger, stop, danger, defiance, aggression, alert, irrational thought.

Red stimulates and has a revitalising effect on the body, raising the pulse rate and stimulating the nervous system. It is lively and friendly but it can also be perceived as demanding and aggressive.

Healing: When you are tired and feeling run down, focus on this colour, it will generate energy. Wear a red scarf or red underwear. Place a glass of water over a red coloured piece of paper for about an hour and then drink. You can also place a red stone in to the bath as you run the water for a more stimulating bath. Red will lift the cellular vibration. Studies have shown that people who choose to wear red are more likely to be extroverted.

Complimentary Colour: Blue

Blue

Intellectual, calming, mental, related to the Throat Chakra, Self Expression.

Positive properties: intelligent, communication, thought, divinity, trust, efficiency, serenity, duty, logic, coolness, reflection, calm, peace, integrity, truth, feminine.

Negative properties: cold, distant, fearful, critical, aloof, lacking emotion, unfriendly, calculating. Very deep blues can enhance depressive thoughts.

Apparently studies suggest that blue is the world's favourite colour as it is the colour of self-expression and the colour of the mind. Blue is essentially soothing and affects us mentally, rather than the physical reaction of red. Strong blues will stimulate clear thought and lighter, softer blues will calm the mind and aid concentration. Consequently blue is serene and mentally calming.

Healing: a peaceful and relaxing colour, blue will soothe distraught nerves and mental anguish. Blue has antiseptic and astringent properties. Blue induces a feeling of security, stimulates feelings of inner peace and is uplifting on a spiritual level. Blue helps you to expand and evolve further into self-understanding and development. Those who wear blue tend to be understanding, calm, and seekers of truth. Blue will help us get in touch with ourselves more, creating an inner peace and tranquillity. Wearing a blue scarf can assist with personal expression and throat conditions.

Indigo Blue: induces spiritual depth and is connected to the Brow Chakra - Self Responsibility, helping the development of intuition and inner wisdom and communication. Connects us to the goddess energy, confidence, beauty and nature, helping to dispel fears, phobias and frustrations. Wearers of indigo blue have a love of beauty and perceive life in a harmonious state, they tend to be understanding, balanced and have a good understanding of the spiritual concepts. Most mystics and clairvoyants wear or use Indigo.

Drinking water enhanced with indigo blue before meditation will assist in a deeper connection.

Complimentary Colour: Red

Aquamarine: expression of universal truth, stillness, dream connections, beauty and sacred sound. Aquamarine is connected to the ocean and the dolphins, brings clarity, harmony, love, foresight, insight and peace. This is the stone of simplification and the ability to go deep within. Aquamarine is an excellent colour for public speakers and writers to wear or work with as it allows the fluid flow of the inner truth. Useful for the thymus gland and for fluid retention in the body.

Yellow

Emotion, feelings, related to the Solar Plexus, Self Worth.

Positive properties: optimistic, confident, powerful, self-esteem, happiness, extraversion, emotional strength, friendliness, creativity, understanding what feels right.

Negative properties: irrationality, fear, emotional fragility, depression, anxiety, suicide, cowardice, disempowerment, low self-esteem, over sympathy.

Yellow is the strongest colour that affects the psyche and is related to the identity and the solar plexus. The right yellow is uplifting and boosts self-esteem. Yellow is the colour of confidence and optimism, connecting with emotional wellbeing. It is related to the identity and an understanding and acceptance of who we are. Yellow awakens and stimulates the mental faculties, assisting with logic and will.

Healing: yellow can be used to dispel depression and anxiety as it promotes optimism and joyfulness. Using the colour yellow inspires communication, expression and mental competency. Too much yellow or the wrong shade can deplete energy and lower self-esteem. Using lemon in water is a great health boost and aids in depression and healthy appetite.

Complimentary Colour: Violet

Gold - is the illustrious depth of yellow, connected to the sun and the masculine, encouraging you to go inward and trust. Auspicious, successful and warm, gold is related to first prize, heightened awareness and ambition, 'Going for Gold'. Gold connects to the divine connection and enhances all other colours. One of the most used properties in Homeopathic medicine, gold has been used extensively throughout time. Gold directly affects the nervous system. It asks you to honour your path.

Mixed Colours in Healing

Green

Balance related to the Heart Chakra, Self Love, combining the properties of yellow and blue.

Positive properties: harmony, balance, reliable, refreshing, fertile, regenerating, renewal, peace, universal love, restoration, reassurance, self-love, abundant, rhythm, nature, acceptance, healing, compassion.

Negative properties: boredom, stagnation, blandness, disease, blockage, resentment, control, jealousy, abandonment, co-dependency.

Green is restful and brings balance to all areas. On a primitive level, when the world about us contains plenty of green there is a feeling of lushness and abundance, indicating the presence of water and survival.

Healing: in green we see the colour of nature, relaxing and refreshing. Green soothes tension in the muscles and nerves. The colour green will promote determination, efficiency, poise and patience. Green assists when there is an imbalance of self-love which may stem from a lack of love as a child, resulting in a sense of abandonment and co-dependency. People who use green in their lives are likely to be orderly and heart centred, dependable and attentive to detail. Green can be used to bring harmony into your life by inducing patience, peace and balance. Eating and drinking green fruits and vegetables is highly recommended for good health. Use with pink to enhance love and heart chakra balance.

Complimentary Colour: Red

Turquoise

The window to the soul and divinity, related to the Heart Chakra. Turquoise holds the blue of the sky and the green of the earth and blends the physical with spirit in unity and oneness.

Positive properties: wisdom, destiny, great spirit, cool, creative, tranquil and peaceful. Turquoise assists with soul connection. Helps to discover your true spiritual self (what really makes you tick). Turquoise boosts the immune system and the digestive system. Excellent for confusion and when feeling ungrounded. Turquoise water aids in detoxification and cleansing. Place the colour under a glass of water, drink half in the morning and the other half at bedtime.

Violet

Spiritual, mystical, related to the Crown Chakra, Self Confidence. Combines the properties of blue and red.

Positive properties: spiritual awareness, intuition, containment, vision, luxury, authenticity, truth, quality, high vibration, divine connection.

Negative properties: introversion, decadence, suppression, inferiority, delusion, depressing, close-minded, secretive, self-denial.

Violet takes awareness to a higher level of thought, to the realms of spiritual concepts. It is the balancer between the physical and psychic. Violet encourages deep contemplation and meditation. It is associated with royalty and quality. Excessive use of purple can bring about too much introspection and the wrong tone can feel cheap and nasty. People who use this colour are likely to be refined, poised and secure within themselves, although they tend be reserved. Violet is linked with the need for spiritual achievement and perfection of the self.

Healing: place a violet scarf over the brow chakra for a deeper relaxation experience and connection to yourself and your baby.

Complimentary Colour: Yellow

Orange

Creativity, related to the Sacral Chakra - Self-Respect. Combines the properties of red and yellow.

Positive properties: fertility, nurturing, physical comfort, food, warmth, security, sensuality, passion, abundance, fun, inner balance, inner knowing, truth and empowerment, acceptance, assertive, compassionate, alive.

Negative properties: deprivation, frustration, frivolity, immaturity, lack, warning, self-denial, lethargy, listless, grief, frivolity and a lack of serious intellectual values.

Since it is a combination of red and yellow, orange is stimulating and reacting, physical and emotional. Orange focuses our minds on issues of physical comfort such as food, warmth, shelter and sensuality. Orange is a 'fun' colour. A balancing colour, similar to red, orange has an enlivening energy. It is stimulating to the nerves and balances the emotional state.

Healing: cheerful and warm, aids fertility, creativity and digestion. Removes fears and inhibitions and aids in expansion of the mind. Orange also allows for new ideas on a mental level and aids in sexual wellbeing. It assists in clearing blockages and fluid flow in the body. People who wear orange tend to be confident, peaceful and considerate, open minded and graceful.

Complimentary Colour: Blue

Pink

Unconditional Love, related to the Heart Chakra, combines red with a tint of white.

Positive properties: soft, gentle, beautiful, tranquillity, love and romance, nurturing, warmth, femininity, love, sensuality, survival, angelic, maternal.

Negative properties: inhibition, emotional claustrophobia, emasculation, physical weakness, aggression, anxiety, restlessness, inability to forgive, overburdened, intolerance, lack of understanding, suffering, oppression.

Being a tint of red, pink also affects us physically, but soothes rather than stimulates. Tints of blue, green and yellow are simply called light or dark. Pink is a powerful colour, it represents the feminine principle and survival, through romance and connection.

Healing: nurturing and physically soothing. Pink absorbs negative energy and stress and heals in a similar way to green through the heart chakra. Relaxes the muscles and slows the heartbeat, however too much pink can be physically draining and disempowering.

Complimentary Colour: Yellow

Grey
Neutral, a mingling of black and white, neither here nor there.

Positive properties: psychological neutral, letting it go, a time to clear.

Negative properties: lack of confidence, indecision, blocking, dampness, depression, hibernation, lack of energy, compromising, anxiety, illness, heaviness, weighed down, confused.

Pure grey is the only colour that has no direct psychological properties, being more an indicator of an emotional block or a feeling that you do not want to face up to something. Grey indicates you need to explore further. It is quite suppressive. A virtual absence of colour is depressing and when the world turns grey we are instinctively conditioned to draw in and prepare for hibernation, deep self-exploration and contemplation. Grey is often the confusion that comes just before the breakthrough. Unless the precise tone is right, grey has a dampening effect on other colours used with it. Heavy use of grey usually indicates a lack of confidence and fear of exposure. Grey affects the equilibrium of the energy centres and can enhance negative feelings. If you have a lot of grey in your wardrobe it may be time to open up and discover your true self, begin by exploring scarfs as an accessory.

Brown
Earthy and grounding, connecting with the Base Chakra.

Positive properties: strong, serious, warm, nature, earthiness, reliability, support, fertile, secure, centred, physical strength, ancient wisdom, endurance.

Negative properties: lack of humour, heaviness, lack of sophistication, drab, dirty, hard work, depressive, stuck, stubborn.

Brown usually consists of red and yellow, with a large percentage of black. Consequently, it has much of the same seriousness as black, but is warmer and softer. Brown has elements of the red and yellow properties and has associations with the earth and the natural world. It is a solid, reliable colour and most people find it quietly supportive, more positive than the ever-popular black which is suppressive, rather than supportive. Different shades of brown will bring different properties. For example adding more yellow creates a bronze effect and the brown becomes illustrious, succulent, enthusiastic and nurturing.

Complimentary Colour: Blue

Black
Mystical, the all knowing.

Positive properties: serious, sophisticated, glamorous, secure, efficient, power, courage, truth.

Negative properties: oppression, coldness, menace, heaviness, terror, shield, mask, void, death, grief, dominance, authority, suffering.

Black is all colours absorbed, therefore it has many interpretations depending on the situation and feeling at the time. Black creates protective barriers as it absorbs all the energy coming towards you and enshrouds the personality. Many people hide behind black, afraid to show their true colours. If this is you I challenge you to start adding colour to your black and observe what you feel. Many people are afraid of the dark, yet it is in the dark you find the light. When you sit in the dark you can go inside yourself with greater ease. Black creates a perception of weight and seriousness. Positively, black communicates absolute clarity.

White
Angelic Light, connected to the Crown Chakra.

Positive: cool, vital, alive, clear, pure, security, clean, simplicity, sophistication, efficient, wise, peace, spirit, oneness, winter, snow, evolvement, self-sufficient, virginal.

Negative: sterile, cold, barren, unfriendly, elitism, lonely, strict, obsessive.

Just as black is total absorption, white is total reflection. White can create barriers, but do not touch! It can be harsh and sterile unless softened with other colours. Visually, white gives a heightened perception of space. Too much white can make other warm colours look and feel garish. White is often softened with other colour shades, there are over 300 shades of white paint to choose from. White is often worn for meditation and spiritual events to allow clear divine communication.

Silver
Silver is aligned with angelic connection and the feminine. The lunar moon energy, go within and discover who you are. Silver has been connected to the goddess energy since ancient times. It is cyclic, flowing, gentle and mothering. Associated with fertility, silver is antibacterial and antiviral. Silver balances the emotional body, is forgiving and compassionate. Silver is associated with the incarnating soul and symbolises when the little one is ready to present.

Light Therapy and Colour
There are many sophisticated light colour healing instruments available, but simply placing coloured cellophane paper over a small torch can have the desired effect. You can use coloured crystals, stones or coloured cards.

Working with clients using this method I have noticed that focusing different colours onto different areas of the body creates different responses. I most often find that those colours that seem to bring discomfort or that the client expresses they don't like are the very colours that need to be explored and worked with.

If you would like to explore the use of colour further I recommend the 'Being in Colour' inspirational cards and healing tools created by Pip Oxlade.

www.beingincolour.co.nz

Vibrational Medicine

Australian Bush Flowers

Australian Bush Flowers are a range of native flower essences developed by naturopath and fifth generation herbalist, Ian White. Ian had used Bach Flowers in his practice for some time, but felt compelled to investigate the potency of Australia native plants. Through meditation and inner guidance he would receive a mental picture of a certain plant, where to find it and what its specific benefit would be. The essences were then developed and trialled.

The essences have a vibrational healing effect, with each flower aligning with specific emotional and physical vibrations in the body. I had the greatest pleasure of studying with a West Australian bush flower practitioner. I was given the opportunity to sit and meditate with the flowers in the wild and the messages and feelings I received aligned with the purpose of the flower. This gave me great insight into the power of these beautiful essences. I began using the essences in my practice and have been astounded by the results. I have included the suggested remedies for specific ailments in the Complimentary Therapies for Discomforts of Pregnancy section. Further information and study can be found on the Australian Bush Flower Site.

http://www.australian-bushflowers.com/
Australian-Bush-Flower-Essences-from-Ian-White

The thirty eight Bach Flower Essences are still readily available and certainly worth checking out. Personally, I am more inclined to use the Australian Bush Flowers as I feel they resonate with the Australasian area. I do however use Rescue Remedy frequently. This remedy is a combination of bach flowers created to assist when you are experiencing anxiety, shock, discomfort, fear and stress. The remedies create a vibration of peace and calm. Particularly good for labour. You can purchase as drops which can be taken orally or as crème which is best applied to the wrists. I have listed the remedies for your interest, with information provided from http://www.bachflowers.com

Impatiens: as the name suggests, for those who lack patience, may tend to be fast thinkers, fast acting and not so patient with others. Recommended for assisting with developing empathy and patience towards others.

Star of Bethlehem: recommended in cases of trauma and shock, past or present, as assists with recovery from trauma and ability to integrate learning into the present.

Cherry Plum: encourages trust in your intuition and the courage to follow it. Recommended for those who worry about doing wrong, who worry about causing themselves trouble by inability to control their thoughts and actions.

Rock Rose: recommended when feeling panic or terror.

Clematis: indicated for those who find it difficult to remain grounded in reality and may have a tendency to retreat into fantasy. Can assist to provide a sense of connection and grounding between fantasy and the physical world.

The Liquid Crystals

Created by Justin Mohkear, The Liquid Crystals (TLC) are geometric vibrational remedies made from the earth's metals, minerals and crystals. Working at the vibrational level, TLC facilitate change and health through vibrational alignment with the body.

Justin describes TLC:

> "The Liquid Crystals are created via an ancient remembered process that embraces Crystalline Integrity, Sacred Geometry, Alchemy, Solar, Luna and Universal energy. The Liquid Crystals have returned to facilitate our planet back to Oneness by Reuniting the Crystalline grids, Above, Below and within Humanity. One Heart, One Voice, One Vision, One Spirit. The Liquid Crystals are Organic, Natural and Holistic. As a vibrational therapy, TLC will not interfere in the action of any other medication or treatment and is perfect for the whole family. Some of the best results we have seen from the Crystals have been in children who respond very rapidly, there are no side effects. TLC can even be safely given to Animals and Plants with great confidence"
>
> Justin Mohikear, www.theliquidcrystals.com

Complimentary Therapies For Discomforts of Pregnancy

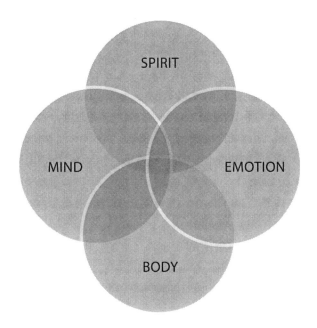

This Complimentary Therapy guide provides easy to use and practical options for natural therapy modalities you may seek to relieve common discomforts of pregnancy. The therapies included here are discussed in greater detail in the previous section 'Complimentary Pregnancy Therapies and Remedies'. Each modality covered in this section is a therapy and so I recommend seeking out a therapist trained in the modality you choose to pursue.

Where highlighted, if you are reading this as an E-Book, click on the links provided and you will be taken to the appropriate diagram or information. Individual detailed reflexology diagrams are included within this section.

This section incorporates the four aspects of healing - Spirit, Emotions, Mind and Body, aligned with Eastern and Western natural philosophy. Therapies included here have been well researched and shown to be safe for use during pregnancy. However it is important that you work in consultation with your maternity caregiver and seek medical advice for any persistent condition.

Acidity

(Acid Reflux see Heartburn)

Your body is naturally attuned to have a slightly alkaline ph. Alkalinity is healthy whilst over acidity can create conditions for disease. A yellow mucus coating on the tongue can be a sign of acidity, as can sour body smell or sour-smelling discharges. Candida infections, vaginal yeast and parasites can also come with over acid conditions. Reducing acidity in the body can reduce the risk of many complications. The easiest way to achieve this is to eat alkaline foods whilst reducing acid foods. There are many references to the alkaline diet online.

I suggest increasing the intake of:

- cherries (fresh when in season or freeze and defrost)
- figs
- celery
- apples, at least two daily (including the peel)
- herbal teas, soy products
- olive, flax and canola oil
- almonds, chestnuts, asparagus, potatoes (fresh from the garden, they become acidic when stored), lemons, and mangoes.
- banana, lemon and honey.

Hydrate - increase clear fluid intake:

- drink meadowsweet tea
- juice cucumber, carrot and celery and drink daily
- drink 500mls Barley water daily. Can be bought at the supermarket or you can soak barley overnight in water and strain.
- consume water (50 percent of your weight in kilos x 30mls) Example: if you weight 80 kilos, times 40 (50% of 80) by 30 = 1200mls per day
- eliminate alcohol.

Refresh your body with a glass of lemonade:

- lemons help clear the body of waste and trigger an alkaline-forming state
- add two teaspoons of honey for an added alkaline boost!

Consider apple cider vinegar therapy:

- add one to two tablespoons of apple cider vinegar to a glass of water and drink. Do this on a daily basis.

Baking soda (sodium bicarbonate) and water:

- in a glass of water, add one to two teaspoons of baking soda. Good for hypertension or oedema.

Reduce fat intake and purines such as organ meat, meats, shellfish, yeast, herrings and mackerel.
Reduce sugar intake and add alkaline foods to acidic foods.
Try the cream tartar remedy:

- add one to two teaspoons of cream tartar in 230mls of water. Alleviates nausea and headache. Cream of tartar is a highly acidic substance that stimulates an alkaline-forming state in your body.

Vegetable Tonic:
Based on physician Henry Bieler's 'Bieler Broth', this vegetable tonic provides an ideal combination of minerals for restoring acid-alkaline and sodium-potassium balance to the body's organs and glands. Vegetarian, cleansing and perfect for the cooler months of the year (Serves 4).

Ingredients:

- 4 cups of spring or filtered water
- 4 medium zucchini, finely chopped
- 425 grams green string beans, roughly chopped
- 1 small bunch of parsley, stems and leaves roughly chopped
- 3 tomatoes, finely chopped
- 2 cloves of garlic
- 2 stalks of celery, finely chopped
- 1 teaspoon sea salt.

Method:

- put all ingredients in a pot. Bring to a gentle boil, lower heat and then simmer very gently for 30 minutes, with lid on.
- strain and use as a broth. Alternatively, leave vegetables in, or even blend to create a thicker soup.

If you have a Vitamix blend for 5-7 minutes to create a soup rather than making a broth.

* Note - A particularly good adrenal tonic for stress-related conditions and general fatigue. A handy vegetable stock to use as a base in other recipes.

Taken from The Food Matters Recipe Book.

Cell Salts:

Nat Phos assists in the elimination of uric acid and governs the acid balance of the body. Indigestion is a sign of lack of this salt.

Homeopathic:

Nux Vomica, Silica, Carbo Vegetabilis, Ignatia. The symptoms guide us to the remedy so need to be examined closely and individualised for a homoeopathic medicine to work best. Please seek out a qualified practitioner.

Reflexology & Su-Jok Points:

Overall massage of the feet and hands can assist with body acidity. Pay particular attention to the detox systems such as the <u>digestive system, liver and lymphatics.</u>

Auricular Therapy:

<u>Massage all over the ears.</u> Pay attention to any points that are tender and massage these more. Use the balance points such as the Shenmen as well.

Acupressure Points:

By massaging the <u>Third Eye (Governing Vessel)</u>, the corresponding body area receives specific therapeutic treatment. It is important to drink plenty of warm water after the massage to help to clear away toxic substances in your body.

Bush Flowers:

Alpine Mint Bush, Vitality essence combination, Crowea, Dog Rose, Pink Mulla Mulla. The remedy will depend on the underlying emotional issue.

Psychosomatic Response:

- not going with the flow, feeling stuck or backed up.
- feeling uncomfortable with the new experience, frustration, helplessness, resistant.

Affirmation:

"I choose to go with the flow, accepting that I am at peace. All is perfect in my world. I let go of fear and I trust."

Liquid Crystal:

<u>Digestive Help</u>.

Allergies / Sinusitis

Often occur due to the heightened antibody production protecting your pregnancy. Upper respiratory problems, sneezing, rhinitis, post-nasal drip, red-inflamed eyes associated with exposure to pollen, grasses, ragweed, dust or other airborne irritants may occur, especially if the diet is inadequate. Gut toxins, stress, erratic blood sugars, asthma, food sensitivities, wheat and dairy foods can exacerbate the condition.

Nutrition:

- antioxidants such as FrequenSea (as a drink and can be applied externally to affected areas), Vitamin C and bioflavanoids, zinc and selenium
- 3000mg fish oils daily
- juice or blend horseradish, garlic, orange, ginger, pineapple, carrots and apricots
- orange and honey - finely chop orange peel, cover with honey. Eat one teaspoon daily for prevention, five teaspoons when hay fever is active.
- reduce carbohydrates and increase protein and vegetables
- probiotics
- herbal formulas (under practitioner guidance)
- avoid dairy foods and food additives.

Homeopathic:

NET Remedy – Allergies (available from a NET practitioner)

Allium cepa - streaming eyes and nose

Arsenicum – sneezing

Gelsemium, Nux vomica – itchy sore ears and eyes

Ferrum phos – inflammation

Ear Candling:

I have had great success with therapeutic ear candling. These candles are very large and TGA approved. Do not use the small 'over the counter' ear candles as they tend to be ineffective and can break into the ear. The candles I use take thirty minutes to burn and are used with a cone and gauze to protect the ear, acting as a vacuum extracting toxins from deep within the sinus and face channels. Seek out a trained practitioner.

http://www.naturaltherapypages.com.au/
connect/casa-del-sole/service/8029

Reflexology:

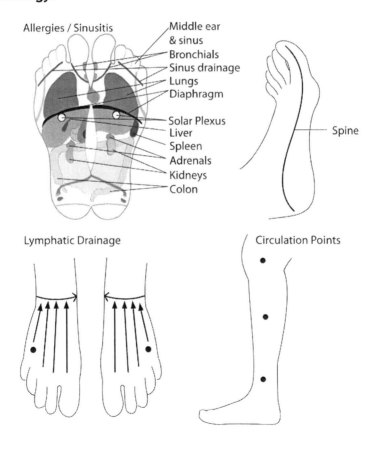

Allergies / Sinusitis
Middle ear & sinus
Bronchials
Sinus drainage
Lungs
Diaphragm
Solar Plexus
Liver
Spleen
Adrenals
Kidneys
Colon
Spine

Lymphatic Drainage

Circulation Points

Facial Massage:

Massage between and across the eyebrows, around the eyes and along the sinus track across the cheek bones. Press into the points that are particularly tender whilst breathing and releasing. See Facial Massage diagram in the section 'Complimentary Pregnancy Therapies and Remedies'.

Su-Jok Points:

Probe along the pad of each finger until the tender trigger point is found. Warm up this point with moxa. Adhere a warming seed, such as a peppercorn, onto the point and massage throughout the day. Also using Moxa warm up the point at the corner of the right side of the nostril in line with the inner corner of the eye.

Auricular Therapy:

- Ear apex
- Endocrine
- Adrenal glands
- Internal and external nose point
- Spleen and kidney

Acupressure Points:

- Elegant Mansion K27 (Kidney)
- Three Mile Point ST36 (Stomach)
- Bigger Rushing LV3 (Liver)

Aromatherapy:

To err on the side of caution, **Do Not** apply oils directly onto the skin during pregnancy. Add the essential oil of lemon, eucalyptus or chamomile into a bath and soak for about twenty minutes. Aromatic oils can be inhaled or absorbed through massage oil to help you breathe better. For inhalation therapy, dilute one drop of ecualyptus and/or lavender essential oil in one cup of steaming water and then inhale the steam.

Lavender and yarrow are good for allergies in general. Eucalyptus, myrtle, lavender, peppermint, rosemary, thyme and tea tree are helpful in treating hay fever. German chamomile, known for its anti-inflammatory effect, suppresses histamine release and should be used as oil with body massage.

Bush Flowers:
Fringed Violet and Dagger Hakea.

Psychosomatic Response:

- denying your own power. What or who are you allergic to?
- examine self worth, denial, life's irritations
- just being pregnant can be an irritation.

Affirmation:
"Nothing irritates me. I live embracing each new moment. The world is safe, I'm safe with life. I'm safe in this pregnancy, my baby and I are perfectly well and healthy. I will be a great mum."

Improving the Immune System:
Place your little finger and ring finger on the tip of your thumb and extend the index and middle finger hold for 10 – 15 minutes whilst meditating on your wellness. Massage the Thymus point several times a day (also known as the heart chakra point). The corresponding thymus point is also on your hand, just below the web between the middle and ring finger, on the foot below the web between the third and fourth toe. The more imbalanced the more painful the points will be.

Colour Therapy:
Green, blue, orange, purple.

The Liquid Crystals:
Allergy Help.

Anaemia

Anaemia is a reduction in the oxygen carrying capacity of the blood. Often due to a deficiency in the quantity or quality of the red blood cells or haemoglobin in the blood. Anaemia in pregnancy can occur at any time, especially if the diet is inadequate. Anaemia can result in extreme tiredness if untreated, possibly leading to a long and difficult labour. Anaemia reduces the pain threshold. I personally have experienced this. I had anaemia with my daughter Vanessa's birth and even though labour was only four hours it felt like one long contraction. This was very different from my son's birth two years previously where I was strong with a good blood count. You need to have a good haemoglobin level prior to birth, preferably twelve or above. An intake of iron loaded foods can be beneficial along with liquid iron such as Floradix or chelated iron with magnesium, zinc and cell salts.

(See also 'Full Blood Count' in Antenatal Visit Assessments)

Nutrition:

Treat the underlying cause by increasing iron rich foods such as macrobiotic food including:

- dark leafy green vegetables, seaweed, sushi, red meat
- juice/blend beetroot (including stem and leaves), carrot, dark leaved vegetables such as spinach, silverbeet and kale, wheatgrass, berries and kelp powder
- avocado (also very good for your baby's teeth, skin and bones)
- kale (possibly the highest ingestible source of vitamin K)
- alfalfa sprouts (an excellent source of iron and vitamin K)
- lots of different types of berries
- apricots, asparagus, celery corn, eggplant and vitamin C rich foods to your diet (see Vitamins under Nutrition)
- do not drink tea or coffee with meals, wait at least an hour before consuming.

Superfoods

- cellular regeneration with FrequenSea, Pure and A.I.M.

The best sources of iron are those that are pre-chelated or liquid. I have assisted women who have haemorrhaged at birth, resulting in a haemoglobin level as low as seven. With pre-chelated iron with liquid supplementation such as Floradix, cell salts, Hemagenics IC from Healthworld, B12 folic acid, Vitamin E and magnesium. Haemoglobin levels were increased to ten within 48 hours.

Homeopathic:

NET Remedy - Fire, Day and Night, Visceral Polarity (available from a NET
    therapist)

Cell Salts:

Calc Phos - stimulates bone marrow for red blood cell production
Ferr Phos - iron absorption
Nat Mur - iron absorption

Improving Circulation:

Vigorously massage the body with a body brush or loofah to bring the circulation to the fore.

Reflexology:

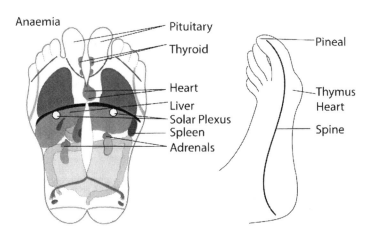

Su-Jok Points:

Using a probe, look for the tender spleen, heart and liver points on the fingers and hands. Warm up these points with moxa as well as massage regularly or adhere to the point a warm seed such as a peppercorn and stimulate regularly throughout the day.

Auricular Therapy:

- Subcortex
- Shenmen
- Adrenals
- Heart
- Spleen
- Kidney
- Small Intestine

Acupressure Points:

- Three Yin Crossing SP6 (Spleen) *** Only to be applied from 37 weeks, after which can be stimulated twice daily.**
- Three Mile Point ST36 (Stomach)

Aromatherapy:

Lemon, Rosemary, Thyme, Ylang-Ylang. To err on the side of caution **Do Not** apply oils directly onto the skin during pregnancy. See aromatherapy section for details of how to use.

Bush Flowers:

Five Corners, Kapok Bush, Bluebell.

Psychosomatic Response:

- the underlying emotional state may be a lack of joy and vitality, tending to find the negative instead of the positive aspect

- worrying excessively, even a fear of living, a sense of not being good enough.

Affirmation:
"I embrace and live life to the full, I am free of fear, I see the positive in all things. I am grateful for my life, for being pregnant and the opportunity to be a mum."
"I am a great mum."

Colour Therapy:
Focus on violet, blue, green and indigo with the colour red. Imagine warming up your body with the red glow, imagine the heat of red flames. Wear red, lie in a red blanket. Rub red based colour therapy or oils onto the colder areas of your body. Bath in red essence.

The Liquid Crystals:
Transition Help or Destress or Cycles.

Anxiety & Stress

Also see remedies for Hypertension and Emotional Balancing. There are many potential stressors during any normal pregnancy, however for some women stress responses can be higher than usual and the need for balance is essential for the wellbeing of both mother and baby. It is well documented how chronic stress and fear influences the baby's health and future stress response for life. Severe stress during pregnancy may also increase the risk of miscarriage or pre-term delivery. Stress is created by our thoughts. Focus on the present rather than the past or future.

Signs and Symptoms:

- anxiety, poor concentration, excessive worry
- insomnia, depression and/or extreme fatigue
- declining vision and/or hearing
- loss of skin elasticity
- palpitations, clammy palms
- digestive cramping, irritable bowel syndrome, food intolerances, indigestion
- muscular tension (eg. shoulders, neck), tension headaches, restless legs, backache.

Assistance may come from:

- breathing is imperative – see the breathing exercise in the Psychosomatic Therapy Section
- reduce lifestyle stressors
- regular exercise
- meditation, yoga, guided visualisation and/or breathing techniques
- set boundaries in relationships, families and work
- learn to say 'I'm not available' and 'no'
- get support from friends, family, colleagues
- tension is created when we hold onto emotion, so allow yourself the time to feel your emotions and concerns, have a good cry, then breathe and get on with day to day activities with enthusiasm
- have regular body massages and reflexology sessions. Touch is very important for the body to clear withheld emotion (see Psychosomatic Therapy).
- make lists, prioritise and focus on one task at a time
- take regular work breaks throughout the day, hug a tree, sit in a garden
- enjoy weekends or holidays away from obligations and worries to help you gain a fresh perspective
- express your creativity - write, garden, paint, sing, take up a new hobby or class.

Nutrition:

- juice/blend berries, grapes, cucumber, tomato, celery, beetroot and carrot mixed with any combination of darg green vegetables. Adding a dash of Tobasco may help to release endorphins (happy hormones).
- eliminate processed chocolate (pure dark chocolate is an excellent stress reducer) coffee, coke and smoking as these contribute to high blood pressure and stress
- increase healthy proteins such as fish, free range chicken, beans and lentils
- reduce carbohydrates and increase EFA/DHA oils (see Daily Fat/ Oil Requirements)
- regular exercise
- reduce pro-inflammatory foods including saturated fats (meats, especially caged poultry, and dairy), refined foods, and sugar
- if you are sensitive to antibiotics best to eat only organic meats to avoid antibiotic residues
- increase foods high in essential fatty acids such as oily fish, avocado, olive oil and nuts
- eat a minimally processed diet rich in antioxidants, phytonutrients and bioflavonoids, I recommend a high raw food diet, balanced with the Paleolithic diet (hunter and gatherer) if you are not vegetarian.

Healthy Foods:

- increase fibre with lots of fresh fruit and vegetables
- natural yoghurt to increase gut bacteria or take probiotics
- reduce bread and pasta
- apples (including the peel) juiced or whole
- half an avocado daily, particularly effective if mixed with an apple, broccoli, corn, eggplant and rolled oats

- oat milk   mix 1 cup of uncooked rolled oats to 1 litre of water and leave in the fridge to cool. Shake the contents and strain. Drink the milk over the course of the day.
- to increase/stimulate the appetite, thirty minutes before a meal eat apricots or globe artichokes and bitter salad, these are a natural bitter digestive tonic. Juiced or pickled beetroot can also stimulate appetite.
- celery is an appetite stimulant when eaten by itself.

Nutritional Formulas:

- increase B vitamins, especially B3
- magnesium
- <u>FrequenSea</u>
- Omega 3 supplementation during pregnancy, and especially DHA, has been shown to support the neurological and immune development in children, with increased hand to eye co-ordination by two years age and less allergies in the first year of life.

Traditional Ayurvedic, Chinese and Western Adaptogenic Herbs:
Available through a herbal or naturopathic practitioner.

Rhodiola and Withania, with Tyrosine, can assist in supporting and restoring adrenal function and may help reduce physical and mental fatigue caused by stress.

Passionflower, in traditional Western medicine, is used for tension, anxiety, irritability and insomnia.

Zizyphus and Magnolia (Honokiol) have been shown to reduce anxiety.

Rehmannia to reduce anxiety with nervous exhaustion, calm and nourish the nervous system and adrenals.

American Ginseng is shown to promote calm by preventing decreases in dopamine, noradrenaline and serotonin in times of stress.

Lavender and hops reduce anxiety and exhaustion.

Most of these herbal products can be sourced as formulas through the Healthworld Metagenics range.

Homeopathic:

Aconite napellus (Acon.) One of the best remedies for rapid onset waves of fear or outright panic. Symptoms are sudden, intense feeling agitated, restless, and fearful. Other symptoms may include dry skin and mouth, thirst; pounding heart. Aconite can also treat ongoing anxiety caused by a past traumatic event.

Argentum nitricum (Arg-n.) Apprehension, anxiety and nervousness, feeling the heat, craving sweet things, 'What if...' thoughts. Anxiety worsens with overheating and tend to feel better in cool fresh air and away from crowds.

Arsenicum album (Ars.) Focusing on issues of security and safety, what will happen in the future, especially at night and when alone. Tend to worry lots and can become overly fastidious, a perfectionist and somewhat selfish in the insecurity. Tend to feel better in company but can become critical of others and controlling in behaviour.

Calcarea carbonica (Calc.) Fear of change and of losing control, insisting on routine. Struggling to keep things the same which can seem stubborn or obstinate. Tire easily on exertion or when walking uphill or climbing stairs. Fear of the dark, insects, spiders and animals, especially dogs, are common.

Kali phosphoricum (Kali-p.) Feeling overwhelmed. Easily, stressed, startled and frightened. Oversensitive and delicate. Easily exhausted and irritability from exhaustion or anxiety. Physical ailments from worry, overwork, and overexcitement. Fear something bad will happen.

Herbal Remedies:

Melissa (Lemon balm), Mistletoe, Bitter Orange, Peppermint, Valerian.

Hops – calming for those who internalize problems and have digestive upsets.

Chamomile – anger, nervous digestion, works especially well for children with focus and attention problems.

Passion flower - feeds the nerves, helps seizures, over-thinking, too many
ideas that don't go away.

Lavender flower - helps to reduce stress and assists in digestion.

Cell Salts:

Kali Phos - all nervous conditions

Mag Phos - muscular tension

Nat Mur - anxiety from grief

Reflexology:

Relaxation Massage, Diaphragmatic Release and breathing exercises. Relax
the adrenals and the endocrine system, use massage crème with relaxing
aromatherapy such as Lavender.

Facial Massage:

A relaxing facial massage with attention to the tightness around the jaw
and around the eyes.

Su-Jok Points:

Relax the adrenals, lungs and heart areas.

Auricular Therapy:

Relax the adrenals, lungs and heart areas.

Acupressure Points:

- Heavenly Pillar
- Heavenly Rejuvenation
- Crooked Marsh on both sides of arm
- Inner Gate on both sides of arm
- Third Eye Point
- Sea of Tranquility

Aromatherapy:

Essential Oil Blends for Stress will help you to relax the mind and forget about things for a while. The following blends are added to 100ml of carrier oil. You can use vegetable oil such as almond, olive or canola.

To 100ml of carrier oil add:

- 10 drops of bergamot oil (bergamot should not be used if you are going out into the sun, as it can cause photo-sensitivity which produces brown patches on the skin)
- 20 drops geranium oil
- 10 drops ylang ylang oil
- 5 drops frankincense oil
- 5 drops cedarwood oil.

Alternatively, you can use the following mix in order to relax aches and pains that are caused by stress. To 100ml of carrier oil add:

- 20 drops lavender oil
- 10 drops rosemary oil
- 10 drops black pepper oil
- 5 drops peppermint oil
- 5 drops cypress oil.

*note that peppermint, rosemary and cypress should be avoided in their concentrated form during early pregnancy, however in this application they are diluted by the carrier oil.

Bush Flowers:

Bush Fushcia, Crowea, Dog Rose of the Wild Forces, Fringed Violet, Old Man Banksia, Angelsword, Black-Eyed Susan. Try one or two at a time to see what works for you.

Psychosomatic Response:

- caught up in the what ifs and the past, finding it difficult to stay in the present
- feeling unsupported and helpless to change the situation, focusing on fear
- allowing the mind to rule, suppressing emotions and feelings.

Affirmation:

"I let go of the past and live in the now. I let go and trust. I am safe and secure. I am fully supported in all that I do and say. I go with the flow and accept change."

The Liquid Crystals:

De-Stress, or Meditation or Balance, Align and Clear.
*See the specific section Stress.

Asthma

During pregnancy you may experience mild symptoms of asthma. Asthma is an airway obstruction characterised by wheezing from bronchial spasm, inflammation and excessive mucus production, sometimes exacerbated by pregnancy. These symptoms may be due to the irritation to your body of pregnancy, your body appearing to have an allergic reaction.

Contributing factors can include chemical sensitivities, food additives, drug sensitivities, household sprays, food sensitivities, toxic reaction to environmental stimuli or toxins from infections creating gut dysbiosis or hyper-immunity. Often things that may not have caused a reaction before may be to blame now. The body tends to become very sensitive during pregnancy to protect the growing baby. Many everyday foods can be highly toxic to the pregnant body.

Nutrition:

- reduce dairy, wheat and processed foods
- drink almond milk daily (50 grams raw almonds, 50 grams honey, 1 litre water). Place the raw almonds in extra water and leave for several hours. Crush the almonds and blend in one litre of water. Filter the formula and stir in one tablespoon of honey, adding a little extra water. Allow formula to sit for several hours and strain. **Do Not** give to children aged under twelve months in case of nut allergies.
- place a cabbage poultice onto your chest. To make a cabbage poultice wash a cabbage leaf, dry off excess water. Place the cabbage leaf on a board and roll with a rolling pin. Place leaf on your chest, hold in place with a cloth or plastic wrap.
- juice/blend one part cabbage and two parts carrot juice daily and add in orange, ginger, garlic, pineapple and chia seeds
- drink warm carrot juice or make up a juice of 2 parts carrot juice, 1 part apple juice and 1 part onion juice
- horseradish is a great asthma preventative
- eat figs, garlic, sorrel, leafy green vegetables

Homeopathic:
Seek out a practitioner as treatment is individualized. An Egyptian study recently found that homeopathic remedies, when individualised to the specific child's symptoms, were effective in reducing the severity of asthma in thirty children studied (Shafei, AbdelDayem & Mohamed, 2012).

Kali phos works to reduces stress and calms the nervous system.

Cell Salts:
Kali Phos – stress induced
Nat Sulph – damp weather
Mag Phos – chest tightness or spasms
Kali Sulph – worse from heat

Reflexology:

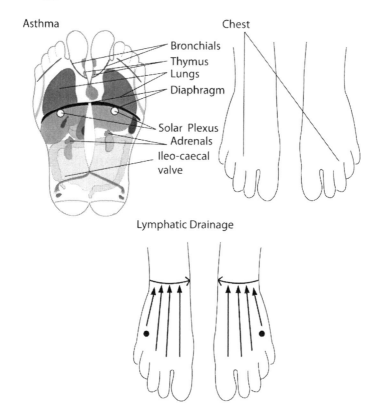

Facial Massage:

Massage to release tension around the heart/emotional area of the face, particularly along the sinus area under the eyes and across the cheeks. Release tightness around the mouth and jaw. Release tension on either side of the eyes between the mental and the emotional zones. Press into the sides of your mouth as firmly as you can stand, rotate inwards and outwards until you feel the release.

Su-Jok Points:

Massage the venus mound on both hands below the thumb. Using the probe explore around the second digit of each finger until you find the tender area of the micro system. Massage and warm up this area with moxa.

Adhere a warming seed to the point and massage throughout the day. Use the colour red to warm up the area.

Auricular Therapy:

- Trachea
- Lungs
- Kidney
- Sympathesis (calms the bronchial muscle)
- Chest and breast
- Spleen
- Large intestine * Only to be applied from 37 weeks.
- Shenmen Occiput
- Adrenal and endocrine points.

Aromatherapy:
Breathe in an infusion of eucalyptus, lavender, tea tree, hyssop. See Aromatherapy for directions.

Bush Flowers:
Bluebell, Red Grevillea, Tall Yellow Top, Grey Spider Flower.

Other treatments can include natural herbal support for respiratory function under practitioner supervision. High anti-oxidants such as those found in superfoods such as Azul or FrequenSea. Essential fatty acids, magnesium and co-factors, Vitamin C, B5, B6 found in hemp oil.

Psychosomatic Response:

- trying too hard to please everyone, wanting to be perfect, difficulty in saying no and standing up for yourself
- bending over backwards to please to the point of exhaustion
- feeling stuck and caged in
- feeling coddled and over protected.

Affirmation:

"I free myself from the past, releasing myself of all feelings of suppression, I breathe in the joy of life. I am free to be me. I let go of all control and allow energy to flow."

Acupressure Points:

Stimulate the points shown. Points will be tender, massage frequently until tenderness decreases.

(1) three finger widths below your collarbone, relieves asthma, breathing difficulties, coughing, tension and congestion in the chest. Also relieves chest tension caused by emotional distress.

(2) below the collarbone, in the hollow next to your breastbone. Good for relieving chest congestion, asthma, breathing difficulties, coughing and anxiety.

(3) one finger width below the upper tip of your shoulder blade, between the spine and the scapula. Relieves asthma, coughing and sneezing, and severe muscle spasms in the shoulders and neck.

(4) inside of your hand, at the centre of the fleshy pad at the base of the thumb. Relieves shallow breathing, coughing and swollen throat.

(5) just below the base of the thumb, in the groove at your wrist. Relieves lung problems, coughing and asthma.

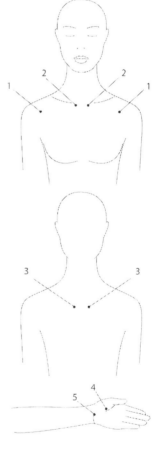

Colour Therapy:

Orange, green, pink and magenta. Warm up your hands by rubbing them together. Feel the warm tingling energy between your palms. Imagine orange flowing between your hands and when you feel they are charged up place them on your lungs with healing intent. Imagine warming sunsets of orange, pink and gold.

The Liquid Crystals:

Stress Help or Balance, Align and Clear.

Backache

As your pregnant body changes the spine can develop a curve. If the posture is not corrected this can result in back ache and sciatic pain (see Core Activation ahead, also see Psychosomatic Therapy). Other causes can be physical damage, stress, over-exertion or lack of nutrients.

Assistance may come from:

- gentle exercise is important, such as yoga and pilates
- chiropractic/osteopathic alignment in conjunction with reflexology, deep tissue massage, relaxation and meditation can assist
- it is important to ensure your back is as pain free as possible before birth.

Nutrition:

- supplementation of magnesium, taurine, selenium, zinc and calcium can all help
- Pure relaxes the muscles and assists in preventing spasms and pain
- juice/blend ginger, orange, berries, wheatgerm, lecithin and chia seeds.

Homeopathic:
Seek out a practitioner as treatment will be individualized and depend on the underlying cause for the back ache.

Cell Salts:
Mag Phos – muscular pain

Calc Phos – tendon support

Kali Phos – tiredness, exhaustion and emotional support

Reflexology:

Backache

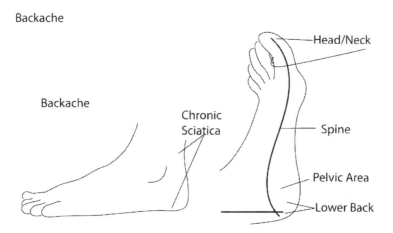

Facial Massage:
Massage the jaw and temple areas and any other areas that are tender.

Su-Jok Points:
Massage down the back of the hand through the main bony structure as shown in the diagram. Place some seeds in the area that is particularly tender. You may find a few seeds taped together work better than just one seed. Massage over these seeds throughout the day to bring relief.

Probe along the sides of the fingers to find the tender points. Adhere seeds and stimulate. Heat with Moxa. Massage along the edge of thumb from the tip to the wrist, especially along the venus pad. The area affected will be sensitive to pressure. Stimulate and massage as frequently as you feel you need relief.

Auricular Therapy:

- Spinal points
- Lumbar and sacral vertebrae.
- Massage along the outer Helix of the ear, paying particular attention to the areas that are tender.
- Kidney, bladder, liver and spleen.
- Pressing the Shenmen hot point relieves pain.

Acupressure Points:

Sea of Vitality B23 (Bladder) - CAUTION - if there are disintegrating discs or fractured bones do not press or apply any pressure. This point may also be very tender if you have a weakness here. In either case, do not apply pressure, instead the light touch of a stationary hand may provide gentle healing. Sea of Vitality is at waist level in the lower back, between the second and third lumbar vertebrae, not on the spine itself. You will find the spot about two to four finger widths away from your spine. This point can relieve lower sciatica and lower back ache and fatigue that may result from back pain.

- Womb and Vitals B48 (Bladder) for lower back ache, sciatica, hip and pelvic tension and hip pain
- Commanding Middle B54 (Bladder) for relief of back pain, stiffness, sciatica and knee pain.

Aromatherapy:

It is more beneficial to blend two or more oils together.

- do not apply essential oils directly on the skin, blend oils or combinations with a carrier oil first

- Chamomile oil helps to control muscle spasms and has pain-relieving and anti-inflammatory properties
- Lavender oil prevents muscle spasms and inflammation, also helps to relieve tension.
- Clary sage is a very soothing oil with anti-spasmodic and anti-inflammatory properties. It has a calming effect if you are anxious and muscles are tensed up from pain. Do not use clary sage during early pregnancy, but it is wonderful during late pregnancy and labour.
- Yarrow has anti-inflammatory and anti-spasmodic properties
- Rosemary is good for relieving back pain as it improves blood circulation
- Ginger oil can ease back pain and helps with mobility. Blend 1 tablespoon sweet oil, 4 drops wintergreen, 4 drops cardamom and 4 drops ginger oil to make a soothing massage oil
- Peppermint is good for muscle soreness
- Frankincense has anti-inflammatory properties and also acts as a mild sedative.

I recommend these aromatherapy blends for relieving back pain:

- peppermint and rosemary
- lavender and frankincense
- chamomile and clary sage.

An aromatherapy bath is a wonderful way to soothe tired, aching muscles and to increase circulation. Add eight to ten drops of essential oils directly to some sea salt (helps the oils disperse). Add to the warm bath water and soak for fifteen to twenty minutes. Adding some Epsom Salts as well helps to relax muscles and provide some necessary magnesium.

The following exercises may assist.

Core Activation Exercises:

Good posture is essential for preventing aches and pains. The key to good posture is the activation of your core muscles. Before any of these exercises are undertaken, breathe in and activate your abdominals and then as you breathe out move into the stretch. Maintain core activation throughout the exercise. Sit on a chair with your posture straight and supported, place one leg up on the other knee and bend forward over the leg, feeling the stretch through the back of the leg. Repeat on the other side.

Squatting hold onto something to support yourself, such as a chair, then squat down and feel the stretch in your thighs. This is also great practice for labour.

Taylor or Lotus Position sit crossed legged (legs in front) with a straight back. You can use your body weight to press into the stretch by leaning onto one knee at a time. You can also press your hand onto the knee and alternate between pushing the knee towards your hand and then pressing the knee away with the hand. Do this on both sides.

Butterfly from sitting cross legged extend your legs out in front of you whilst bending forward from the waist. Join the balls of your feet together. As you become more flexible your feet will join together at the bottoms also. Lean into the stretch, leaning towards your feet whilst holding onto your toes with your hands. The more flexible you are the more you will be able to reach your head to your toes. Do not bounce, just gently release and stretch.

Psoas Muscle:

Your psoas muscle connects your spine to your thigh and activates when you walk, run and sit. A tight psoas can feel like an ache just outside of your groin, in your hip. A shortened psoas muscle can cause a tightening in your lower back. Having a relaxed and toned psoas muscle assists in preventing back pain in pregnancy and allows flexibility during birth by allowing the pelvis to open up and provide greater room for your baby to be released.

A good way to test the psoas is to sit on the edge of a massage table or a strong coffee or dining table and allow your legs to hang over at the knees. Now pull your knees to your chest with your arms and roll back onto the table. You may need someone to support you as you roll back. Once you are on the massage table continue to hold one knee to chest while allowing the other to float to the table and hang over at the knee. If your thigh is slightly above the table and you can put your hand between thigh and table, this indicates a tight psoas. If the psoas is relaxed your thigh will make good contact with the table and a right angle will be created at the knee.

Stretching the Psoas stand at the end of the table and extend one leg up on the table. Maintaining a soft knee on the standing leg, ensure your feet are facing the table. Feel the stretch along the extended thigh. You can extend this stretch by leaning into it from the waist as you breathe out.

Runner's Lunge this classic stretch requires holding a kneeling position for a minute on each side, so find a thick mat to pad your knee. Kneel on all fours on your mat, then bring your right foot forward to between your hands. Lean your hips forward to create a stretch where your left leg meets your hip. Breathe in this position for sixty seconds. To intensify this stretch, place your hands on your knee and lift your torso to upright. You can also extend your left knee farther back to increase the stretch, but keep your hips square with the front of your mat to focus the stretch in your psoas.

Egoscue Release (recommended by posture expert Pete Egoscue)

Lie on your back with your knees bent and your feet flat on the floor in line with your hips. Support your back with a cushion as you get bigger with the pregnancy. Notice the amount of curve in your lower back. Extend your right leg on the floor and rotate it inward until your knee and toes point upward. Breathe easily for up to twenty minutes. You may feel the arch in your lumbar spine flatten slightly, which is a sign that your psoas has released. Now switch and activate the other side (Egoscue & Gittines, 2000).

Pilates Toe Taps

Lie on your back with a towel-roll or pilates roller under your sacrum. Lift your legs into a tabletop position - knees are bent with the calves extended in line with the knees at 90 degree angle so your shins are parallel to the floor. Take a breath in to prepare, engage your abdominal core and then as you breathe out slowly allow one leg to float to the floor. Tap your toes on the floor and then float the knee back to your start position. Repeat this pattern, alternating legs for about two minutes.

* Must ensure the core is engaged thus the abdominal muscles are firing, not the legs which are completely relaxed.

Foam Roller Release

Lie face down on a mat and place a foam roller under your hips where your hipbones stick out. Place your elbows and forearms on the floor for support. Roll forward and backward a few inches, creating massage pressure on your psoas muscles. To intensify this massage, cross one leg over the other to shift more body weight onto one psoas at a time.

Fit Ball Exercises:

Knee Stretch lay belly-down on your Fit ball with your hands on the floor. Extend your body and legs into a push-up position. Walk your hands forward until your thighs are off the ball. Exhale as you tuck your knees toward your chest. Allow your back to round up. Inhale as you extend your legs behind you. Continue this piston action for ten to twenty repetitions. Make this exercise harder by increasing your ball size or starting with less of your body in contact with the ball. As you can probably imagine, this exercise becomes less possible as your pregnancy progresses.

Wall Squat while standing with your feet hip width apart, place a smaller ball between your lower back and a wall. Press your back firmly into the ball. Exhale as you squat, rolling your back against the ball. Lower until your thighs are at a 90 degree angle to the wall and hold this position for three to five slow breaths. Exhale again as you return to upright. Repeat this exercise ten times. You can vary this movement by changing your foot position from toes forward to feet facing outward in a wide 'V' shape.

Big Stretch choose a Fit ball that you can sit on with your thighs parallel to the floor. Sit on your ball and walk your feet forward as you drape your back onto the ball. Fully extend your legs as you reach your arms back by your ears. You should feel a stretch in your psoas when you extend your legs. Breathe in this position for three to five minutes. You can intensify this stretch by using a taller ball, but you will need to stay in control to relax into this stretch.

Sciatica:

The sciatic nerve runs from the lower back down the legs to the feet. Pressure on this nerve during pregnancy can cause pain and inflammation. Contrary to commonly held beliefs, you are not more prone to sciatica in pregnancy. Most women feel tightness and discomfort in their hips and pelvic girdle that can be released with pilates or yoga exercises. Sciatic pain is a more intense pain that is often associated with a burning sensation and needles and pins running down the leg to the feet.

Testing

You can do this test with your partner or practitioner. Lie on your back and relax your body and legs. Your partner lifts one leg at a time. You must not assist. Let go of the leg and let it hang heavy but straight. As your partner lifts your leg up slowly whilst bending at the hip notice if any area is particularly uncomfortable or painful. If so indicate to your partner and get them to stop at the pain. The pain may be on the upward or on the downward motion.

Now your partner gently presses into the foot whilst holding the leg in place.

Partner - Place both hands around the foot and press towards the hip, the leg is being pushed into the hip joint for about a minute. This is incredibly relaxing and can release sciatica very quickly. Now test again.

Sciatica and Psoas release on the feet

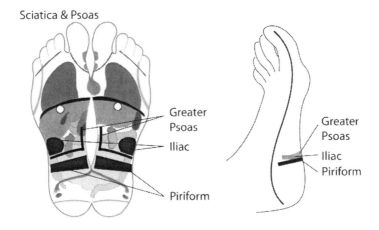

Sciatica & Psoas

Greater Psoas
Iliac
Piriform

Greater Psoas
Iliac
Piriform

Bush Flowers:

Waratah, Paw Paw, Sunshine Wattle.

Psychosomatic Response:

- your spine is the main support for your body. If you are not feeling supported in life then the most likely place for this negative energy to be stored will be in your spine.

Tune into your back and become aware of how heavy the baggage is that you are carrying. Imagine taking off a backpack and throwing it in the garbage, imagine feeling safe, warm and satisfied.

Affirmation Upper Back:

Upper back represents lack of emotional support, holding back love, feelings of not being loved. Shouldering responsibility, taking on other peoples stuff. Say to yourself 'Not my Pig, not my Paddock'.

"Life supports me, I fully support and approve of myself."

Affirmation Middle Back:

Middle back represents feeling someone's on your back, feeling trapped, stuck in past issues, guilt. Overly sensitive, stuck in the past, heart protection, holding onto past pains and not forgiving self. Focused on what's wrong rather than what's right.

"The past is the past I live in the now, freeing myself to move forward with love."

Affirmation Lower Back:

Lower back represents lack of support financially, money fears, who or what doesn't support you? Financial insecurity, feeling unable to support self, lack of external support, feeling a victim.

"It is safe to trust the process of life. Financially my needs are met, I'm safe."

Colour Therapy:

Gold, green.

The Liquid Crystals:

Sore Back Help.

Blood Pressure (see Hypertension)

Candida

Candida can be common in pregnancy due to hormonal changes resulting in a different ph balance in mucous membranes, such as the vagina, making them more susceptible to infection. Contributing factors may be caffeine, toxic exposure, high sugar processed food diet, wheat and dairy sensitivity, low gut flora, stressed gut, high yeast intake, low nutrient intake, long term antibiotic use, long-term steroid use, recreational drugs or low immunity. It is preferable that you and your partner are treated. Your partner may not show symptoms but can still be a carrier and so able to re-infect you. Implementation of a comprehensive detoxification program of the gut and liver is virtually the only procedure needed to manage candidiasis. This may assist with correcting gut flora, correcting digestion, repairing gut permeability and improving liver detoxification. However detoxification can only be undertaken once you have finished breastfeeding. In the mean time instigate either the anti-candida diet, blood type diet or insulin zone system.

Nutrition:
Under practitioner supervision anti-bacterial/anti- viral herbs can be prescribed.

- garlic
- fish oils
- St. Mary's Thistle
- broad spectrum anti-oxidants
- FrequenSea
- Five Japanese Mushrooms
- Coriolus Gifolus
- low level Zinc therapy
- high-potency probiotics formula

- herbal teas such as dandelion, ginger and nettle boost the immune system and support the liver
- juice/blend orange, green vegetables, parsley, basil, celery, garlic, lemon, avocado, cucumber and cabbage leaves.

Supplement Treatment:

Short term control includes using 1,000 micrograms of Biotin two to three times a day. When symptoms settle use once daily for at least 2 weeks. Biotin is a B vitamin that controls sugar and carbohydrate metabolism. If this is not sufficient, add the trace mineral Molybdenum 150 micrograms twice a day.

I recommend Metagenics Gammagenics which contains Gamma Oryzanol (rice bran oil) and Pau D'arco. Promotes normal healthy immune function and is particularly effective for candida (follow this link for details on how to order).

Homeopathic:

Treatment is individualised and response is usually quick. Candida is linked to grief from separation and feelings of abandonment. This could be your own issues coming up as a result of your own birth experience.

Argentum nit – digestive disturbances and sugar cravings. Anxiety and nervous conditions.

Pulsatilla– nervous crying women with creamy changing vaginal discharges, changeable moods.

Sepia - extreme vaginal itchiness, accompanied by a yellow or greenish discharge.

Alumina - watery discharge with itching.

Helonias - white curd like discharge.

Borax - runny egg white discharge.

Pulsatilla - yellow discharge but no irritation.

Kreosotum - yellow discharge with irritation.

Mercurius vivus - greenish discharge more irritating at night.

Herbs for Hormonal Balance:

- Blessed Thistle - to help the liver balance hormones
- Vitex - to balance oestrogen and progesterone levels

Cell Salts:

Nat Phos - acidity, creamy discharges

Calc Sulph - toxicity, yellow discharges

Nat Sulph - liver support, yellow discharges

Reflexology:

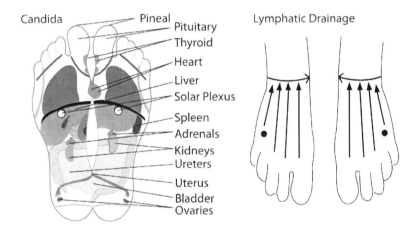

Candida — Pineal Pituitary — Thyroid — Heart — Liver — Solar Plexus — Spleen — Adrenals — Kidneys — Ureters — Uterus — Bladder — Ovaries — Lymphatic Drainage

Su-Jok Points:

Massage the <u>reproductive areas</u> gently. Place a red band or paint red on the reproductive area at the base of the little finger. Can also find the most tender point and place a seed here for stimulation.

Aromatherapy:

Male: Combine one drop of tea tree and of patchouli to a bowl of warm water and wash under the foreskin or glans penis twice a day. Dilute patchouli in 30mls vegetable oil and apply daily.

Female: Yoghurt Method - 100g of whole-milk natural, white unpasteurised yoghurt with live acidophilus culture. You can add acidophilus or ultra-probioplex to the yoghurt to increase its effectiveness, make sure it is an NCFM strain. Add five drops of chamomile, lavender, tea tree stir well. Place this into the vagina either through using a spatula or a tampon applicator. You may prefer to submerge yourself in a bowl of warm water with the mixture added, ensuring the mixture enters the vagina (though this is not as effective).

　Do not Douche.

Vinegar Rinse
Two teaspoons apple cider vinegar (no added sugar) to one cup of warm water. Wash vagina and vulva with the solution several times daily until no more discharge is present. Do not douche.

Tea Tree Oil
A few drops of tea tree oil in one cup of warm water. Apply as in vinegar rinse above.

Coconut Oil
Coconut oil, one of the easiest fats to digest as it contains medium-chain triglycerides, has been found by researchers to halt the growth of the candida yeast that triggers thrush, yeast infections and leaky gut.

Garlic Suppository
Dip one clove of garlic into oil and allow to soak for a while, then place into vagina. Change twelve hourly. Repeat for up to five days. Discharge may increase at first. Or add two drops of lavender, rosemary and tea tree to the solution then add to a bath with one tablespoon of rock salt.

Bush Flower Remedies:
Spinifex, Kangaroo Paw.

Psychosomatic Response:

- self doubt, feeling scattered, hazy, frazzled, stressed, trapped
- angry at not getting what you want but not wanting to change or take positive action
- trust issues.

Affirmation:

"I appreciate everything I have and all that is done for me, I am worthy of the best."

Colour Therapy:

Visualise your vagina, uterus, fallopian tubes and ovaries bathed in a beautiful pink magenta ray. Imagine them cleansing and regenerating as you recall how special and magical this part of your body is that it can create another human being without you doing anything. Allow yourself to forgive those who have hurt you and tell your female parts that you forgive them and love them too. Other colours to work with and wear are orange, green and pink.

The Liquid Crystals:

Cycles or Crocoite.

Carpal Tunnel Syndrome

Numbness or burning on the palm surface of the first three digits of the hand may develop in late pregnancy. The cause is unknown, although it may be due to increased pressure on the nerves from fluid. Numerous clinical studies have demonstrated a direct relationship between oral Vitamin B6 therapy, magnesium and the relief of the symptoms of carpal tunnel syndrome.

Nutrition:

- high anti-oxidants are recommended such as those in FrequenSea which scavenge free radicals in joint tissue. FrequenSea can be taken as a drink and applied externally on affected areas.
- Pure
- address acid levels with an alkaline diet
- juice/blend anti-inflammatory vegetables such as berries, broccoli, ginger, oranges, grapefruit, chia seeds, cucumber and tiny drops of chilli to increase endorphins (the natural painkillers).

Homeopathic:

Choose the homeopathic remedy which matches your symptoms, or see a registered, qualified homeopath. Use a 30c strength of tablet, available from health stores and homeopathic pharmacies, and take one tablet every two to three hours as required. Try:

Apis - if tingling and numbness radiates up your arm and you have swollen wrists and fingers. Also if the pain is in the first and second fingers of your left hand, and lessens if you move your wrist, but gets worse when you are hot and feel weepy.

Causticum - if you have tingling and numbness in your fingers, fingertips and thumb, but there is limited swelling. Also if the pain is worse when you wake up, and you are sensitive to cold.

Lycopodium - if you have tingling and numbness in all your fingers except the little finger, with or without wrist swelling. Also if you feel worse at night and on waking, are restless and anxious but hide how you're feeling.

Calcerea carb - for tingling, numbness and swelling in your wrists and first three fingers. Also if you feel anxious, sluggish and have difficulty concentrating, or feel cold but sweat a lot in certain areas of your body.

Herbal Remedies:

Drinking strong chamomile tea may help to reduce inflammation.

Ginger is also good for circulation and has anti-inflammatory properties, easing aches and pains during pregnancy (Bone et al., 1990).

You could also try placing green or white cabbage leaves on your wrists to draw out excess fluid and relieve the swelling. The leaves should be wiped clean but not washed, and may be cooled in the fridge but not in the freezer. Wrap the leaves around your wrists to make a compress. Leave them until they become wet, then repeat with fresh leaves until the pain is reduced.

Cell Salts:

Calc Fluor – connective tissue
Calc Phos – tendon support
Ferr Phos – inflammation
Mag Phos – muscular pain

Vertical Reflexology:

Imagine a vertical line coming down from the base of your fourth toe. Feel along this line for about 2cm (0.8 inch) until you find the most tender spot. Press the centre of this spot as firmly as you can bear with your thumb. If you can't comfortably reach the point, ask someone to do it for you. Use constant pressure until the tenderness has dispersed. Repeat this process about four or five times until the point you are pressing feels less tender. This may temporarily ease the pain in your wrists and is a useful technique when pain hits in the middle of the night.

Massage:

Massage the hands and circulation points as shown on the arm and hand reflex diagrams that follow. Gently massage your hands and wrists, moving up towards your armpits, then your shoulders, neck and upper back.

Facial Massage:

Check for mouth and jaw tension. <u>Massage the heart zone ar</u>ound the eyebrows and eyes as the arms are the extension to the heart.

Su-Jok Points:

Find the most tender points on the hand and finger areas relating to the <u>arms and hands</u>. Use pepper seeds to warm up the area or warm up with red colour. Stimulate as often as possible to release.

Auricular Therapy:

Massage the arms and hand areas on the ears. Massage wherever it feels tender often throughout the day.

Reflexology:

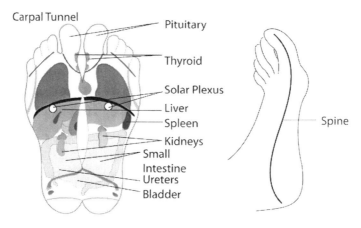

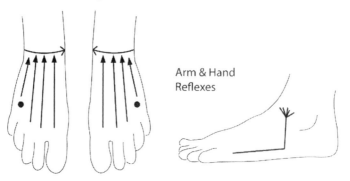

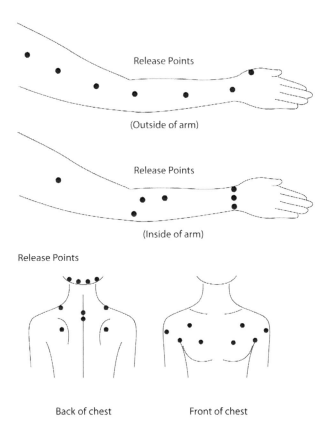

Aromatherapy:

Cypress and lemon can be used as a compress to reduce swelling. Add two drops of each essential oil to warm or cool water and soak a cloth in it. Wrap the soaked cloth around your wrists. It is not safe to use juniper berry oil in pregnancy, even though it is often used to reduce swelling, as it may affect your kidneys.

Acupressure Points:

- Big Mound P7 (Pericardium)
- Active Pond TW4 (Triple Warmer) Stimulating the nerves using acupressure causes the nerve impulses to flow through the joint and releases natural anti-inflammatory chemicals into the body.

- <u>Inner Gate P6</u> (Pericardium)
- <u>Outer Gate TW5</u> (Triple Warmer)
- For the last two pressure points again bend the elbow, but this time extend the arm across the front of the body like it is in a sling. One point is at the outside of the elbow crease and the other is three finger widths from that point in a straight line going toward the thumb. To find this last pressure point feel for the most tender area.

Recommended Exercises:

- Clasp one wrist with your other hand and massage it with a circular movement. This should ease congestion and encourage the movement of fluid.
- Gently stretch your hands and arms. Try not to do any movements that are painful. It may also help to hang your hands over the edge of your bed during the night.
- Place your hands in ice-cold water or use a bag of frozen peas against the painful area on your wrist. Gently exercise your fingers and wrists to help move the excess fluid, and keep your hands raised whenever possible.
- Squeeze a tennis ball 25-100 times with each hand.
- Keeping your elbow straight, extend your left arm in front of you with the palm facing upwards. Gently, use the fingers of your right hand to bend the wrist of your left palm in the upward direction. Hold the position for 15-30 seconds till you feel the stretch in your forearm. Repeat the same with the right hand.
- Again, extend your left arm in front with elbow straight. Gently bend the wrist forward with the right hand in such a way that the fingers point downwards and the stretch is felt in the forearm for 15-30 seconds. Repeat with the other hand.
- On your hands and knees, keep your arms straight with the palms of your hands flat on the floor. Keeping arms straight, turn your

hands so that your fingers face towards your knees. You will feel this stretch up your inner forearm and at the wrist.
- Wrist circles - draw clockwise circles in the air keeping the tips of the second and third finger close together.
- Clap your hands as this works the upper arms.

Bush Flowers:
Bottlebrush, Crowea, Southern Cross. The choice of Flower will depend on the underlying emotional condition.

Psychosomatic Response:

- ask yourself what are you trying to numb down, how are you blocking the energy flow in life?
- holding onto grief and sadness from the past – what can't you handle?

Affirmation:
"I choose to create a life that is joyous and abundant, I am at ease."

Colour Therapy
Take a moment to pause and tune into your hands and wrists, imagine releasing all the restraints and shackles from them. Bathe them in yellow light and liquid gold, dry them off with pink and green.

The Liquid Crystals:
Transition Help.

Constipation

Constipation can be due to Candida albicans, lack of exercise, emotional stress, low fibre intake, bile insufficiency, low fluid intake, food allergy or intake of processed food.

Assistance may come from:

- emotional release trigger point therapy
- relaxation techniques
- rest
- reflexology and osteopathy
- yoga pelvic rocks.

Traditional herbs for clearing constipation and improving regularity are unsafe for pregnancy. They can tax vital organs with extended use, and in progressing pregnancy the organs are already working hard. The more nutritive food-type plants are still a good option for treating constipation.

Superfoods:

- Pure - taking 3-4 mls usually has the desired effect
- FrequenSea and Azul are excellent in providing balance to the colon.

Nutrition:

- Aloe Vera 30 - 50 mls daily, does tend to be dose dependant, so continue to increase the dose each day until effect achieved
- Slippery Elm, liquorice, probiotics, fluids with lemon, dandelion tea, psyllium seeds and linseed
- eat lots of whole fresh fruit and vegetables, grains and other high fibre foods
- increase water intake

- iron supplements may cause constipation. Use chelated iron for better results and less side effects
- eat daily 15 almonds (preferably roasted), one apple with peel, one cup of green beans
- drink almond milk (see recipe under Asthma)
- eat cabbage regularly
- soak prunes overnight in half a glass of water and the juice of one lemon. In the morning eat the prunes and drink the juice. Prunes can also be eaten dried or whole.
- juice/blend two dandelion leaves, cabbage leaves, green apple, grreen vegetables, prunes (stones removed), figs, rhubarb and cherries or berries.

Sorrel Bouillon Recipe

- 40gms Sorrel, 20gms lettuce, 20gms leek, 5 gms butter 750mls water
- Melt the butter in saucepan and place in vegetables. Sauté for a few minutes then add water. Bring to the boil and allow to simmer for a short while. Strain and allow to cool.
- drink daily.

Blackberry Root Powder – take 1 tspn on an empty stomach. Blackberry is a powerful medicine full of wonderful minerals and salts.

Bulk fibres in powdered form can be added to a glass of juice or tea, including oat bran, celery fibre, wheat bran, flaxseeds, prunes and psyllium husk powder.

Flax seeds can be added to baked goods or eaten with grains and salads. Fibre helps absorb water and keeps constipation at bay.

Homeopathic:
Take one dose and see what the effect is.

Pulsatilla 30C - only take one dose.

Bryonia - indicated for constipation with a feeling of dryness in the rectum and large dry stools that are hard to push out, with sticking or tearing pains.

Lycopodium - you may benefit from this remedy if you have frequent indigestion with gas and bloating and many problems involving the bowels. Rubbing the abdomen or drinking something warm may help to relieve the symptoms. A craving for sweets and an energy slump in late afternoon and early evening are strong indications for Lycopodium.

Nux vomica - 'Wants to but can't' is a phrase that brings Nux vomica to mind. This remedy is often helpful to people who are impatient, tense, and ambitious, who work too hard and exercise too little, indulge in stimulants or alcohol, and are partial to sweets and spicy food. Headaches, chilliness, and constricting pains in the bowels or rectal area often accompany constipation when Nux vomica is needed.

Sepia - A heavy sensation in the rectum, remaining after a bowel movement, may indicate a need for this remedy. Stools can be hard and difficult to pass, although they may be small. The person often has cold hands and feet, and is weary and very irritable. Exercise may bring improvement, both to constipation and to mood and energy level. Sepia is often useful to women who develop constipation just before or just after a menstrual period.

Cell Salts:
Flax or psyllium fibre is desirable
Kali Mur - to remove mucus
Nat Mur - excessive dryness
Nat Phos - to remove acidity
Nat Sulph - to support the liver

Reflexology:

Points along the gut and colon can be stimulated to help elimination.

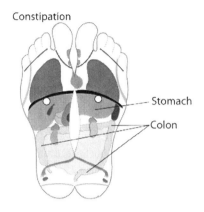

Constipation

Stomach

Colon

Facial Massage:

Release around the mouth and jaw, massage all zones.

Su-Jok Points:

Massage across the fullness of the palm in a clockwise direction towards the fingers as if you are moving along the large intestine. Using the probe massage along the first digit of each of the fingers closest to the palm until you locate the point that is tender. Massage this point vigorously. Apply a seed to the point and massage throughout the day.

Auricular Therapy:

Digestive system, Shenmen, any point that is tender.

Acupressure Points:

Warm up the pressure points indicated with moxa.

- Crooked Pond LI 11
- Three Mile Point ST36

Aromatherapy:

Three times daily massage over the lower abdomen in a clockwise direction with a mixture of fifteen drops rosemary, ten drops lemon and five drops peppermint, diluted in vegetable oil.

Bush Flowers:

Vitality Essence, Wild Potato Bush, Spinifex, Silver Princess, Red Grevillea.

Psychosomatic Response:

The bowel and colon are related to elimination of that which is no longer necessary. Constipation is related to holding on and the need to control the material world. Problems in this area may indicate:

- holding on too tightly to people, material things, or the past
- guilt, bitterness, doubt, cynicism, envy
- over-controlled attitudes, feeling cut off, lonely, or left out
- unwillingness to let go, repressed rage, fear of rejection, long standing repressed emotions
- financial worries and feelings of scarcity can restrict the movement of the bowels
- fear of rapid change.

Affirmation:

"Life flows through me easily, I let go and let live, I am free to be me."

Colour Therapy:

Imagine waves of orange, yellow, brown and blue in a peristaltic wave.

During Facial Massage find the cleft in the middle of your chin. Place your middle finger on that spot, rotate it several times as strongly as possible then rotate the other way. Repeat this process several times. Visualise green light energising and moving the bowel. If you have a green light shine it onto this area.

The Liquid Cyrstals:
Transition Help or Digestive Help or Motivate Help.

Cramps and Spasms (muscle cramps and spasms)

Usually caused through poor diet, incorrect posture, standing for long periods on cold floors, under or over taking of specific nutrients, lack of exercise or circulatory problems. Use mineral-rich natural foods and the supplements listed below. Eliminate tobacco, alcohol, coffee and soda drinks. These are harmful and rob your body of minerals and other nutrients.

Nutrition:

- Pure, containing 92 rapid acting minerals and a high dose of magnesium with cofactors such as taurine and calcium phosphate is the most effective source of minerals I have found to assist in the fast relief of spasm, pain and inflammation. I have received excellent feedback from clients about the benefits of this product.
- glucosamine enhances the production of connective tissue, cartilage and bone. In combination with manganese, it is able to stimulate the repair of damaged joints and help reduce joint pain.
- increase calcium intake aswell.

Homeopathic: You may use 6X, 30X, 6C or 30C potencies.
Calcera carb - calf cramps at night in bed.
Cuprum metallicum - muscle twitch, particularly hands, feet or restless legs.
Cimicifuga - calf cramps, restless or trembling legs.
Magnesia phosphorica - muscle spasms with stiffness and sore feet.
Veratrum album - stiffness and cramping starts in hands and feet and spreads to other muscles, carpal tunnel during pregnancy.

Herbal Remedies:

Valerian combined with magnesium supplement take as necessary during the day, too much may cause diarrhoea.

Cramp Bark as a tincture, 20 drops usually is enough.

St. Johns Wort in low doses to relax and assist restless sleep.

Cell Salts:

Calc Phos - digestive cramps

Kali Phos - nerve cramps

Mag Phos - muscle cramps

Ferr Phos - inflammation

Nat Phos - over-acidity

Silicea - connective tissue integrity

Night Cramps can be caused by too much milk (over 1200mls per day). The phosphorus in milk may depress ionisable calcium levels, resulting in muscular cramping.

Try taking calcium and magnesium cell salts, take Vitamin E, increasing dosage daily until results are achieved along with Hemp oil. Aerobic exercise such as walking/swimming daily will improve circulation.

Reflexology:

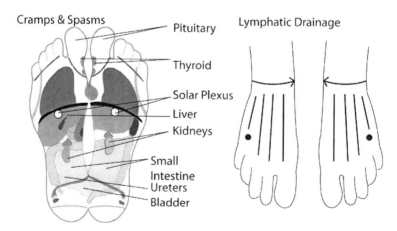

Cramps & Spasms

Pituitary

Lymphatic Drainage

Thyroid

Solar Plexus

Liver

Kidneys

Small Intestine

Ureters

Bladder

Facial Massage:

Massage <u>across the cheeks, release around the mouth and jaw</u> particularly where it feels tight.

Aromatherapy:

For leg cramps create a foot bath by combining five drops geranium, ten drops lavender and two drops cypress to water.

Bush Flowers:

Grey Spider Flower, Bottlebrush, Black-eyed Susan, Crowea, Tall Mulla Mulla.

Psychosomatic Response:

- feeling restless and tired, demanding, wanting things now.

Affirmation:

"I am relaxed and at peace in my mind."

Colour Therapy:

Imagine orange, green and blue coloured light dissolving the tension and relaxing your muscles.

The Liquid Crystals:

<u>Sore Back Help</u> or <u>Stress Help</u>.

Depression

(See <u>Postnatal Depression</u>)

Taking high superfood nutritional formulas throughout pregnancy and post birth will assist greatly with the prevention of depression. Having regular body massages and reflexology with the opportunity to talk through any issues is a great help too.

Scientists from Brown University found that people who practise mindfulness meditation are better able to effectively manage chronic pain and depression symptoms due to the mental exercises improving their ability to control which alpha rhythm sensations they paid attention to. Participants learned how to regulate and become less responsive to negative sensations, including those involved in depression.

http://www.frontiersin.org/Human_Neuroscience/10.3389/
fnhum.2013.00012/abstract

Nutrition:

Hippocrates stated that "Food is our medicine, and medicine is our food." Believe it or not this may be the best medicine when battling depression. The first step is to restore gut health, following suggestions in the nutrition section. This can be assisted through:

- balancing the ratio of omega 6 to omega 3 essential fatty acids. Increase the intake of omega 3 fats by supplementation of EPA/DHA oils. Aim for 2g-4g per day.
- reduce grains, legumes, processed sugars and dairy as these tend to exacerbate the inflammatory response in the body, contributing to depression
- eat plenty of vegetables, particularly dark green vegies high in folate, to feed the good gut flora and help your digestive system heal from the inflammation
- eat foods high in selenium such as quality meats, seafood, nuts, and seeds
- tryptophan deficiency has been associated with depression. Sources of tryptophan include seaweed, phytoplankton and sea algaes, dark green vegetables, water cress, soya beans, mushrooms and bananas.
- Vitamin D deficiency has also been linked to depression, especially during the winter months. Aim to get adequate sunlight or supplement with Vitamin D.

- juice/blend berries, grapes, cucumber, tomato, celery, beetroot and carrot mixed with any combination of dark green vegetables. Adding a dash of Tobasco may help to release endorphins (happy hormones)
- eat daily half an avocado, broccoli, apricots, lettuce juice and rolled oats.

Supplementation:

- A.I.M. contains excellent levels of Vitamin D with transfer factor
- cod liver oil contains healthy levels of vitamin A
- B-complex vitamins, especially B3, has been shown to be of great benefit
- 600mg-800mg of magnesium, preferably magnesium glycinate because it is highly bioavailable
- take L-tryptophan (amino acid) 500mg daily with vitamin C and a B-complex

Homeopathic:
Careful choice is required with your practitioner.

Ignatia amara - depression after trying to suppress feelings of grief, despair or emotional upset.

Natrium carbonicum - gentle, unselfish people who care deeply for their family and friends. Tend to hide their feelings from others, which does not help their condition. Can isolate themselves and may listen to sad music.

Natrium muraticum - bottled up feelings. Trying to be stoic and controlled. Tend to cry alone. Tends to be depression as a result of grief or loss. Can become separate and isolated.

Cimicifuga – feeling like a dark cloud is overhead but can't explain why. Sleeplessness.

Phosphoric acid – depression from emotional worry with confusion. May be emotional, sleepy, apathetic but not able to express what's going on.

Pulsatilla - feel a sense of self pity, sadness and loneliness. Very expressive, crying, sobbing, needing nurturing. Pulsatilla is a useful remedy for depression due to hormonal changes after childbirth or menopause. Often crave sweet foods and put on weight.

Sepia – hormonal depression linked to oestrogen dominance (childbirth). Angry and yelling, isolating self, apathetic, confused, detached, mood swings. The remedy is used for postnatal depression, loss of libido and menopausal symptoms, especially when accompanied by a sagging feeling in the pelvic area. Women lacking in sepia who have a history of miscarriage between five and seven months gestation, those who already have children, may be more likely to suffer from a sepia state and require homeopathic supplementation.

Herbal Remedies:

There has been some concern regarding taking herbal formulas with anti-depressants. I advise taking them with caution and consult your doctor if you feel better and wish to start to come off the drugs.

St. John's Wort - effective for mild and moderate depression.

Melissa (Lemon balm) – depression with sleep problems. Mild mood elevator.

Rhodiola – nervous depression, immune weakness, energy without stimulation. Improves circulation and increases oxygen to the head.

Korean Panax Ginseng – depression from extreme fatigue where you are too tired to sleep. Improves energy. Can be too stimulating at times.

Cell Salts:

Kali phos – nervous conditions and depression

Nat mur – for grief, depression and sadness

Nat sulph – for negativity, anger, suicidal feelings and liver support

Reflexology:

Stimulate the circulatory and adrenal systems, heart, lungs, pituitary and thyroid.

Su-Jok Points:

Stimulate and warm up tender points with moxa on the hand and fingers, especially the <u>heart and head regions</u>. Apply seeds for stimulation. Each case will be individual.

Auricular Therapy:

- <u>Anti-Depressant 1</u>
- <u>Master Cerebral</u>
- <u>Point Zero</u>
- <u>Shen Men</u>
- <u>Autonomic</u>
- <u>Master Oscillation</u>

Acupressure Points:

Working on these points stimulate a state of well being by increasing happy hormones. You do not have to use all of these points, using just one or two of them whenever you have a free hand can be effective.

- <u>Gates of Consciousness</u>
- <u>Heavenly Pillar</u>
- <u>Sea of Vitality</u>
  Sea of Vitality B23 (Bladder) – CAUTION – if there are disintegrating discs or fractured bones do not press or apply any pressure. This point may also be very tender if you have a weakness here. In either case, do not apply pressure, instead the light touch of a stationary hand may provide gentle healing. See your doctor first if you have any questions or need medical advice.
- <u>Third Eye Point</u>
- <u>Elegant Mansion</u>
- <u>Letting Go</u>
- <u>Sea of Tranquility</u>
- <u>Three Mile Point</u>

Aromatherapy:

The study 'Orange Scent Reduces Anxiety, Boosts Mood' (Lehrner et al., 2000) found that the aroma of orange essential oil reduces anxiety and generates a more positive mood and a higher level of calmness in women exposed to it in a dental office waiting room. Combine a few drops of Clary sage, Basil, Rose, Lavender, Sandalwood and Ylang Ylang essential oils to a carrier. Apply around the neck area or to the heart chakra.

- add the combination to pure water and use as a body spray
- add the pure oils to an aromatherapy atomiser
- add to sea salt then soak in a bath or foot bath.

Bush Flowers:

Personal Power Essence or Vitality Essence. Individual essences will depend on the underlying emotion.

Psychosomatic Response:

- pressure to survive, lack of hope, overwhelmed, hopeless
- suppressed anger or sadness, feeling like a victim
- unable to forgive and let go
- stuck in the past, replaying the story over and over.

Exercise has been shown to be very beneficial in creating happy hormones. Try to find thirty minutes a day.

Affirmation:

"I am full of confidence, inner strength and wisdom. I let go of the past and celebrate the now. Every day in every way I am becoming stronger and happier. I am at peace. I am clear."

Focus on your strengths, what are you good at? What do you enjoy doing? Find time to do these things. Celebrate the little things. Pat yourself on the back for just showing up every day, acknowledge little improvements each day. Look in the mirror and become your own best friend. Talk to you, coach you, boost yourself up.

Colour Therapy:
A 2005 study also found that ambient odours and colours, particularly orange, reduced anxiety and improved mood in patients waiting for dental treatment. Use colours orange, purple, violet and yellow.

The Liquid Crystals:
De-Stress, or Meditation or Balance, Align and Clear.
*See the specific section Stress.

Link:
http://blog.naturaltherapyforall.com/2013/06/25/antidepressants-may-pose-great-risk-to-the-unborn-expert-says/

Diabetes – Gestational

Gestational diabetes refers to the glucose intolerance and hyperglycaemia associated with pregnancy and other hyper-oestrogenic states. Without treatment it can cause a very large baby, perinatal morbidity and mortality. Half of those women affected will go on to develop impaired glucose tolerance or non-insulin dependent diabetes, with a dramatic increase in the risk of cardiovascular disease. Exercise and nutrition help diabetes. Exercise promotes the entry of glucose into the cells and so can lower a diabetic's glucose levels. Too much exercise can bring on an episode of hypoglycaemia if levels are borderline. Walking, with plenty of hydration, is one of the safest methods of exercise.

Nutrition:

- Pure provides magnesium, chromium, selenium, zinc and high anti-oxidant

- FrequenSea has been researched to effectively balance blood sugar levels
- following the insulin zone and blood type diet can be beneficial
- http://www.rawfor30days.com/
- one cup of lightly steamed beans daily has been associated with reducing blood sugar levels and lessening the need for insulin
- one key to stabilising blood sugar is the required 75-100 grams of protein daily, eaten in six meals throughout the day
- avoiding white processed foods such as bread and pasta. One bowl of pasta is equal to one glass of sugar.
- carbohydrates break down into sugar, so limit portions.

There are also specific nutritional medicines that are very successful for this condition but must be organised through your practitioner.

Over-eating early in pregnancy may put your children at risk of diabetes and heart disease in later life. Phil Owens (Adelaide University, Department of Obstetrics and Gynaecology, 2000) has shown that the amount eaten by mothers at crucial stages of pregnancy determines the ability of offspring to produce Leptin. Leptin is a hormone which regulates appetite and fat. Secreted by fat cells into the blood, Leptin acts on the brain to control appetite and energy expenditure. People who are obese or suffering diabetes tend to have high levels (The Australian Sept. 1999).

One study found that for people with type 2 diabetes two grams of cinnamon a day over twelve weeks significantly reduced diastolic and systolic blood pressure (Akilen et al., 2010). Another study found that drinking 250mgs of cinnamon resulted in a thirteen to twenty three percent increase in antioxidants connected with lowering blood sugar levels and regulating blood pressure (The Center for Applied Health Sciences, Ohio).

My client Mel, 32weeks, received a phone call to say she had tested positive to the Glucose Tolerance Test and it was suggested she begin taking Insulin. Mel in her wisdom suggested they wait a week and see what she could do herself. On her next visit I worked the Endocrine System and Stress points on her feet. Connecting in with her I felt a sense of agitation and nervousness from her baby who felt very active. When I expressed this to her and suggested she may have some fears around mothering that needed to be discussed, she expressed a lot of emotion around not being able to connect to this baby because of having experienced two miscarriages before. Psychosomatically diabetes is linked with lack of self-esteem, the sense of 'life isn't sweet enough'. I worked through this with Mel, helping to change her thoughts and beliefs, and assisted her to connect with her baby and make a commitment to leave work in order to shift into motherhood and help to prevent further complications.

Mel also said that she did not eat enough or regularly. So we put a healthy eating plan into action with more protein and more healthy raw foods. I also started her on FrequenSea, as it has been tested to be very effective in balancing blood sugar levels. It is a superfood that crosses the cell membrane, immediately reducing insulin resistance. Mostly throughout the day Mel's blood sugar levels were ok but she tended to get a high very early in the morning, probably due to the lack of food overnight. I suggested she drink a high energy protein milk drink before bed and make up the juices suggested in this section. I also suggested that if she woke during the night to take a shot of FrequenSea to sustain her. By doing this Mel's blood sugars stabilised without the need for further treatment.

Changing her eating habits by eating highly nutritious healthy food every 2-3 hours plus implementing some of the suggestions here changed Mel's health status and prevented her from experiencing serious complications and high intervention. How I wish these type of suggestions would be instigated in the medical system rather than resorting immediately to pharmaceutical treatment.

Homeopathic:

Note: due to complexities of this condition it is essential to consult a practitioner.

Helonias - particularly exhausted women and for gestational diabetes mellitus. Ten drops three times a day.

Herbal Remedies:

Nature's Way Blood Sugar -includes GTF Chromium, with other vitamins and herbs, part of the glucose tolerance molecule that is an important cofactor for insulin. Formula: Vitamin A, Chromium, Cinnamon, Fenugreek, Nopal Optunia, Bitter extract, Gymnema Sylvestre extract, Gymnemic Acids, Bilberry.

Two herbs helpful for diabetes and safe during pregnancy are Buchu and Uva Ursi. The dosage is as a tea. Boil a heaped teaspoon of Uva Ursi in 470ml of boiling water for thirty minutes (low boil to prevent evaporation). Remove from heat and add an ounce of Buchu Leaves (from Africa). Do not boil. Steep and sip throughout the day.

Cell Salts:

Use for hypoglycaemia - pancreatic weakness, low blood sugar. Shakiness when hungry.

Ferr Phos - inflammation, stress on the pancreas

Nat Phos - blood sugar balance, over-acidity, digestive conditions

Nat Sulph - liver and pancreas support

Su-Jok Points:

Warm up and stimulate the endocrine system points and specifically the pancreas on the hand and fingers. Use warm seeds such as pepper seeds applied to tender points for extra stimulation. Warm up stomach 36 on both legs and J12 point just above the naval using moxa.

Auricular Therapy:

Main points:

- pancreas
- endocrine
- lung
- stomach
- kidney

Associated points: Sanjiao, Shenmen, heart, ear root of nerve vagus.

Reflexology:

I have treated women with a positive glucose tolerance test effectively with reflexology, specific phyto nutrients, herbs and mineral formulas to help balance blood sugar levels.

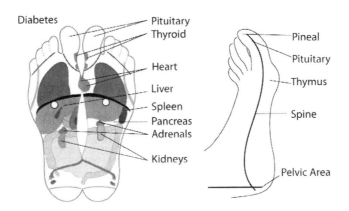

Acupressure Points:

- Three Yin Crossing SP6 * **Only to be applied from 37 weeks, after which can be stimulated twice daily.**
- Bigger Rushing LV3
- Bigger Stream K3 * Only to be applied from 37 weeks.
- Stomach 40

Aromatherapy:

Tangerine, mandarin, grapefruit, geranium, chamomile roman, rose bulgar, rose maroc, jasmine, ylang ylang, lavender.

Bush Flowers:

Old Man Banksia, Wild Potato Bush, Mulla Mulla, Dog Rose, Fringed Violet, Paw Paw, Peach-Flowered Tea Tree + Sunshine Wattle.

Psychosomatic Response:

Balancing the sweetness of life, being able to give and receive love. Uncertainty, worry, mental confusion, anger, hostility, bitterness/resentment can take the sweetness out of one's life (and blood).

- can be related to issues of rejection and abandonment from cellular memory in the womb at birth
- feeling unaccepted, self pity and/or sorrow, feeling deprived of the sweet things in life
- inability to handle/assimilate the sweetness and beauty of life, loneliness, trying to hold onto life too tightly.

Affirmation:

The recommended affirmation is:

"I embrace joy in my life and I am full of sweetness and love."

Another helpful affirmation can be:

"I experience the sweetness of life every day."

Colour Therapy:

Activate your hands by visualising warm streams of orange and yellow light flowing between your palms. When they feel warm and tingly hold your hands palms facing your solar plexus (diaphragm) with the fingers touching at the tips, imagine powering up this area. Then imagine sending this orange light to your pancreas where deeply healing can take place.

The Liquid Crystals:

Transition Help or Stress Help or Sensual Help.

Diarrhoea

Diarrhoea can be of concern in pregnancy as the smooth muscle of the bowel is similar to the smooth muscle of the uterus. If the bowel spasm is strong enough it can stimulate the uterine muscle to contract, resulting in premature labour. Hence the historical use of bowel stimulants to induce overdue pregnancies, such as castor oil or a very hot curry. Ensure you rehydrate with mineral salts and if diarrhoea persists after 48 hours please seek medical advice.

Nutrition:

- grate two apples including the peel, expose them to the air until they go brown, then consume
- over-ripe bananas can assist too, especially if you sprinkle a little blackberry root over them
- take one teaspoon of blackberry root in a small amount of water
- carrot and pineapple can assist
- see electrolyte rebalancing formula under nausea and vomiting
- juice/blend cabbage leaf, ginger, pineapple and mint. Can also add orange, cucumber, apple or paw paw. Add honey or maple syrup to taste.

Homeopathic:
Seek practitioner advice for your specific symptoms.
Sepia Ignatia, nux vomica - diarrhoea
Arsenicum & Veratrum Album - vomiting and diarrhoea
Chamomilla - settles the digestive system

Cell Salts:
Mag Phos - muscular pain or cramping
Kali Phos – nervous conditions, calms the emotions
Nat Mur – iron absorption, excessive dryness, assists with long held grief and holding onto emotions

Reflexology:

See <u>constipation</u> but use relaxing, gentle pressure not stimulating point work.

Su-Jok Points:

Sedate the <u>digestive system, especially the bowel</u>, press into the most tender point and hold to sedate.

Auricular Therapy:

Sedate the <u>digestive system points</u> as well as the Shenmen, heart, stomach and lung (stimulating the vagus nerve).

Acupressure Points:

- <u>Three Mile Point</u>

Aromatherapy:

A massage oil with essential oils rubbed over the abdomen area can assist.

Add 2 drops each peppermint, lavender, chamomile, eucalyptus and geranium oil to 10ml of a carrier oil (vegetable oil) and massage this into the abdomen.

Bush Flowers:

Will depend upon the emotional issue underlying the condition. Emergency essence can assist with calming down the body's reaction.

Psychosomatic Response:

- discomfort with life's decisions, anxious and wanting to run away
- fearful, nervous, insecure, feeling unable to ask for help, confused.

Affirmation:

"I am at peace, I have all the answers inside. I am supported in everything I say and do. I can do this I trust the process of life. Giving birth is easy."

The Liquid Crystals:

Digestive Help.

Infantile Diarrhoea

Diarrhoea must be checked quickly in babies as they are very prone to dehydration.

- Cook a small amount of carrot and water, puree and mix with water until the right consistency for the age of your child. You can add extra boiled water so that it can be given by bottle for a younger baby. Or for children less than three months dilute the puree with milk.

Fatigue

Also see Insomnia and Tiredness. It is perfectly normal to feel tired during pregnancy, especially in the first three months due to the physical and emotional changes taking place. It is important that you get enough rest, including if possible a daily nap. Do your best to retire early. Research supports the theory that your body rests best when you go to bed before ten pm. You should find your energy levels rise during the second trimester. Once you reach about 32 weeks you may find yourself slowing down as you become heavier and begin to withdraw in readiness for the new arrival. Resting well late in pregnancy helps you gain energy for labour. Fatigue is a symptom not a disease therefore treatment will depend on the underlying emotional and physical issue.

Nutrition (see Superfoods in Nutrition section):

Diet and nutrition play an important role in creating and maintaining energy levels. Follow the guidelines outlined in the Nutrition section.

Energy creating foods:

- juice/blend green vegetables, especially kale, spinach and parsley. Add carrot, beetroot, apple and wheatgrass if available.
- almonds/almond milk, combined with apple juice
- apricots, globe artichoke, carrots, celery, figs, avocado and kiwi fruit
- introduce 1 cup of steamed beans into your diet

Superfoods:

- FrequenSea, A.I.M. Fish oils.

All things green (containing chlorophyll) are super foods.

Homeopathic:

There are many and varied reasons for fatigue so treatment will depend on the individual situation. I prescribe Kali phos (Kali phosphoricum) for exhaustion in labour. Often one dose is enough to restore energy enough to continue on and birth. It is also good for nervous exhaustion caused by stress or overwork, or both as may be the situation during labour. During labour and birth, everything is very intense and the right homeopathic remedy should make a difference within five to ten minutes.

Cocculus - good for the mother during sleepless nights

Ignatia – sleeplessness

Arnica - for muscular aches and pains

Arsenicum – restless, tense and anxious

Coffea - overactive mind

Manganum - for energy in the morning

Sepia - after giving birth

Gelsenium and Staphysagria – emotional stress.

Herbal Remedies:

Drink lemon balm (lemon balm leaves steeped in boiled water for 10 minutess) and yarrow tea (buy commercially). Valerian, chamomile, relaxation blends, Peppermint tea can be stimulating.

Cell Salts:

Ferr Phos - inflammation, assists iron absorption and blood circulation

Mag Phos - muscular pain or cramping

Nat Phos - over-acidity

Silicea - connective tissue integrity, acts as a muscle relaxant

Calc Phos - stimulates bone marrow for red blood cell production

Nat Mur - iron absorption

Kali Phos - blood and calms the emotions

Reduce Stress (see Stress section)

Enlist support, do not be frightened to ask for help. Take time to rest. Check for anaemia and introduce the suggestions from the anaemia section.

Reflexology:

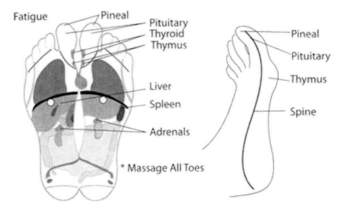

Facial Massage:

Massage all facial points paying particular attention to those areas that are tender.

Su-Jok Points:

Stimulate and warm up all the <u>thyroid and endocrine points</u> on the macro (hand) and insect (finger)system.

Acupressure Points:

- <u>Gates of Consciousness</u>
- <u>Heavenly Pillar</u>
- <u>Sea of Vitality B23</u> (Bladder) - CAUTION - if there are disintegrating discs or fractured bones do not press or apply any pressure. This point may also be very tender if you have a weakness here. In either case, do not apply pressure, instead the light touch of a stationary hand may provide gentle healing.
- <u>Third Eye Point</u>
- <u>Elegant Mansion</u>
- <u>Letting Go</u>
- <u>Sea of Tranquility</u>
- <u>Three Mile Point</u>

Aromatherapy:

A combination to revitalise and give you a lift:

- 8 drops lemon oil
- 2 drops eucalyptus oil
- 2 drops peppermint oil
- 1 drop cinnamon leaf oil
- 1 drop cardamom oil (expensive, so optional)
- 2 ounces vegetable oil

Combine ingredients and use as a massage oil, add 2 teaspoons to your bath, or add 1 teaspoon to a footbath. Without the vegetable oil, this combination can be used in an aromatherapy diffuser, simmering pan of water, a potpourri cooker or it can be added to 2 ounces of water for an air spray. The cardamom oil is optional, but, oh, does it enhance this massage oil! Use it as often as you like.

Bush Flowers:
Vitality Essence, Banskia Robur, Crowea, Detox Essence, Fringed Violet.

Psychosomatic Response:

- out of alignment with life purpose
- not going with the flow and forgetting to accept life changes
- over nurturing, giving out more than you are giving to self.

Find time to nurture you through massage or reflexology. I rarely see my clients with fatigue because they receive fortnightly reflexology sessions, which is like a rejuvenating tune up.

Affirmation:
"Life is abundant. I am able to flow and embrace the joy of life."

The Liquid Crystals:
Stress Help or Sleep Help.

Fibroids

The liver's ability to perform its vital role in regulating the amount of oestrogen in a woman's blood may be affected by consumption of alcohol and caffeine. Practitioners of Chinese medicine attribute uterine fibroids to an over-accumulation of blood in the uterus, brought on by the stagnation of blood and qi. According to Chinese medicine, the excess blood solidifies and turns into tumours.

To eliminate and prevent the stagnation of blood and qi, Chinese medicine practitioners prescribe Fu Ke Zhong Zi Wan, a herbal formulation that includes Chinese angelica, bupleurum root, peony root and other herbs. If you wish to try this Chinese medicine, consult your nearest Chinese practitioner for proper administration of herbs.

Assistance may come from:

- restricting the diet to your blood type
- restricting estrogenic foods such as fats, dairy and meats
- eliminating xanthenes (tea, coffee, chocolate and cola) which stimulate fibroid growth
- rest and positioning for pressure symptoms.

Nutrition:

- prioritise vegetables and vegetable juices, especially carrot juice, which inhibits tumour growth
- whole grains, vegetarian protein sources, fresh fruits, high-iron food and seafood
- add top quality prenatal supplements
- superfoods such as FrequenSea
- traditional Chinese Medicine remedies can be of great benefit too.

Homeopathic:

Silica - stimulates the body to reabsorb fibrous tissue.
Pulsatilla - for heartburn.
* Take care and only use under professional advice

Herbal Remedy:

Herbs to be used for treatment after pregnancy or discontinued if pregnancy is suspected.

Angelica tincture - warms, reduces mucus, increases uterine strength and
is an immune stimulator.
Damiana - harmonises menstruation, strengthens the mind.

Horsetail (shave grass) - reduce bloating, as a diuretic and to strengthen kidneys, bones and reproductive system.

Sage tincture - warming, endocrine tonic, dries up mother's milk and reduces sweating.

Rosemary - **DO NOT USE** when there is high blood pressure. Used to aid circulation, memory and concentration.

Cell Salts:

Calc Fluor - nutrition, calcium and connective tissue support, scars

Kali Mur - excess mucus

Nat Sulph - regulates hormones, liver support

Silicea - dissolves scar tissue, connective tissue support

Reflexology:

After pregnancy, regular work of the reproductive system, lymphatic system and endocrine.

Su-Jok Points:

Seed or point work to the uterine points, warm up with moxa.

Auricular Therapy:

Reproductive areas, pancreases, endocrine, lung, stomach and kidney, Sanjiao, Shenmen, heart, ear root of nerve vagus.

Acupressure Points:

- Bigger Rushing LV3

Three Yin Crossing SP6 * Only to be applied from 37 weeks, after which can be stimulated twice daily.

Most of the treatments for Fibroids will need to happen after pregnancy as it is difficult to treat Fibroids whilst pregnant.

Aromatherapy:

To a carrier oil of pure coconut oil add ten drops each of ginger oil (for warming and increasing the circulation to break down the fibroid), marjoram oil (to reduce muscle cramps) and rose oil. Massage daily to the lower abdomen over the uterus.

Bush Flowers:

She Oak, Bush Iris, Mountain Devil, Slender Rice Flower, Sturt Desert Rose.

Psychosomatic Response:

The uterus is all about giving birth to new and creative ideas. Fibroids can be a sign that there are blockages and a lack of letting in of life.

Can be a result of:

- unresolved issues with a relationship, particularly with men
- sexual repression, holding onto old wounds and pain regarding sex and/or relationships
- feeling unrecognised and/or misunderstood
- repression and/or guilt regarding sex
- fears or anxieties related to childbearing and motherhood
- issues related to receiving, vulnerability and femininity.

Affirmation:

"I release the pain of previous relationships, I embrace my femininity and create a wonderful life."

Colour Therapy:

Imagine vacuuming out your uterus with yellow, orange and pink rays of strong energy. Allow the colours to spin and churn through the uterus, cleansing and clearing. Place your hands on your growing uterus and give great thanks for the growing child within and the wonderful magic it is performing. Release any pain or hurt that may be stored in the fibroid. Allow yourself to forgive.

The Liquid Crystals:
Cycles or Menses Help.

Fluid Retention (see Oedema)

Haemorrhoids (also called Piles)

Haemorrhoids occur due to blockages and pressure build up in the veins around the perineal area. Can be caused through frequent constipation, dehydration, low fibre diet, an increase in progesterone, pregnancy and liver congestion.

Lifestyle Changes:

- eat dinner early, before 8.30 pm, and rest the gut for twelve hours after
- first thing in the morning, on an empty stomach, drink one to two glasses of warm water with lemon
- drink Aloe Vera juice.

Nutrition:

- gentle liver and gut cleansing foods (not detoxification) such as dandelion, green vegetables, green tea, St Mary's thistle
- correcting gut flora with probiotics and reducing toxic foods and binding carbohydrates such as wheat products, refined foods and sugar
- increase fibre rich vegetables and fruits, Aloe Vera, Slippery Elm, specific liver nutrients and herbs
- high anti-oxidant formulas such as Bioflavonoid with Vitamin C and ForeverGreen AZUL and FrequenSea

- juice/blend celery, cucumber, watermelon, watercress or cabbage leaves, carrot, green vegetables, garlic, onion and chia seeds.

Homeopathic:

Combine Lachesis, Muriatic Acid, Arnica, Aesculus hippocastanum, 1 tab every morning and evening. Help may also come from:

Sepia – pelvic congestion from the pregnancy
Collinsonia – associated with pregnancy constipation, bleeding or straining
Nitric acid – pain during and for some time after stool
Nux vomica – straining for stool but no result, itching

Cell Salts:

Kali sulph – haemorrhoids with constipation, or yellow diarrhoea
Nat sulph – bruised like pain, burning after elimination (stool), itching bottom
Silicea – straining, ineffectual stools, itching during stool, connective tissue support

Reflexology:

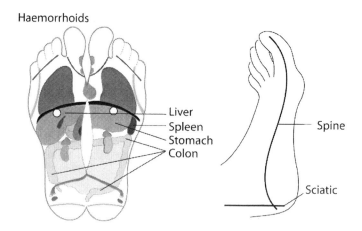

Haemorrhoids

Liver
Spleen
Stomach
Colon

Spine

Sciatic

Facial Massage:

Release around the <u>sacral chakra, mouth and jaw.</u>

Su-Jok:

Warm up the acupressure points <u>Three Yin Crossing</u> (*** Only to be applied from 37 weeks, after which can be stimulated twice daily**), <u>Bigger Rushing</u> and <u>Stomach 40</u> on the legs with Moxa.

Massage the anus point in the webbing on the back of the hand or foot at the third and fourth finger/toe.

Auricular Therapy:

- <u>Haemorrhoid point</u>
- <u>Constipation point</u>
- <u>Anus</u>
- <u>Large intestine, liver, spleen, bladder and adrenals</u>
- <u>Shenmen and ear apex</u>

Acupressure Points:

Same as <u>constipation</u>.

Aromatherapy:

Mix fifteen drops of geranium and five drops of cypress in lavender oil and massage up the legs to enhance circulation. You can make this into a cream or using KY gel and rub into anal area, which will alleviate as well as prevent haemorrhoids.

Bush Flowers:

Bottlebrush, Dagger Hakea, Black-Eyed Susan

Recommended Exercises:

Ensure with all exercises that you engage the core muscles in your abdomen and do not place pressure on your spine or neck. Arms and legs should be relaxed as you engage your glutes (buttocks) and core.

Lie on your back, palms of your hands facing downward at your sides, legs straight and touching each other.

- breathe in and engage your core – imagine you are pulling your navel back to your spine. Make sure you are using your abdominal core and not your back or leg muscles.
- as you breathe out, using your abdominal muscles, move your legs gently up at 30 degrees and stay in this position for a few seconds
- breathe in, then on the next breath out lower your legs gently down to the ground, coming to the normal position
- rest for 2-3 minutes and repeat this exercise. Do this for 3-6 times
- if you have a tender back do this with one leg at a time. This exercise massages the digestive system.

Scissor exercise – whilst the legs are lifted begin to scissor your legs up and down in the same position whilst pressing into the ground with the palms, again ensuring your core is engaged.

Boat pose - lie on your stomach, arms folded so hands rest on each other and your forehead rests on your hands. Legs straight out behind you.

Inhale and engage your abdomen.

- with the out breath lift your head whilst relaxing your shoulders towards your feet, then lift your legs up towards the head, creating a curve in your body. The strength is held by the abdomen. You should not feel this in your back at all. If you do, you are doing this incorrectly.
- **do not over extend** - it is better to use small movements that engage your core than to try to use large movements that are using the incorrect muscles. Repeat three times.

Pelvic Rocks - lie on your back with the knees bent and feet on the floor. Take a breath in and engage your core.

- as you breathe out gently rock your pelvis towards your tummy, scrunch your tummy and pull your pubic bone towards your abdomen

- breathe in, then as you breathe out relax and rock your pelvis towards the floor by pushing the pubic bone down towards the floor
- do this a few times.

This is wonderful for massaging the internal organs and the lower back and is great for period pain. Once again, you should not feel any strain in your back.

Psychosomatic Response:

- 'life is unfair', critical of self and others
- loss of direction and confidence, holding onto outdated family beliefs and fears.

Affirmation:
"There is time and space for everything I want to do."

Colour Therapy:
Imagine orange, brown and green healing rays of light, clearing and releasing any held on guilt or discomfort. Squeeze the muscles of your anus and as you release and focus on letting go. Energise your hands by rubbing them together and imagine orange light coming out of your palms. Sit on your hands and send this healing energy to your anus. Imagine or feel the tingling and healing energy.

The Liquid Crystals:
Transition Help or Stress Help.

Headaches

There are usually three reasons for a headache - dehydration, hunger or tiredness. Listen to your body. If the headache is unusual or persists after rest or treament, please see your medical professional as it could be a sign of high blood pressure or pre-eclampsia.

Nutrition:

- drink at least two glasses of warm water with lemon first thing in the morning
- eat small amounts frequently as your body's metabolism increases during pregnancy and many women suffer from low blood sugar levels which can create headaches
- lack of fluids and constipation will trigger headaches. Rectify these situations (see constipation)
- add one to two teaspoons of cream tartar to 230mls of water. Cream of tartar is a highly acidic substance that stimulates an alkaline-forming state in your body and can alleviates a headache.
- juice/blend green vegetables, broccoli, alfalfa, carrot, celery and berries to taste.

Homeopathic:
Depends on the symptom and the events contributing to the headache. A combination of St. John's Wort, Chamomile, hops and lemon balm will often make a headache disappear. Make an infusion with equal parts of each herb.

Belladonna – throbbing headache
Bryonia – feeling pressure and need to lie still
Gelsemium - dull stress headache, may feel like a band around the head
Sepia – migraines that start over your left eye, may extend to nape of neck, tend to be worse during a period and during pregnancy.

Cell Salts:
Nat Mur – excess fluid, iron absorption, where there is grief
Mag Phos – spasms, muscles
Kali phos - stress and overstrain

Reflexology:

Massage the feet, paying particular attention to the big toes as these represent the head and neck. Gently massage any areas that are tender until discomfort diminishes.

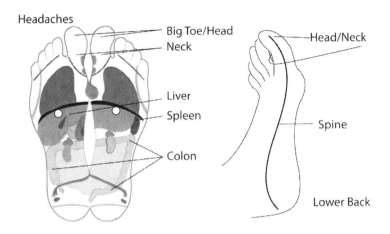

Su-Jok Points:

Establish the associated painful point on the top of the thumb or tops of fingers, use seed therapy, colour, magnet or massage to reduce the pain or warm up with moxa.

Auricular Therapy:

Massage or apply a magnet to tender points on the ear. Use point work to sedate the congested point.

Acupressure Points:

Third Eye

Drilling Bamboo

Facial Beauty

Gates of Consciousness

Heavenly Pillar

Bigger Rushing

Above Tears

Facial Massage

Emotional Release Points and Acupressure Points:

1. **Third Eye GV24.5 (Governing Vessel)** between the eyebrows in the groove where bridge of nose meets forehead. Balances the pituitary gland, relieves hay fever, headaches, ulcer pain and eyestrain.

2. **Drilling Bamboo B2 (Bladder)** the indent either side where bridge of nose meets the ridge of eyebrows. Relieves eye pain, headaches, hay fever, eye fatigue and sinus pain.

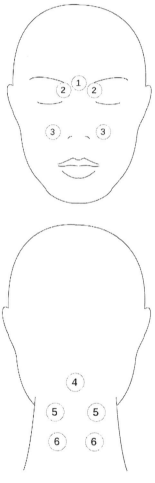

3. **Facial Beauty ST3 (Stomach)** at the bottom of your cheekbone, below the centre of your pupil when you are looking straight ahead. Relieves eye pressure and fatigue, nasal and head congestion, eyestrain and toothaches.

4. **Wind Mansion GV16 (Governing Vessel)** back of your head, in the centre, at the large hollow below the base of your skull. Relieves eye pain, ears, nose and throat as well as mental problems, headaches, vertigo and stiff neck.

5. **Gates of Consciousness GB20 (Gallbladder)** below the base of your skull, in the hollow between the two vertical neck muscles. Relieves headaches and migraine, dizziness, stiff neck, neck pain, eyestrain and irritability.

6. **Heavenly Pillar B10 (Bladder)** back of your head, half an inch below the base of the skull, on the muscles half an inch outwards

from your spine. Relieves stress, burnout, exhaustion, insomnia, heaviness in the head, eyestrain, stiff neck and sore throats.

Aromatherapy:
For headaches associated with neck tension slowly massage the neck and shoulder with lavender and rosemary oil.

Bush Flowers:
Black-Eyed Susan, Boronia, Bottlebrush, Crowea, Dagger Hakea, Emergency Essence, Five Corners, Paw Paw, She Oak, Sturt Desert Rose.

Psychosomatic Emotional Release:
As mentioned in Psychosomatic Therapy, your posture can have an effect on your overall health. Thus it is very important to check your posture throughout the day. If your head is forward of your body, this compresses your neck and chest, making it difficult to breathe. Psychosomatically the head forward posture indicates that mentally you are ahead of your body, your thoughts are creating stress. See Postural Integration.

Psychosomatic Response:

- self criticism, lack of faith in self, lack of self recognition
- too much mind activity to allow you to relax. Time to meditate and learn relaxation techniques.

Affirmation:
"I love and approve of myself. I accept that I am perfect the way I am."

Colour Therapy:
Lying in a relaxed position, focus on your breathing. Imagine you are breathing through the area that feels tight and sore. Imagine indigo, green, white and yellow rays of light dissolving away the stress and tension. Place

a cool, moist cloth in one of these colours on your head and imagine you are breathing in the colour.

The Liquid Crystals:
Headache Help.

Heartburn

Heartburn is the reflux of gastric contents into the oesophagus and can be very uncomfortable in pregnancy. It is very common in the last trimester due to the baby squashing and pushing the organs upwards. Avoid hot and spicy foods, caffeine, smoking, chocolate, high fat diet, alcohol, acidic food and aspirin.

Contributing Factors:

- stress
- overeating
- irregular eating habits
- bending, lying down or physical exertion too soon after eating
- obesity
- alcohol
- cigarette smoking
- some drugs or medications such as aspirin, antibiotics, etc.
- poor posture, resulting in squashing of the diaphragm
- avoid foods which relax the sphincter such as tomatoes, citrus fruits, garlic, onions, chocolate, coffee, tea, alcohol and peppermint.

Prevention:

- maintain reasonable weight
- relax and enjoy the eating experience

- avoid drinking immediately before meals and drink little during meals as this dilutes the digestive effect in the gut
- eat slowly, chew each mouthful well
- eat meals frequently but in small amounts and at regular timings
- avoid heavy meals, spicy, greasy, sugary and acidic foods. Stick to a bland, high-fibre diet.
- drink lots of fluids and exercise daily
- raise the head of the bed 2-4 inches with a stable support or sleep upright but try to lie on your left side as this is better for your baby
- avoid bending over or lying down when your stomach is full. This increases abdominal pressure and makes gravity work against you, thus increasing the likelihood of heartburn.
- do not lie down immediately after eating. If it is necessary to lie down after eating, lie on the left side. In this position the stomach remains lower than the oesophagus.
- recognize signs of stress and identify the causes (see Stress)
- undertake a good exercise program with yoga or pilates
- take adequate rest.

See Your Doctor if:

- after taking an antacid to relieve heartburn there is no relief within 15 minutes
- along with heartburn, there is difficulty in swallowing, breathlessness, sweating, dizziness, nausea, vomiting, diarrhoea, extreme abdominal pain, fever or black or bloody stools
- the discomfort around the chest region is aggravated by exercise and relieved by rest
- the heartburn is chronic, occurring daily or almost daily
  CAUTION: Take Antacids as a last resort as they can mask or aggravate some ailments.

- do not take antacids before consulting your doctor if you have high blood pressure, irregular heartbeat, chronic constipation or diarrhoea and vomiting
- pregnant and nursing mothers should consult a physician before taking any medication, including antacids.

Assistance may come from:

- Pure
- ensure you are taking in enough fluids
- following the blood type diet to reduce exposure to antigens that may increase the severity of the condition
- drinking cold milk can relieve the pain of heartburn but is not a remedy. Milk can actually worsen the effects of heartburn as once in your stomach the fat, calcium and protein in milk cause increased acid secretion.
- although mints are often credited with alleviating heartburn, they actually relax the sphincter, making heartburn more likely
- hot compresses over your stomach may help to improve blood supply and relax muscles

Nutrition:

- FrequenSea, or Azul calms the gut
- keep meals small and frequent
- high fibre diets
- probiotic formula with acidophilus may help as well as natural yoghurt
- eating avocado, paw paw or pineapple can settle the stomach
- infuse one teaspooon grated apple or grapefruit peel in boiling water, cool then sip to settle acid stomach
- drink a small glass of potato juice
- juice/blend red apple, pear, celery, alfalfa sprouts, carrot, cabbage leaves, chia seeds and cherries.

Homeopathic:

Iris Vesicolor, Robina, Arsenicum, Carbo veg, Pulsatilla, Magnesia Carbonica if dairy intolerance.

Cell Salts:

Calc Phos - nervous digestion to correct acidic stomach

Mag Phos - muscular spasms of the stomach

Nat Phos - over acidity

Nat Sulph - pancreas, liver support

Nat Phos 6x homeopathic remedy great for reflux in babies too. Made from simple baking soda, completely safe for a baby any age.

Reflexology:

Press or sedate these points, do not stimulate. Points may be tender, a gentle touch is preferable.

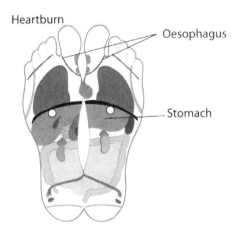

Su-Jok Points:

Sedate the tender stomach and oesophagus points on the hands and second digit on all the fingers. Each finger is different so explore individually until you find the sore point.

Auricular Therapy:

- Stomach, oesophagus, spleen and liver
- Shenmen, Adrenals.

Acupressure Points:

- Three Mile Point
- Sea of Vitality B23 (Bladder) - CAUTION - if there are disintegrating discs or fractured bones do not press or apply any pressure. This point may also be very tender if you have a weakness here. In either case, do not apply pressure, instead the light touch of a stationary hand may provide gentle healing.
- Grandfather Grandson SP4 (Spleen) relief of abdominal cramps, stomach ache, indigestion and diarrhoea.
- Inner Gate

Aromatherapy:

- add one drop of peppermint oil to a teaspoon of honey and dissolve in warm water
- use a massage crème containing peppermint and eucalyptus oil to massage into the chest area
- peppermint, lemongrass, ginger, parsley, raspberry leaf teas are all very helpful
- mix half teaspoon of slippery elm with half a cup of warm water and sip slowly after meals.

Note: From a naturopathic perspective antacids containing sodium and aluminium should not be used as they tend to disrupt the normal flora of the gut leading to longer term problems.

Bush Flowers:

Dog Rose, Paw Paw, Crowea, Black-eyed Susan, Bluebell, Helmet, Old Man Banksia.

Psychosomatic Response:

- difficulty expressing feelings, repressed emotions, fear, anger, stress, conflicts and over working
- finding life difficult to digest, 'burning up' inside, had a gut full, wounded heart
- the stomach is the seat of the emotions.

Affirmation:

"I express myself clearly, I am respected and listened to. I express my emotions, I relax and take time out, I am free of anger and guilt.'

Colour Therapy:

Relax and focus on your stomach. Imagine purple and golden yellow rays clearing and calming the irritation and pain. Take in deep breaths and now imagine green, yellow and blue are cooling and calming, settling the burning feeling.

Liquid Crystal:

Digestive Help.

Herpes Simplex

A recurrent viral infection affecting the skin or mucus membranes.

- Type 1 commonly causes herpes labialis (fever blister or cold sore).
- Type 2 is usually genital and transmitted sexually.

Contributing Factors:

Stress, fatigue, systemic infection, lowered immunity, TH2 dominance, sun exposure, trauma, low lysine diet, high arginine foods such as almonds, peanuts, chocolate and turkey may contribute to this condition.

A study of the herpes simplex virus (HSV) in pregnancy and its effects on newborns tested 8538 women for the presence of antibodies against HSV. The only babies in the study who contracted neonatal herpes were born to women who acquired genital herpes near the onset of labour (New England Journal of Medicine, 1997, Vol. 337 No. 8).

Babies are most likely not at risk of infection during pregnancy, but if the mother's immune system drops and she has an outbreak of lesions at the time of the birth, then the baby is at a higher risk of infection. Therefore the objective is to build the immune system so you can avoid the risk of a breakout before delivery, enabling you to attempt labour and vaginal birth rather than requiring a caesarean section.

Ways to Build Your Immune System:

- take probiotics

Immune boosting blend:

- juice/blend coconut milk, raisins, chai seed, almonds, rhubarb, banana and stone fruits (stones removed)
- eat 1-2 apples (including peel) every day along with garlic, dandelion leaves and calendula flowers as part of a fresh leafy salad
- blend 10% cabbage juice with 90% pure paw paw crème and apply to the affected area

Specific Supplementation:

For best effect take the following from 35 weeks onwards:

- zinc
- *Andrographis paniculata* (King of Bitters) and *Uncaria tomentosa* (Cat's Claw) may contribute to improved immunity, regulation of cytokine production and natural killer cell function, assisting in the improved clearance of infective microorganisms
- I have used Coriolus mushroom extract with great success. Mushroom polysaccharides may exert remarkable actions on various elements of the immune system.
- *Grifola frondosa* (Maitake) may assist in increasing helper T-cells, activate macrophages, memory T-cells, NK lymphocytes and stimulates interleukin immune response
- A.I.M. contains transfer factor and like colostrum contains a wide variety of immunologically active factors including cytokines, peptide fragments, oligosaccharides, growth factors and immunoglobulin
- Pure and FrequenSea.

Homeopathic:

Best to consult a practitioner as an assessment of your physical, emotional and psychological make up needs to be considered to determine the most effective remedy for you. The following may be beneficial:

For cold sores:

Natrum muriaticum - for eruptions that occur at the corners of the mouth during times of emotional stress, tend to be worst during the day, can appear watery, puffy and burning

Rhus toxicodendron - for eruptions of many small blisters that itch most intensely at night, may feel tingly and sting

Sepia - for outbreaks that do not improve with other homeopathic
   remedies, this remedy is most appropriate for those who tend to lack
   energy and don't tolerate cold weather
Cantharis - for large blisters smarting and burning, bleeding
Hepar sulph - pus and worse to touch

For genital lesions:

Graphites - for large, itchy lesions in individuals who are overweight
Natrum muriaticum - for eruptions that occur during periods of emotional
   stress, symptoms that tend to be worst during the day
Petroleum - for lesions that spread to anus and thighs, symptoms tend to
   be worst in winter, improving during summer

Source: Herpes simplex virus http://www.umm.edu/altmed/
articles/herpes-simplex-000079.htm#ixzz2W3DVFUGP
University of Maryland Medical Center

Herbal Remedy:

Lemon balm - a cream to apply to sore lips to reduce redness and swelling
Aloe - aloe gel to help genital herpes lesions heal
Rhubarb cream - a topical cream made from rhubarb and sage may be
   effective in healing cold sores.

Cell Salts:

Calc Sulph - toxicity
Nat Mur - for grief, depression and sadness
Nat Sulph - for negativity, anger, suicidal feelings and liver support

Reflexology:

As with any infection, focus on the lymphatic system, spinal reflexes, liver,
spleen and detoxification areas. Sedate the reproductive area to assist in
preventing a breakout.

Su-Jok Points:

Reproductive areas, Liver and Spleen

Auricular Therapy:
Reproductive areas, Shenmen, Balance point

Acupressure Points:
Need to boost the immune system .
Bearing Support
Sea of Tranquility
Three Mile Point
Crooked Pond
Outer Gate
Sea of Vitality B23 (Bladder) - CAUTION - if there are disintegrating discs or fractured bones do not press or apply any pressure. This point may also be very tender if you have a weakness here. In either case, do not apply pressure, instead the light touch of a stationary hand may provide gentle healing.

Aromatherapy:

- add a drop of geranium oil to a cotton bud dipped in oil and apply directly to the sore
- combine geranium, lavender, thyme and lemon oil in a carrier oil and massage into the neck and throat area
- peppermint oil, although reported to have stopped the herpes virus from reproducing in test tubes, has not adequately tested on humans yet.

Bush Flowers:
Sturt Desert Rose, Billy Goat Plum, Spinifex.

Psychosomatic Response:

- sexual repression, self-punishment, deep dislike of self
- partnership disharmony or anger, sexually angry with partner, not feeling honoured

- rejection, repressed feelings, long term anger from sexual abuse.

Affirmations:

"I embrace the beauty of who I am, I accept myself for who I am unconditionally right now."

The Liquid Crystals:

Cycles or Crocoite.

Hypertension (high blood pressure)

High blood pressure is defined as blood pressure of 140/90 or greater, measured on two separate occasions six hours apart. During pregnancy a rise in the diastolic (lower number) of fifteen degrees or more, or a rise in the systolic (upper number) of thirty degrees or more, warrants closer observation. Hypertension can create capillary spasm and a lowering of oxygen to the placenta. Severe blood pressure can result in placental haemorrhage and death of placental tissue. Hypertension by itself is not a criterion for pre-eclampsia, but has added significance if you have other symptoms such as fluid retention and protein in the urine.

Blood pressure tends to drop in the second trimester of pregnancy, so it is good to know your regular blood pressure prior to pregnancy. This is particularly important if your blood pressure is normally considered low (hypotension), as a rise may be less obvious in those with hypotension.

'Pregnancy Induced Hypertension' is caused by low blood volume. Although pregnancy actually increases the blood volume by 50-60%, poor nutrition leading to lack of healthy salt, protein and calories can cause the blood volume to stop increasing, to plateau or to even drop. Your body reacts to the lowered blood volume as it would to haemorrhage, restricting blood flow to only essential internal organs. This restriction is caused by the kidneys releasing renin, which constricts the capillaries, resulting in a rise in blood pressure. Increasing your healthy salt (such as Himalayan, sea salt or kelp salt), protein, and calorie intake will increase blood volume, normalising blood pressure.

Please note that home monitors are not always as accurate as those used in clinics or hospitals. Home readings should therefore not replace prenatal visits, nor should a 'normal' reading mean you can ignore other symptoms of pre-eclampsia. It is best to take blood pressure on the same arm and at the same times daily.

Relaxation is very important. Invariably I take a blood pressure on my mums prior to reflexology and it's on the high side, then following the session it has lowered considerably. Reflexology has been well researched as having an excellent effect on hypertension.

Nutrition:

- eat small amounts of protein every hour, such as a handful or two of nuts (not peanuts), cheese cubes, trail mix, canned fish, a hard-boiled egg, a slice of cold meat, a cup of yogurt, or 1/4 cup of cottage/ricotta cheese
- juice/blend cucumber, celery, parsley, fennel, garlic, onion, apple, orange and chia seeds
- juice/blend oat, nut or rice milk, banana or berries, pineapple and chia seeds.
- eliminate chocolate, coffee, coke and smoking
- reduce carbohydrates and increase EFA/DHA oils (see Nutrition)
- eat cucumber, one clove of garlic and three apples a day (including the peel)
- include onions, beans, broccoli, carrot, kiwi and small amounts of spicy food in your diet
- eat three figs a day to assist low blood pressure
- in a glass of water, add one to two teaspoons of baking soda. Good for hypertension or oedema.

Add the following foods to your diet for added blood pressure reducing properties.

Ginger – stimulates circulation, inhibits production of inflammatory cytokines and suppresses the creation of leukotrienes. Together these actions help maintain arterial blood flow and promote cardiovascular health (Balch & Rister 2002).

Garlic – studies suggest that fresh garlic has more potent cardio-protective properties than processed garlic or powder. Be careful with garlic supplements as the concentrations are quite strong and garlic can thin the blood and interact with drugs.

Cinnamon – one study found that for people with Type 2 diabetes two grams of cinnamon a day over twelve weeks significantly reduced diastolic and systolic blood pressure (Akilen et al., 2010). Another study found that drinking 250mgs of cinnamon resulted in a thirteen to twenty three percent increase in antioxidants connected with lowering blood sugar levels and regulating blood pressure (The Center for Applied Health Sciences, Ohio).

Onions - contain quercetin, an antioxidant flavonol found to prevent heart disease and stroke. Research published in the Journal of Nutrition reported that subjects with hypertension experienced a decrease in their blood pressure by 7mmHg systolic and 5mmHg diastolic.

Olives -Polyphenols in extra-virgin olive oil was credited for the significant reduction of blood pressure.

Cardamom – high blood pressure has been shown to be effectively reduced by taking 3grams of cardoman powder daily (Indian Journal of Biochemistry and Biophysics)

Oregano - contains the compound carvacrol, which has been shown to be effective against blood pressure.

Changing your diet is an important part of lowering high blood pressure. Studies have found that the DASH diet (Dietary Approaches to Stop Hypertension), promoted by the National Heart, Lung, and Blood Institute of the National Institute of Health (NIH, USA), can reduce high blood pressure within two weeks. The DASH diet includes fruits and vegetables, low-fat dairy foods, beans and nuts, with sodium limited to 2,400 mg per day.

http://www.dashforhealth.
com/?gclid=CNnj-ZihlL0CFUEgpQod3ggA4w

Nutritional Supplements:

Pulse-8 Larginine with L-Arginine and eight heartfelt super ingredients.
http://casadelsole.fgxpress.com/farmers-market/

CoQ10 (Coenzyme Q10) - there is some evidence that the supplement CoQ10 may help to reduce high blood pressure. Two twelve week trials resulted in a significant reduction in systolic blood pressure.

Inulin - a natural sweetener which is also a good source of soluble fibre, that may help lower blood cholesterol and glucose levels.

Acái - acái berries have been found to be some of the highest antioxidant foods on the planet. The antioxidants they provide have beneficial effects throughout the body, not just the heart.

Pomegranate –provide superior antioxidants that inhibit LDL oxidation, which supports arterial wall strength while enhancing the activity of the enzyme responsible for converting L-arginine to nitric oxide.

Red Wine Extract - Science has proven grapes are a signature food high in antioxidants, anthocyanins and polyphenols (resveratrol) - beneficial for the heart and reduces LDL oxidation.

Fish Oil / Krill Oil - Preliminary studies suggest that fish oil may have a modest effect on high blood pressure. Although fish oil supplements often contain both DHA (docohexaenoic acid) and EPA (eicosapentaenoic acid), there is some evidence that DHA is the ingredient that lowers high blood pressure (see Nutrition).

Calcium, Magnesium, and Potassium - sources see PURE and cell salts.

Homeopathic:

Viscum Album-30 (5 drops three times a day) as needed. Other common remedies include Acetic acid, Apocynum, Arsenic alb, Helonias, Kali carb, Kali chlor, Phosphorus, Thlapsi bursa pestoris.

Also try:

Argentum nitricum - if blood pressure rises with anxiety and nervousness, can assist with 'Stage fright' or anticipation of a stressful event such as the birth.

Herbal Remedy:

An infusion of Shepherd's Purse (Herba Bursae Pastoris) and hops (Humules Lupulus) drunk two to four times daily can have a relaxation effect.

Hawthorn - in a randomized controlled trial, after sixteen weeks participants taking hawthorn supplement had a significant reduction in mean diastolic blood pressure.

Agrimony (batch flower remedy) 2 drops three times in a day. It is very safe for pregnancy.

Passionflower - the recommended dose is 2 - 4 capsules daily, or 15 drops of the tincture three times a day (Wise Woman Herbal for the Childbearing Year, Susan Weed).

However, in my experience the best results occur with a combination of reflexology, cell salts and increasing protein, and the other aspects of the Brewer Diet alongside the use of the Passionflower. Susan suggests up to half a cup a day of beet juice, and combining one grated raw beet with one grated raw apple for a tasty and healthy snack that can help relieve elevated blood pressure and pre-eclampsia.

You can also read one or more of Dr Tom Brewer's books and consult with your midwife to decide what the best path is for you and your baby.

Herbs to Avoid:

- Licorice
- Asian Ginseng

Reflexology:

Massage the big toe up and down as well as the point in the inside corner near the webbing. Relaxing and sedating the solar plexus point is very important to assist with blood pressure. Blood pressure is psychosomatically connected to holding onto a long standing emotional issue that is preventing you from moving forward, and in pregnancy can be related to the change of identity and the emotional stress involved. The solar plexus is the chakra of identity. Massaging and releasing this chakra on the feet, hands and face can be greatly beneficial.

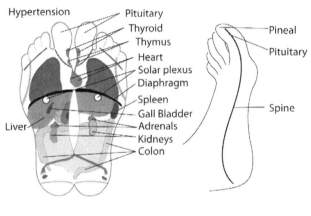

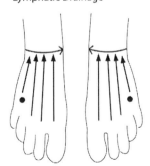

Lymphatic Drainage

Cell Salts:

Cell Salts can be of great benefit, especially magnesium phosphate. Cell salts have been found to be very effective for mothers with borderline high blood pressure posing the question of induction. I encourage you to visit your reflexologist prior to your obstetric visit for a deep relaxing reflexology session and magnesium phosphate cell salts. This has worked many times to prevent women from being induced in labour. Given hourly during labour cell salts may prevent blood pressure complications too. During many labours I have combined cell salts and reflexology to balance hypertension.

Calc Fluor - relaxes the connective and muscle tissue
Ferr Phos - assists iron absorption and blood circulation
Silicea - connective tissue integrity, acts as a muscle relaxant
Kali Phos - blood and calms the emotions

Facial Massage:
Massage along the solar plexus area, nose and cheeks, in the emotional zone, releasing around and under the eyes. Release the jaw and mouth.

Su-Jok:
Warm up and massage the heart points on each hand, on the base of the venus mound below the thumb. Warm up and stimulate the brain zone on one or both thumbs, paying particular attention to the most sensitive points. Warm up the four points on the outside of the wrist in line with the little fingers. Massage and stimulate the kidney and spleen points as well. Use seed therapy, eg a peppercorn, on the most sensitive heart points of each finger and massage through the day.

Auricular Therapy:

- Shenmen
- Subcortex
- Heart, liver, spleen and adrenals

Acupressure Points:

- Crooked Pond
- Three Mile Point

- <u>Bigger Rushing</u>
- <u>Bubbling Spring</u> & <u>Joining the Valley</u>

Aromatherapy:
Gentle massage using the following essential oils can have a beneficial effect on high blood pressure.

Combine a few drops of each in a carrier oil:

- Clary sage
- Lavender
- Marjoram
- Melissa
- Ylang-ylang

However these oils must be avoided:

- Hyssop (contains pinocamphone)
- Rosemary (very stimulating)
- Sage (contains thujone)
- Thyme (hypertensive - increase blood pressure)

Bush Flowers:
Bluebell, Crowea, Five Corners, Hibbertia, Little Flannel Flower, Mountain devil, Mulla Mulla.

Isometric Hand Grips Exercises:
This exercise can be beneficial in lowering blood pressure. Roll up two face cloths or hand towels. Hold one in each hand. Squeeze hard on the towels to get a sense of how strong your squeeze is. Now reduce this pressure to about thirty percent. Squeeze and relax. It is very important not to over squeeze, the aim is to stimulate the deep muscles. Squeeze for two minutes and rest for three minutes. Repeat four times for a total of twenty minutes, three times a week. Incorporate guided breathing, a deep breath in and out with each squeeze.

Psychosomatic Response:

- seething inside, feeling hurt, wanting revenge, holding onto hate, rage and anger
- experiencing too much pressure and demands
- wanting to be liked, over pleasing, pushing past your limits

Emotional trigger point therapy focusing on the solar plexus helps to identify fears that aren't being expressed. Meditation and relaxation exercises can help you access and resolve these fears. A client with BP of 200/100 who was not responding to medication achieved a lowered BP of 130/70 from sessions where I focused on massaging her solar plexus to help her identify and release her fears.

Affirmation:

"I trust in the process of life. I let go and allow the flow of life. I trust my body. I trust this pregnancy and that my body knows how to birth."

The Liquid Crystals:

Transition Help or Stress Help or Meditation.

False Hypertension Linked With Caesarean:

One study suggests pregnant women may undergo unnecessary caesarean sections because they have 'white-coat hypertension', or high blood pressure that happens only when they are around doctors, and that almost one third of pregnant women have such false high blood pressure.

"Believing it is real hypertension, doctors usually treat it with blood pressure lowering drugs, which can compromise a woman's ability to have normal contractions and in the study led to apparently unnecessary caesareans."

Dr. Gianni Beliomo, Researcher, Assisi Hospital, Italy

Midwifery Today, 1999 (Issue 44).

The study reported that of the 144 pregnant women who had high blood pressure during their third trimester:

- 42 had white-coat hypertension, of which 19 underwent caesareans (a rate of 45 percent).
- of the 102 women with true hypertension 42 underwent caesareans (41 percent)
- at 23 percent, caesarean rates were much lower for the comparison group which comprised 103 women with normal blood pressure.

Indigestion (see Heartburn)

Insomnia and Tiredness

Everyone suffers from sleepless nights occasionally. Research suggests practicing relaxation techniques can have an eighty percent positive effect as that of deep sleep. Trying to force your body to sleep can have a detrimental effect as this creates anxiety. If you are finding it difficult to sleep get up, meditate, do something relaxing rather than tossing and turning, then go back to bed when you feel tired.

Assistance may come from:

- FrequenSea
- a relaxing foot massage prior to bed has been shown to be of great benefit, have your partner massage your feet or massage your own
- ensuring your body is supported and comfortable, practice some yoga relaxation positions to find out which ones support you best. Most women prefer to sleep on their left side in the 'flying fish position', which is lying on your left side with the right leg bent up and supported by a pillow.

Nutrition:
See Fatigue.

Homeopathic:
Passiflora 10drops in water before bed. Add Gelsemium if there is an emotional issue. Belladonna is excellent for fear of nightmares.

Herbal Remedy:
Mix equal parts of valerian, hops, skullcap (Scutellaria Lateriflora) and chamomile. Take about an hour before retiring. The tincture is more effective than the infusion, along with raspberry leaf.

- honey is a very good sleep inducer, take one teaspoon after the evening meal and another later in the evening
- Pure at bedtime as a muscle relaxant
- do not eat or drink stimulants such as coffee, chocolate, alcohol or energising herbals teas/oils such as peppermint, lemon, grapefruit or ginger after 5pm. Instead drink relaxing herbal drinks such as chamomile or warm, nurturing drinks like warm milk and honey.

Cell Salts:
Mag Phos - relieves cramps and aids muscle relaxation
Calc Phos - stimulates bone marrow for red blood cell production
Kale Phos - reduces stress

Reflexology:

Needs to be relaxing and soothing not stimulating.

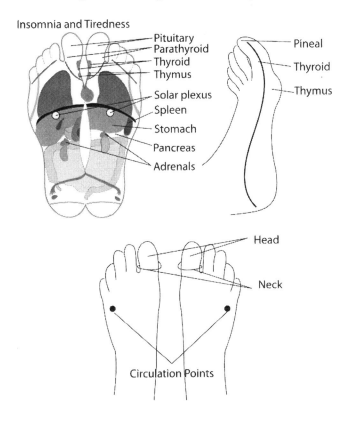

Insomnia and Tiredness

Pituitary
Parathyroid
Thyroid
Thymus

Pineal

Thyroid

Thymus

Solar plexus
Spleen
Stomach
Pancreas
Adrenals

Head

Neck

Circulation Points

Acupressure Points:

- Wind Mansion
- Gates of Consciousness
- Heavenly Pillar
- Inner Gate
- Spirit Gate
- Third Eye
- Calm Sleep
- Illuminated Sea

Aromatherapy:
Put a few drops of lavender oil, Roman chamomile and clary sage together on your pillow. The aroma will have a sedating effect. Add a few drops to Sea Salt and mix into a warm bath. Do this a couple of hours before bedtime as a bath can be stimulating due to the heat increasing circulation and bathing before bed can have the opposite effect.

Bush Flowers:
Blackeyed Susan, Crowea, Boronia, Emergency Essence, Green Spider Orchid + Grey Spider.

Psychosomatic Response:

- can't relax, feeling unsafe, unable to let go
- over thinking, over planning, wanting to control
- unable to disassociate mind from heart, feeling scattered and fearful, not trusting own instincts and intuition
- harbouring feelings of guilt and resentment
- unable to accept and be in the moment.

Practicing the breathing technique outlined under psychosomatic therapy can be very beneficial, especially before going to bed. It is your mind that is keeping you awake. By focusing on your body, your breath and your intuition (inner tutor) the mind becomes occupied and cannot take you off on a story. It is only a story because you are not experiencing it now, it is fictitious, created by the imagination of the mind.

Before you go to sleep rather than running through things that may be of concern for you spend some time focusing on the things you are grateful for from the day just gone. This can be as simple as the fact you have running water, clean sheets, a warm comfortable bed to sleep in and a beautiful bonny baby to look forward to meeting. When you focus on the positive in life you lift the vibration of every cell in your body.

Repeat the word peace over and over. Doreen Virtue (angel intuitive) recently conducted a study looking at the vibration of words. The more positive and loving the word the higher the vibration. Peace has the highest vibration of any word, negative words had very little vibration and worry had the lowest.

http://www.healyourlife.com/author-doreen-
virtue-and-grant-virtue/2010/11/wisdom/
inspiration/your-power-words

Worry is a useless place to be as it cannot achieve anything except stress and tire your body. When we learn to surrender and allow events to unfold we accept life as a journey that must be experienced not orchestrated. Rather than worrying about what could go wrong, close to falling asleep focus your mind on what it is you would love to see as the best outcome in your life. This then becomes the last thing your conscious mind is focused on before you drift off to sleep, thus whilst you sleep your mind is occupied with positive, creative thoughts.

Affirmation:

"I lovingly release the day and slip into peaceful sleep, knowing tomorrow will take care of itself."

Colour Therapy:

Gently relax and begin to breathe in, imagining you are breathing in a ray of uplifting green and blue light. A relaxing mudra is to place your little finger and ring finger on top of your thumb whilst extending the index and middle finger. Lie down quietly whilst holding this pose with your fingers, breathe and visualise the blues of the ocean and the gentle lapping of the waves on the beach. Feel the yellow warmth of the sun dissolving away the tension in your body. Feel the lightness of your body surrounded in the beautiful colour rays of gold, white, blue and green. You will sleep like a baby.

The Liquid Crystals:

Sleep Help or Stress Help or Meditation.

Itchy Skin

Itchy skin is an uncomfortable state at any time but can be more so in pregnancy. Many mums suffer from this irritation. The skin is a large organ that acts as a detoxifier through the sweat glands and lymphatic system. During pregnancy it becomes quite stretched and overheated. The itch can occur due to your body attempting to detox excess oestrogen, and may also be due to an overactive liver. Use only natural organic products on the skin and drink lots of water. Try adding oatmeal to your bath and soothing oils. Coconut oil is wonderful for the skin and may prevent stretch marks.

Nutrition:

- FrequenSea
- A.I.M.
- juice or blend horseradish, garlic, orange, ginger, pineapple, carrots and apricots.

Homeopathic:
Dolichos + Staphysagria, Ignatia

Herbal Remedy:
I recommend dandelion tincture (Taraxacum officinale), dandlelion tea or a gentle liver tonic to help boost the liver's function. As the liver is nurtured and strengthened the itching will stop, or at least lessen considerably.

- Yellow Dock (Rumex crispus) is also a good treatment for itching and is mildly cathartic (help empty the bowels) and diuretic, which is useful for removing toxins from the stressed liver.

The condition may be due to the increased immune Th2 response that occurs to protect your pregnancy. Sometimes the side effect of this is a hypersensitive state that can result in allergic symptoms. Taking probiotics can help counter this effect.

Cell Salts:

Ferr Phos - low grade inflammation and heat

Kali Phos - nervous conditions

Kali Sulph - hormonal issues and sweating

Silicea - inflammations associated with hot flashes and heat in general

Reflexology:

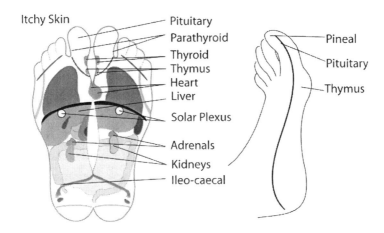

Su-Jok Points:

Work the <u>spine on the bony back surface</u> of the hand and fingers.

Auricular Therapy:

<u>Overall immune system boost.</u>

Acupressure Points:

- <u>Skin Condition</u>

Aromatherapy:

Add to a few drops of coconut oil one or two of the following oils. Massage into the skin. Trial and error will let you know which ones work the best for you.

Do Not use the oils directly, always dilute in oil.

Sandalwood is beneficial for dry, itchy skin and can be used in combination with frankincense, geranium, clary sage, lavender, neroli, lemon or jasmine.

Ylang Ylang balances the skin's natural oils, making ylang ylang soothing to dry, itchy skin and one of the most used oils in skin care.

Geranium essential oil is valued for its ability to balance the production of sebum, keeping the skin smooth and supple. Also an effective treatment for a variety of skin conditions, including dermatitis, eczema and itchy, dry skin.

Chamomile essential oils are beneficial for dry, itchy skin and may be a useful treatment for eczema, dermatitis and rashes. Both types (German and Roman) of chamomile essential oils blend well with other skin-friendly essential oils, including bergamot, tea tree, lavender, ylang-ylang, rose and grapefruit.

Lavender is a beneficial treatment for a variety of skin conditions, including eczema and dry, scaly skin. Nearly any essential oil blends well with lavender, including geranium, nutmeg, pine, clary sage and cedarwood.

Bush Flowers:
Red Grevillea, Blackeyed Susan.

Psychosomatic Response:
Itchy skin is related to your sensitivity and feelings, issues related to letting things go, accepting change, which is what pregnancy brings.

- skin irritation may indicate fear, anxiety/restlessness, lack of fulfilment, feeling irritated about something or someone and/or anxiety regarding one's relationship to oneself and the world.

I recommend massaging, breathing and releasing the solar plexus, sacral and heart areas on the body, face, hands and feet as you breathe in the joy of life.

Affirmation:

"I am at peace right here right now. I love being in my body and accept the life path I have chosen at this time and trust that all will be wonderful."

The Liquid Crystals:

Transition Help or Stress Help or Meditation.

Morning Sickness & Nausea

Most common in the first trimester, associated with hormonal changes. Also thought to be due to the body excreting toxins, preparing your body for the growth of the baby. There is some thought that excessive nausea may be associated with an allergic reaction to the growing baby, as the body feels like it is carrying a foreign object. It may also be associated with the level of acceptance of the pregnancy by you, the mother.

In my experience, those mothers who come to me for preconceptual care tend to experience less nausea and vomiting. This leads me to support the theory that dietary insufficiencies may be a contributing factor. Nutritional formulas and body care in early pregnancy can reduce the effect quite markedly. Many of the women who come through my clinic are so well that they often state this seems surreal as they are not suffering the problems their friends are.

Assistance may come from:

- Vitamin B6 (50mg per day), Magnesium (100mg), B complex, Vitamin C (25mg daily)
- Vitamin K (5mg daily) supplements may help nausea
- kale (possibly the highest ingestible source of vitamin K)
- massage the acupuncture point under the chin, wrist or hand point
- sedate the stomach reflex point on the feet

- adding one to two teaspoons of cream tartar in a glass of water settles nausea and alleviates headache
- grate beetroot and combine with natural yoghurt
- raspberry leaf tea with ginger tea

An electrolyte-balancing tea for nausea in pregnancy (makes one litre):

½ cup lemon juice, 1/3 cup honey, 1/4 teaspoon salt, 1-2mls Pure then add water to make one litre. Take spoonfuls at regular intervals.

Juicing/blending is an excellent way to get phytonutrients and assist your gut to settle. Try refreshing blends such as pineapple, cucumber, watermelon, parsley, apple, alfalfa and chia seeds.

Recent Case - I found the following nutrient combination to be very effective recently with a client who was pregnant with twins and suffering from Hyper-emesis to the extent she had to be hospitalised and stabilised with intravenous fluids. I began treatment with the liquid phyto-nutrient formula FrequenSea plus an Electrolyte formulation and Pure. Within 48 hours the vomiting reduced by half, to just daily by the end of one week, finally settling completely after two weeks. The mother also received reflexology twice weekly, concentrating on sedation of the stomach and GUT points, which proved to be very effective. She went on to birth at full term without complications with both twins weighing 3000 grams, quite remarkable for twin pregnancies.

Homeopathic:

- Homoeopathic V.T.S. drops - 15 drops on tongue three times a day or hourly if necessary.

Nux Vomica - for nausea, especially in the morning and after eating. Use if irritable, impatient, chilly, also if there is dry retching, stomach cramping and constipation.

Ipecacuanha - intense nausea felt all day with retching, belching and excessive salivation. Worsened when lying down or moving. Vomiting does not relieve nausea.

Pulsatilla - indicated if nausea is worse in the afternoon and evening (may be in the morning as well) with lack of thirst. You may experience cravings for a wide variety of foods.

Lacticum acidum - nausea at its worst when you first wake in the morning. Eating often helps you to feel better and your appetite is likely to be good.

Asarum - for persistent nausea and retching.

Colchicum - intense nausea that is worsened by the smell and sight of food. Retching and vomiting, likely to feel sore and bloated in your abdomen.

Sepia - intermittent nausea but stomach feeling empty. At its worst in the morning. Eating does not relieve the discomfort and you may vomit after. Nausea may be more intense when lying on your side.

As you can see there are many forms of nausea and homeopathic remedies that can assist. For best results I would recommend you see a practitioner.

Herbal Remedy:

- Raspberry leaf tea or capsules two to three times a day
- Peppermint tea
- Ginger tea with cloves, cardamom and cinnamon (especially in the traditional Chinese formulation)

Ginger tea during pregnancy can help to settle nausea. One study of a group of pregnant women found nausea during the first trimester was reduced by eighty five percent compared with nine percent for those taking a placebo (UMMC 2012).

Mix equal parts of spearmint (Mentha spicita), borage (Borrago officinalis), lemon balm (Melissa officinalis), chamomile (Anthemis nobilis) and raspberry leaf (Rubus idaeus). Make an infusion and sip.

Or

Mix equal quarter part dandelion root (Taraxacum officinale) and quarter part cloves (Eugenia caryophilla) with half part grated ginger root (Zingiber officinale). Make as a decoction and sip throughout the day.

Or

Mix half part meadowsweet, quarter part black horehound and quarter part chamomile. Drink as a tea three times a day or as needed.

- try filling gelatine capsules with ginger root powder and swallow
- other herbs of benefit are Digestant, Basil, Alfalfa, and Golden Seal

Reflexology:

See Acidity and Heartburn in this section. Use a light touch to gently massage and sedate.

Facial Massage:

Massage the temple area, release around the heart and emotional zone (points 3 and 4). Massage the jaw and mouth. Release points below the eyes on the cheek bones (point 4).

Su-Jok:

Sedate and warm up the stomach and oesophagus area on the venus mound below the thumb also massage middle digit of each finger paying particular attention to any area that feels tender. Press and sedate these points with your fingers or use seed therapy.

Auricular Therapy:

- Stomach, Spleen, Liver and Abdomen
- Sympathesis

- <u>Subcortex</u>
- <u>Mid-ear</u>
- <u>Shenmen</u>
- <u>Diaphragm</u>

Acupressure Points:

- <u>Intermediary</u>
- <u>Inner Gate</u>
- <u>Three Mile Point</u>
- <u>Bigger Rushing</u>
- <u>Severe Mouth</u>
- <u>Heavenly Appearance</u>

Aromatherapy:

The stomach may be settled with one drop of peppermint or spearmint, mixed with oil and used to sedate the gut reflexes on the feet or use in a diffuser.

Bush Flowers:

Crowea, Dagger Hakea, Dog Rose, Paw Paw.

Psychosomatic Response:

The ability to discern, choose, digest and properly assimilate life's experiences, recognising what is beneficial and what is not. The stomach is a very sensitive organ which reflects even our most subtle feelings.

Problems in this area may indicate:

- emotional upsets, worries, anxiety, fear, discontent, impatience
- repressed feelings
- inability/resistance to assimilate and process life's experiences
- difficulty accepting the pregnancy, especially if the pregnancy has been unplanned.

Affirmation:

"I trust this life process, I am safe and trust my own ability to be the best I can be to bring only good to myself and my baby."

Colour Therapy:

Relax and focus on your stomach. Imagine purple and golden yellow rays clearing and calming the nausea and discomfort. Take in deep breaths and now imagine green, yellow and blue are cooling and calming, settling the stomach.

The Liquid Crystals:

Digestive Help or Transition Help.

Oedema

Your hands and feet may become puffy and swollen as your baby's birth approaches. The larger baby becomes the more pressure your uterus (womb) puts on blood vessels in your pelvis. The most affected is the Inferior Vena Cava (the large vein that receives blood from your lower limbs) on the right side of the body. Circulation slows due to this pressure causing blood to pool and fluid is forced into tissues of the extremities, feet and hands.

Most women gain fluid during pregnancy, some more than others. In all three of my pregnancies I gained around ten kilos of fluid without it being a problem.

By the third trimester between fifty and eighty percent of healthy pregnant women will develop oedema. Hot weather can make oedema worse. It is important to observe how much fluid retention you are experiencing.

If you feel that you are particularly swollen, tighter than usual around the ankles and hands, then please get checked out. Oedema is one of the signs of pre-eclampsia if accompanied by high blood pressure so have your BP checked often.

Nutrition:

- reduce salt intake
- Vitamin B6
- juniper tablets
- FrequenSea
- Hemp oil - Increase essential fatty acids EPA-DHA to at least 3000 milligrams a day either from good quality fish oils or hemp oil **this is very important
- Pure
- add one to two teaspoons of baking soda to a glass of water
- avoid artificial sweeteners and caffeine
- reduce carbohydrates
- buckwheat strengthens the circulatory and lymphatic systems
- juice/blend watermelon, pineapple, orange, parsley, celery, dandelion leaves, ginger, horseradish, cucumber (Lebanese) and mint leaves.

Assistance May Come From:

A compress of green or white cabbage leaves can be used as often as needed to help draw out excess fluid and relieve your discomfort. Simply wipe the leaves clean but do not wash them. Cool leaves by placing in the fridge (not the freezer). Wrap the cooled leaves around the most swollen parts of your legs and feet. Leave on the area until they become moist, replace with freshly cooled leaves and continue until the pain is reduced. You can do this as often as you need to.

Daily exercise such as yoga and pilates may also help.

Homeopathic:

Pulsatilla + Natrum muriaticum may help with excess fluid. Take one or two 30c strength tablets under your tongue four times a day for five days. See a qualified, registered homeopath if there is no improvement after this.

Arsenicum album - is worse evenings between 10pm and 2am, feeling of the stitch, heavy, perfectionism, burning restless feet, improves with warmth.

Herbal Remedy:
Dandelion Tea.

Use a combination of the following herbs in capsule or powder for general leg swelling, and adjust as your condition improves. The herbs are specific for each underlying cause. Therapeutic dose is equal to one capsule of each herb three times a day or 15 drops of a herbal tincture three times a day.

- red root helps with lymphatic and liver congestion
- juniper berries support the urinary system and produce a diuretic effect
- hawthorn berries support heart circulation and blood pressure as well as nerve support
- dandelion root and leaf provide liver and kidney support as well as a diuretic effect.

Cell Salts:
Nat Mur - removes extra fluids, indicated where legs swell but no pitting of skin, where there is grief and symptoms are worse in heat and mornings around 11am

Nat Sulph - when leg swells with pitting of skin (press and finger mark stays for a few seconds to minutes) and symptoms are worse in damp and cold weather and around 4-5 am

Silicea - oedema with cramping, icy cold sweating and worse in the cold and changes in moon phases

Facial Massage:
Massage through the emotional zone and down towards the mouth. Release around the mouth and jaw, massaging in a downward approach to encourage drainage.

Reflexology:

Reflexology is so effective for this condition that often after working one foot the woman will need to wee to remove the fluid that has been stimulated out of the body. Many women are astounded to find the side of the body relating to the foot that was just massaged has less fluid retention compared to the other. Get adequate rest and avoid unnecessary standing. Lymphatic drainage massage is a lighter, gentler foot massage.

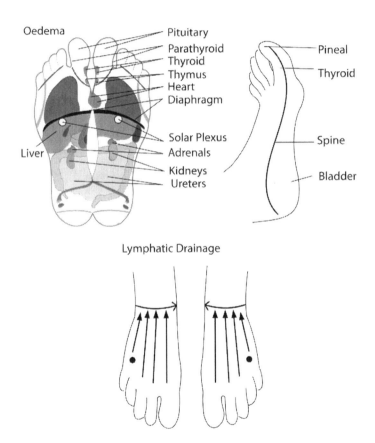

Lymphatic Drainage

Su-Jok:

Massage all of the <u>main area of the hands</u> working towards the bladder point between the third and fourth finger. Pay attention to areas that are sensitive, massage the fingers downwards towards the palm in the same way.

Auricular Therapy:

- Shenmen
- Subcortex
- Brain stem cortex Heart, kidneys, liver, spleen and adrenals

Acupressure Points:

- Shady Side of the Mountain
- Three Yin Crossing * Only to be applied from 37 weeks, after which can be stimulated twice daily.
- Illuminated Sea
- Blazing Valley

Aromatherapy:

Add lavender and chamomile oils to a carrier oil and use to massage the legs and feet. Cypress oil is also good for circulation and varicose veins.

Bush Flowers:

Bluebell, Flannel Flower.

Psychosomatic Response:

Circulation, fluid and lymphatics are related to the water element and the ability to flow with life. It is based on the principle of a river which flows wherever it can, up and over, around, it finds a way. We can flow in the same way when we allow life to flow through us, letting go of that which doesn't serve us. This brings nourishment to cells, tissues and organs. Restriction of emotional energy such as feeling uptight, restricted, over-burdened, confused and scared will produce a corresponding restriction of lymphatic flow.

Affirmation:

"I flow with life with ease and allow life to be. I am fulfilled and happy. I trust the flow of creation. I trust my body to birth easily."

Colour Therapy:

Rub your hands together and imagine pink and green energy flowing through and around your fingers. Imagine massaging these colours around your kidneys, calves and ankles. Imagine a silver light energising your body and moving the fluids around your body in a balanced way.

The Liquid Crystals:

Transition Help.

Pre-eclampsia

Pre-eclampsia, or toxaemia of pregnancy, is a syndrome characterised by hypertension and proteinuria (protein in the urine), which is often accompanied by oedema. Pre-eclampsia affects approximately ten percent of all pregnancies to varying degrees and is a major contributor to maternal mortality, premature birth, intrauterine growth restriction and perinatal mortality.

It is the most serious condition of human pregnancy that is medically known, affecting both mother and baby. Pre-eclampsia usually arises during the second half of pregnancy, and can even occur some days after delivery. Most antenatal screening is focused on catching this syndrome before it develops by observing for the presence of the following symptoms:

In the mother:

- high blood pressure (hypertension)
- leakage of protein into the urine (proteinuria)
- thinning of the blood (coagulopathy)
- liver dysfunction

As Pre-eclampsia is a collection of symptoms it is best to treat each symptom as they arise using the suggestions in this section. Pre-eclampsia affects mother and baby. Increasing hypertension can create spasming of the arteries and reduce the blood supply to the baby, which may result in a lack of growth for the baby. Conservative management and careful monitoring is usually the choice through rest and observation to give the baby the best opportunity to continue its development in the womb.

Pre-eclampsia is usually associated with first-time pregnancies and oddly in women who are having a first time pregnancy to a new partner. The University of Nottingham School of Medicine (Broughton Pipkin, 2001) investigated the possibility of a link between the father as well as the mother related to pre-eclampsia and concluded that there is a paternal as well as a maternal component to the predisposition to pre-eclampsia. There is a slight risk for women who have experienced pre-eclampsia once to experience it again in subsequent pregnancies, but this is rare.

How Can I Best Prevent Pre Eclampsia?
Nurture and look after yourself with good phyto-nutrients and relaxing body work such as maternity reflexology. Of all the women I have seen over many years in practice, none have experienced pre-eclampsia. This may just be the luck of the draw but I believe it is due to the care these women receive, fortnightly reflexology sessions, the taking of high nutrient super-foods and being able to deal with any emotional issues or fears as they arise.

Nutrition
I recommend:

- FrequenSea 50mls a day provides high bio-available nutrients and the highest readily absorbable source of anti-oxidant
- A.I.M. two tablets daily provides Vitamin D, Transfer Factor and co-factors for the immune system
- Pure 1-2mls daily for essential minerals that assist in maintaining good vasodilation for improved blood flow
- essential fatty acids (EPA-DHA) 3000mg – 6000mg a day reduces the production of thromboxane (a powerful vasoconstrictor

and aggregating factor), thereby reducing blood pressure and improving blood flow to baby.

There is also the simple not yet proven method by Dr. Tom Brewer.

Eat 80-100gms of protein a day, with plenty of fresh fruit and vegetables, salt to taste, drink to thirst (ensure the salt you use is high quality sea salt).

The blood type diet can be of benefit as well. Researchers at Magee Women's Research Institute and the University of Pittsburgh, School of Medicine have found that vitamin C deficiency, even to a mild degree, leads to poor vascular elasticity and function, a key symptom of pre-eclampsia. FrequenSea is a great source of antioxidants. Maternity Reflexology has many beneficial effects.

Reflexology:

See also Hypertension and Oedema.

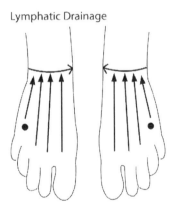

Lymphatic Drainage

Auricular Therapy:

See Hypertension and Oedema

Acupressure Points:

Refer to the points to massage for Hypertension and Oedema

Bush Flowers:

Dagger Hakea - shifts deep resentment

Black Eyed Susan - for those on the go

Crowea - worry and anxiety

* See Oedema and hypertension for other suggestions.

Psychosomatic Response:

Understand that many issues that the body faces are based in the emotional body. It is very important to address any fears or emotional challenges you may be facing and to shift these with Psychosomatic Therapy or NET therapy.

It is also very important to look at the mind-body connection. Maybe its time to stop, relax, smell the roses and be a mum.

Please refer to this section under Hypertension & Oedema

The Liquid Crystals:

Transition Help or Stress Help or De-Stress.

Restless Legs

Restless legs is common in late pregnancy due to the increased load on muscles and your nervous system. Exercise legs by walking daily 15-30 minutes daily. See muscle cramps and spasms.

Nutrition:

- drink celery juice daily
- increase green leafy vegetables
- many of my clients have found great relief from taking PURE and extra magnesium
- almond milk is high in magnesium and minerals
- juice/blend cucumber, beetroot, pineapple, carrot, lettuce, spinach and chia seeds

Reflexology:

See <u>Cramps and Spasms</u>.

Stretch Marks

Caused by weakening of the elastic tissue commonly associated with pregnancy, excessive obesity, muscle growth and rapid growth spurts. Note that once stretch marks have occurred, it is unlikely that any treatment will cause them to disappear completely. I have found massaging with pure coconut oil to be greatly beneficial.

Assistance may come from:

Ka Huna (<u>http://vimeo.com/55418689</u>) or deep tissue massage with pure coconut oil is wonderful for maintaining great skin elasticity and health.

Nutrition:

- zinc
- magnesium
- fish oils
- avocado
- Pure, FrequenSea
- coconut oil
- Vitamin E
- almond milk
- Any combination of juiced/blended vegetables and fruit is going to have great benefits for your skin. Once you begin using raw foods you will notice your skin becomes tighter, cleaner and brighter <u>http://www.rawfor30days.com/</u>
- juice/blend carrot, beetroot (including tops), celery, cucumber, all green vegetables, citrus and berries.

Homeopathic:

Thiosinaminum is prescribed for scar tissues and keloids after an operation and can be effective for stretch marks appearing on your abdomen due to pregnancy.

Arnica may assist.

Cell Salts:

Calc Fluor - for marked whiteness of skin or scar tissue 6x (Biochemic) 4 pills three times a day. Add Silica if there are hard elevated edges of ulcers, surrounding skin purple and swollen.

Calc fluor - elasticity

Kali phos - muscles, muscle spasm, nerves

Aromatherapy:

Combine to pure almond, wheat germ or coconut oil a few drops of borage seed, lavender, tangerine or carrot oil and massage into tummy daily.

Bush Flower:

Bottlebrush, Isopogen, Five corners, Billy Goat Plum, Fringed Violet, Jacaranda.

Psychosomatic Response:

- feeling overstretched, pressure from stress and high expectations
- challenged by change
- frustration and lack of protection, feeling exposed.

Affirmation:

Release feelings of being uptight, too firm, controlling, non-flexible, fear and anxiety.

"I am flexible and expanding with joy."

The Liquid Crystals:

Transition Help.

Urinary Incontinence

Often over the years of my midwifery practice I have heard the comment that women who birth naturally have a high incidence of urinary incontinence following delivery. A survey of 1008 women from an antenatal clinic in northwest England found that fifty-nine percent of the women reported stress incontinence during pregnancy, thirty one percent following delivery. Ten percent had daily episodes of incontinence during their pregnancy, and two percent of all women reported daily incontinence following delivery. Stress incontinence was found to be higher amongst women experiencing more pregnancies.

No difference in the prevalence of stress incontinence was found between women who had a normal delivery and those having an instrumental delivery. A caesarean section was found to be associated with a lower incidence compared with a normal spontaneous delivery (Mason et al., 1999).

Avoiding episiotomy is very important as women with episiotomy have a high incidence of urinary incontinence that is not associated with muscle failure but due to misalignment of the sphincter muscle after stitching. There are so many small muscles in the perineal area that it is a very difficult task to align these muscles effectively.

A large scale study conducted in Australia in the early 1990's called HOOP (Hands off or Poised) discovered very little indication for episiotomies.

Of course there is going to be a slight difference in the pelvic floor muscles after birthing a baby but this can be treated easily through regular pelvic exercise.

I recommend pilates and the following exercise:

Exercise:

1. go to the toilet and pee. Stop urinating midstream (this uses your pelvic floor). If you are unsure of how to contract the correct

muscles, place a finger inside your vagina and squeeze, feeling a tightening sensation around your finger.

2. take yourself to a quiet room and sit in a comfortable and easy yoga pose. Make sure your back/spine is straight.

3. pull up your perineum by contracting your entire pelvic floor, just as if you are trying to stop urinating midstream. At the same time, contract the muscles around your anus as if you are trying to stop yourself from passing wind. Hold for three seconds.

4. release and relax all muscles you have contracted during Step 3 for a count of ten.

5. repeat steps 3 and 4 nine more times, holding the contractions for three seconds each time.

6. over the next three months do this daily and gradually increase the time spent in step 3 to ten seconds.

Homeopathic:

A combination of Belladonna 6x, Cantharis 6x, Causticum 12x, Equisetum hyemale 6x, Petroselinum sativum 6x, Plantago major 6x, 12x, 30x, 200x, Pulsatilla 12x and Sepia 12x.

Cell Salts:

Calcium fluoride

Potassium phosphate

Sodium phosphate

Sodium sulphate

Silica

Use of the tablets:

You can take a combination or 1 to 3 tablets at a time.

High dosage - 1 tablet every one to ten minutes

Reflexology:

Massage gently the reproductive and urinary system, especially the area around the inside of the inner heel just before the arch (the slightly puffy area).

Nutrition:

- eat cucumber, horseradish, almond milk, cabbage, artichoke, green beans, carrot, celery, cucumber, garlic and onion
- drink 3 cups of corn silk tea
- drink 3 cups of couch-grass tea daily
- drink 25mls of celery juice with carrot and parsley, combine with two tablespoons of apple cider vinegar, one tspn of honey and one whole lemon, add water to taste

Prevention is best with good nutrition and immune building support.

- juice/blend celery, cucumber, watermelon, tomato, beetroot, carrot, dandelion and cabbage leaves, ginger, garlic, red onion, parsley and pineapple

Immune boosting blend:

- juice/blend coconut milk, raisins, chai seed, almonds, banana and stone fruits (stones removed).

Prevention is the best policy:

- it is best to wee before and after intercourse to flush out unwanted bacteria
- increase fluid intake
- olive leaf, dandelion tea, Vitamin C and other anti-oxidants are beneficial, as well as probiotics and gentle detoxification.
- herbs such as Barosma betulina (Buchu) and Zea mays (Cornsilk), nutrients like potassium magnesium aspartate, quercetin and vitamin B6 can help with the regulation of water and electrolyte losses, renal circulation, and resistance to stone formation, infection and injury

According to a recent study cranberry juice can prevent cystitis and other urinary tract infections from occurring because cranberries contain isolated compounds called condensed tannins or proanthocyanidins. Researchers suggest the compounds are capable of preventing Esherician coli (E coli) from attaching to cells in the urinary tract, and that a 300ml glass of high-concentration cranberry juice consumed daily would help prevent E coli urine infections (Professional Care Mother and Child, 10: 1).

Homeopathic:
Staphysagria twice daily, Cantharis, Mercurius Corrosivus and Formica Rufa, Apis Ferrum Phos.

Herbal Remedy:
Horsetail (Shave grass) as a diuretic and healthy for the urinary tract

Nettle - anti-inflammatory, full of minerals, has a drying effect
Uva ursi - use only for a few days to treat symptoms of Urinary Tract Infection

Cell Salts:
Ferr Phos - inflammation
Kali Mur - mucus and inflammation
Mag Phos - spasms, muscles
Nat Phos - over acidity

Reflexology:

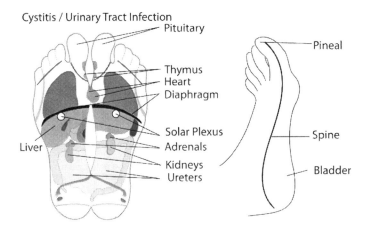

Cystitis / Urinary Tract Infection
Pituitary
Pineal
Thymus
Heart
Diaphragm
Spine
Solar Plexus
Adrenals
Liver
Kidneys
Bladder
Ureters

Su-Jok Points:

Massage and stimulate the <u>bladder area on the hand</u> and each finger. Pay particular attention to the little fingers, warm up these points with Moxa and use warm seeds such as pepper and the colour red.

Auricular Therapy:

<u>Sedate the urinary system, bladder and Shen Sheim.</u>

Aromatherapy:

Combine one to two drops of three or four of the following into a massage oil for your feet or for a bath - rosemary, thyme, sage, savory, pine, niaouli, marjoram, oregano, hyssop, basil (use sparingly), clove, cajuput, cinnamon, lavender, fennel, cumin, coriander, cypress, eucalyptus.

Bush Flower:

Dagger Hakea, Bottlebrush.

Psychosomatic Response:

- factors can include anger, resentment, past abuse, holding on to emotions, control, frustration, feeling 'pissed off' with partner or self.

Affirmation:

"I am flowing with the joy of life releasing all past issues as I go."

Colour Therapy:

Imagine you are holding a yellow energy ball between your palms. Massage this ball and you will begin to feel a tingling sensation between your fingers. Now imagine massaging this ball of energy into your bladder. Feel a healing warmth, then as it begins to feel lighter and less irritated imagine the colour becoming green and refreshing.

The Liquid Crystals:

Transition Help or Stress Help.

Varicose Veins and Circulation

The weight of the growing baby and extra circulating fluids can sometimes result in varicose veins and haemorrhoids. During pregnancy, these conditions can indicate a more serious complication, especially when accompanied by oedema and/or hypertension.

Usually if the blood pressure and urine screenings remain normal the varicosity is likely to disappear after birth. In the meantime, for the final weeks of pregnancy and following birth, you can use herbs traditionally used for such discomforts.

Contributing factors such as constipation, lack of exercise, vitamin E deficiency and a lack of Omega 3 must be addressed along with circulation exercises.

Assistance may come from:

- Witch Hazel crème/ointment specifically made for varicose veins
- exercise
- reflexology

Nutrition:

- Pure
- kelp
- pineapple juice
- Vitamin C and bioflavonoid
- juice/blend all berries, especially blueberries and blackberries, with ginger, garlic and grapefruit.

Homeopathic:
Aesculus Hippocastum, Arnica, Hamamelis, Fluoric Acid, Sepia.

Herbal Remedy:
Choose herbs high in bioflavonoids, which act to support connective tissue.

Use a combination of the following herbs in capsule or powder for maximum benefit. Adjust as your condition improves. Therapeutic dose is equal to one capsule of each herb three times a day, or one liquid dropper full of a herbal tincture three times a day.

Hawthorn – author herbalist Jill Rosemary Davies recommends the use of hawthron in her book 'In a Nutshell; Hawthorn' as a safe treatment in pregnancy

Guta kola – helps peripheral circulation, better memory and concentration

Gingko biloba extract promotes circulation and vein integrity, memory and concentration

Butcher's Broom - is used long-term to strengthen veins and used for haemorrhoids.

Astringents

Astringents are herbs that have the quality of drying, shrinking, and binding tissues. They help reduce inflammation, swelling, and secretions. Astringents can be used internally, externally at the site of stress, and in baths. The water element gives comfort and relief.

How to Use Astringents:

Liniment combine extracts of selected herbs and use topically. Apply several drops to a cloth or cotton ball and saturate the appropriate area.

Poultice add extracts to powdered bentonite clay to make a paste. Apply to the affected area and allow to completely dry. Poultices can be removed when dry and freshly reapplied.

Compress made from a strong tea of the chosen herbs, a compress is a cloth soaked in cooled tea (a warm infusion tends to aggravate conditions) and directly applied where it is needed.

Bath full-body or sitz baths allow herbal essences to be taken into the body through the pores of the skin. External areas needing attention are sufficiently reached as well. Infusions, decoctions of the appropriate herbs, or tincture doses can be added to a bath.

Make up a compress and apply directly to the varicosity or add the following herbal astringent tinctures to a bath or sitz bath. The following astringent herbs can be remarkably effective for external treatment of varicosities:

- blackberry root (rubus villosus)
- witch hazel bark (Hamamelis virginiana)
- oak bark (Quercus)
- yarrow (Achillea millefolium).

Cell Salts:

Calc Fluor - connective tissue weakness, leg ulcers, swelling and hardness

Calc Sulph - weakness of legs, leg tender to touch, feet slightly swollen and tender

Ferr Phos - inflammation in general, swelling with or without fever

Reflexology:
See <u>Hypertension</u> and <u>Oedema</u>

Facial Massage:
<u>Massage and release areas of tightness.</u> Stimulate along the mouth and jaw line, around the eyes and emotional zones

Su-Jok Points:
Stimulate the <u>circulatory, heart and lymphatic systems.</u>

Auricular Therapy:
<u>Heart, lungs, circulation system, Shen sheim</u>

Acupressure Points:

- <u>Gates of Consciousness</u>
- <u>Three Mile Point</u>
- <u>Active Pond</u>

Aromatherapy:
Add a few drops of lemon oil to massage oil and gently massage. Add five drops each of essential oils cypress and lavender to your bath to help with varicosity in legs and labia.

Bush Flowers:
Five Corners, Tall Mulla Mulla, Paw Paw, Red Grevillea

Psychosomatic Response:

- difficulty in receiving love
- blocking and stagnation of energy
- feeling fearful, helpless and unsupported
- overwhelmed, burdened.

Affirmation:

"I connect with love, wellbeing, peace and happiness. I allow life to flow with ease. I am full of love and vitality."

Colour Therapy:

Alternate the healing energy of red and blue over the affected area. Imagine massaging the colours into the area and wear these colours to enhance the healing. Also visualise purple violet rays of healing energy moving through your circulatory system.

The Liquid Crystals:

Communication Help or Stress Help or Transition Help.

Pregnancy Complications

The majority of pregnancies will progress safely, happily and without any major problems or emergencies, but for some there may be complications. To be on the safe side and for your own peace of mind, you should be aware of any potential complications and the corresponding danger signs so that you can seek medical care if necessary.

If you experience any unusual symptoms or if you have concerns about any of your pregnancy symptoms contact your doctor as soon as possible to arrange a check-up.

Unstable Pregnancy

Ectopic Pregnancy

In normal pregnancy the fertilised ovum implants itself in the uterus, however in an ectopic pregnancy it implants in another area, most commonly the fallopian tube. As the embryo grows, it pushes against the fallopian tube and gradually weakens the walls, resulting in bleeding and ultimately a burst fallopian tube.

Thankfully there are warning signs for an ectopic pregnancy and along with any other unusual symptoms these must be reported to your doctor immediately to enable quick treatment.

You may be alerted to an ectopic pregnancy by abdominal pain (usually felt on one side), possible bleeding, feeling faint or fainting and shoulder pain in the same side of the body as the abdominal pain.

If detected early, the fallopian tube can be saved before rupture occurs, however the embryo cannot be saved. An acute ectopic pregnancy will result in a burst fallopian tube, for which surgery is required. Depending on the extent of damage to the tube, it may need to be removed. After experiencing an ectopic pregnancy you can successfully become pregnant again, depending on your individual circumstances. Even with one tube there is still a high chance of pregnancy success. If both tubes are damaged IVF may be attempted.

Incompetent Cervix

The cervix is sealed closed in normal pregnancy, holding baby in the uterus. An incompetent cervix is when the cervix begins to open before the term of the pregnancy (usually in the third of fourth month), resulting in early labour. This can lead to rupture of the amniotic sac and miscarriage.

This condition is rare, but may occur if the cervix has been damaged during previous pregnancies or surgery. This condition is usually picked up after one or two miscarriages. Unfortunately it can't be diagnosed before pregnancy. If a previous miscarriage is thought to have been caused by an incompetent cervix, preventative measures can be taken for your next pregnancy. Rest is recommended and the cervix can be sutured closed until labour begins at term.

Miscarriage

The loss of a baby before twenty weeks is termed a miscarriage while after twenty weeks or a birth weight of at least 400 grams the loss of the baby is called a stillbirth. The causes of miscarriage are not always known. Miscarriages usually occur in the first trimester, sometimes before the pregnancy has even been suspected. Five out of six conceptions miscarry before six weeks. Approximately thirty percent of all pregnancies end in miscarriage. In most cases a period may be late and heavy and the conception and miscarriage may not have been noticed.

Research indicates that good pre-conceptual care for both partners results in less miscarriage and more successful viable pregnancies. It is imperative that both you and your partner seek preconceptual treatment to assist in creating healthier sperm and ova. If you are vegetarians, consider increasing protein rich foods into your diet. An increase of as little as ten percent can improve conception as can a weight gain of one to two kilos if you are underweight.

It is vital that you both avoid nicotine, alcohol, caffeine and chemical toxins in and around your home. Having a hair analysis can assist in recognising any chemicals that may be causing a problem. Taking ForeverGreen's ZMP 400 can assist in eliminating chemical toxins from the body. Women who suffer from recurrent miscarriages often have an immune irregulatory related to an excess in T-helper 1. There are specific herbal formulas that can assist this, one being Polydpodium extract, best sourced through a Naturopath or herbalist.

Types of Miscarriage

If bleeding occurs at any stage in your pregnancy you must see your doctor. Bleeding is the most common symptom of miscarriage. Miscarriage can be caused by many factors including:

- genetic problems due to chromosomal defects
- environmental factors such as smoking, alcohol and other recreational drugs
  - hormonal abnormalities
- pre-existing disease or illness
- uterine abnormalities or other medical conditions in the womb
- bacterial and viral infections.

Experiencing a miscarriage doesn't mean you aren't likely to conceive again, however miscarriages can increase in frequency with age and with the number of previous pregnancies. Small numbers of women can experience up to three or more miscarriages in a row and approximately fifty percent may still go on to have a successful pregnancy, even though they will have suffered emotional pain, frustration and disappointment on previous occasions.

Subclinical Miscarriage happens early usually within the first couple of weeks with the mother only experiencing a late period or heavier bleed than usual.

Missed Miscarriage occurs in the first trimester around six to eight weeks. Often the women is very aware of the pregnancy but then suddenly notices the symptoms seem to be diminished, on ultrasound there is no heart beat. The body will spontaneously abort in a few days or a dilatation and curette may need to be undertaken.

Clinical Miscarriage generally occurs in the first or second trimester up to twenty four weeks and involves stronger symptoms such as cramping, bleeding and symptoms of labour.

Mid-Trimester Miscarriage less than ten percent of miscarriages occur this way. Can be due to foetal abnormalities, infections, chromosomal activities or cervical incompetence. This tends to take on labour symptoms with mild contractions, rupturing of waters developing into strong contractions and the need to deliver the baby.

Stillbirth occurs when a baby dies after twenty weeks pregnancy. The baby is usually given a birth certificate and funeral.

Self Help Guide

Although the conception may be a healthy one, sometimes conditions affecting the mother may cause miscarriage. Research has found that by correcting these conditions, the mother may be able to continue the pregnancy, have a normal labour and delivery and produce a healthy child. Some of these factors involve correcting structure through chiropractic adjustment and using nutritional supplementation to correct imbalances caused through lack of specific nutrients, particularly magnesium and zinc.

While most people generally understand the need to grieve for the loss of a stillborn baby (after 20 weeks), often others do not understand that a miscarriage can also cause great grief and depression. If you have experienced miscarriage, talk to others who have been through the same experience. This is a time to ask for help, seek out a therapist. I have found emotional release work excellent following a miscarriage, it allows a time for grieving and saying goodbye whilst clearing the way for a healthy pregnancy next time.

The following are some suggestions that may assist in preventing miscarriage:

- refrain from sexual relations or any sexual stimulation when any spotting has occurred. Note that some women continue to spot at the time of what would have been their normal menses throughout their pregnancy without risk to their pregnancy. It seems to be a habitual thing the body continues with.
- take three grams of Vitamin C or other antioxidant formula daily to strengthen the immune system and capillary walls. I recommend FrequenSea.
- 1000mg magnesium combined with an excellent source of associated nutrients is important to maintain hormonal flow and reproductive health. Avoid all over the counter medications or medicinal herbs, without correct professional advice.
- take Omega-3 3000 mgs daily

If spotting has occurred complete bed rest is advisable for the next three days.

- when spotting ceases and there is no signs of cramping then gently begin to resume normal activities
- continue to rest daily for a couple of hours with feet up. Extra rest is essential.
- avoid hot baths, showers and spas. Do not use electric blankets or a heated waterbed as these may increase bleeding. Remove all potential sources of electro-magnetic radiation (such as electrical appliances) from the bedroom area.
- avoid lifting, especially toddlers and pets.

Remember rest will help to re-balance the body but it will not prevent a miscarriage if nature has intended this outcome.

If you have had several previous pregnancies then the uterus can become a little lax. The following may assist:

- elevating the foot of the bed can assist with alleviating pressure on the cervix
- magnesium and co-nutrients can assist in strengthening the muscles and cervical walls.

If heavy bleeding occurs contact medical assistance as soon as possible. Feel free to contact me for professional support, or in the event of miscarriage I can assist you, or you may wish to contact your local Naturopath for appropriate pre-conceptual help to encourage a healthy pregnancy next time.

Healing After a Miscarriage

Herbal Remedy

A favourite recipe is equal parts of licorice root, sarsaparilla, blessed thistle, black haw (or cramp bark), and squaw vine (partridge berry). If you are able to source the dried herb then mix equal parts of each and steep in boiling water to make a strong tea. Take in the following way:

Week 1 - one cup a day
Week 2 - one cup every other day; then progress to three days between cups, and finally choose a day for your last cup.

Placenta Praevia

In a normal pregnancy the placenta implants itself in the top part of the uterus. In placenta praevia the placenta implants itself close to or across the cervix and can get in the way of the baby's passage at birth. After two months of pregnancy this may indicate placenta praevia. This occurs in about five percent of pregnancies. The cause of placenta praevia is unknown, but it is more common in women who have had several children, which may indicate that placental scarring in the uterus from previous pregnancies plays a role.

At 18-20 weeks, the placenta is situated low in the uterus either close to, or covering the cervix. As pregnancy progresses however, the lower part of the uterus (known as the lower uterine section) elongates to help mould the baby's head and the placenta may naturally migrate up the side of the uterus clear of the cervix. In ninety five percent of cases the placenta will be clear of the birth canal by 37 weeks of pregnancy.

If you have bleeding after the twentieth week of pregnancy (possibly after sex) or haemorrhage in the last two months of pregnancy. Placenta praevia can be diagnosed by ultrasound and treatment involves bed rest.

You will most likely be informed at your 18-20 week scan that the placenta is lying low, but the chances of it moving up are high. Normally you are able to continue your normal everyday activities. A repeat ultrasound should however be arranged at around 28-32 weeks of pregnancy to determine if the placenta has moved away from the cervix.

A placenta which is praevia may cause vaginal bleeding in later pregnancy. Also in some cases the baby may need to be delivered by caesarean section. So in this situation extra care and monitoring of your baby and the placenta may be required. Your birth carer will discuss with you the best way to manage this situation and advise you of any precautions.

Placental Insufficiency

A healthy placenta is vital for maintaining a healthy baby. Placental insufficiency results in below average growth and development of the baby. A mother who has taken good care of herself by increasing her nutritional supplies through supplementation is less likely to experience this condition.

An insufficient placenta can prevent your baby from gaining essential nourishment. Symptoms for placental insufficiency may include below average weight gain, below average foetal development, or slow growth of the uterus. An ultrasound examination will determine if growth of the baby is adequate. Another useful sign is the activity of the baby in the last few months of pregnancy. Some maternity care providers suggest using a kick chart, explained in the 'Routine Procedures' section of this book. Close monitoring of your baby is imperative.

Placental Separation

Sometimes the placenta can separate from the uterus, either partially or completely. There is a slightly higher risk for women who have had several children, but the cause is unknown. Again taking good care of yourself and increasing superfoods throughout your pregnancy can reduce the risk. In mild cases, slight blood loss occurs and the condition is treated with bed rest and monitored by ultrasound, however labour may be induced if the pregnancy is close to term.

The condition is acute when more blood is lost and a large amount of the placenta separates from the wall. As usual, if you notice any unusual symptoms, such as bleeding or pain, advise your doctor or specialist straight away.

Emotional Balancing, Changing Your Harmful Habits

Stress

For many pregnancy is a wonderfully joyful time but for others it can be a very stressful state. Trying to juggle work, home and other children can be difficult when pregnant. The sheer nature of pregnancy can make you very tired in the first three months, particularly if there is nausea and morning sickness, which for some can last all day.

Dr. Thomas Verny states that:

> "a mother's anxiety-provoking hormones can flood her baby's system, making him worried and fearful. The developmental significance of emotional dependency between mother and child beginning in utero suggests that postnatal bonding is a continuum of security that, if missed, can cause a lifelong primal wound"
>
> Carista Luminare-Rosen, Ph.D.,
> Parenting Begins Before Conception,
> Healing Arts Press, 2000

Women who are anxious during pregnancy tend to have lower birth weight babies, probably because blood flow to the uterus is impaired. Researchers at Queen Charlotte's and Chelsea Hospital in London had 100 pregnant women complete questionnaires on anxiety levels during their third trimester. Anxiety scores were compared with results from colour Doppler ultrasound to measure uterine blood flow.

Of the women who were most anxious, twenty seven percent had an abnormally high uterine artery resistance score. This high resistance to blood flow has previously been shown to be associated with poor obstetric outcomes, especially impaired foetal growth and pre-eclampsia. Of the women who were least anxious only four percent had an increased resistance (Nursing Times, Jan. 27-Feb. 4, 1999).

Significant stress at work and home can lead to increased chances of preterm births, low birth weight infants and possibly less healthy children. Pregnant women who stand for long hours or work in a stressful environment for more than forty hours a week can increase the risk of having a preterm birth or of developing pre-eclampsia. Women who have stressful life events during pregnancy can be more likely to have preterm births.

In experiments on monkeys, the infants of mothers who were stressed during pregnancy showed increased abnormal social behaviour and had poorer motor abilities and shorter attention spans (Childbirth Forum, Summer 1997).

Stress can be extremely detrimental to your health. Today's lifestyle results in most people experiencing some level of stress. Psychosocial stress, defined as a lack of social support, has become prominent in western societies of the 21st century.

> "If we continue to do medicine in pieces, we will succeed in making one set of symptoms go away only to await the next and never truly deal with underlying health."
>
> Lonsdorf, Butler & Brown 1999, p.41.

Our response to stress is really our survival mechanism. Every thought, feeling or emotion we experience can cause stress. Stress is the negative feedback system of the fight and flight reaction. The reason that humans have survived as long as they have is due in some part to this response mechanism.

If we experience fear then our body needs to respond in such a way that we can either run from or stop and face the danger. Your brain concentrates on heightening the senses of sight, hearing and smell so that your mind can process thought faster and life saving decisions can be made in time. Adrenaline, sugar and other stimulants surge through your body. Blood is diverted from relatively unimportant functions such as the stomach, immune system and reproductive system to rush to those organs necessary for preparing your body to take action, including the musculoskeletal system, heart and lungs.

Once the danger is over breathing pattern returns to normal under the guidance of the parathyroid hormone (PTH), produced and released by the parathyroid gland. PTH regulates the amount of calcium, phosphorus and magnesium in the bones and blood. Minerals calcium and phosphorus are crucial for healthy bones. Blood-borne calcium is also needed for the proper functioning of muscle and nerve cells. When calcium levels in the blood are too low, the parathyroid glands release extra PTH, which leeches calcium from the bones and stimulates calcium re-absorption in the kidney. Alternately, if the level of calcium in the blood is too high the glands drop hormone production.

Problems can occur if the parathyroids are overactive or underactive. Stressing out over a long period of time puts too much pressure on the adrenals and the para-thyroids, eventually creating adrenal exhaustion. This can lead to hormonal imbalances, fertility problems, anxiety, depression, chronic fatigue and pregnancy stress and complications.

Humans no longer need this fight and flight response to survive against nature as was originally intended, but our minds create so many stressful thoughts that it is activated almost daily.

Your Mind

Your mind can be overpowering and at times very active, to the point of preventing rest and relaxation. The mind creates thoughts based on information from past experience, a bit like a data base of memory. The challenge is to become aware of what thoughts your mind is creating and whether they pertain to the present or relate to the past or future.

Your mind bases thoughts about new situations or events upon the experiences of the past, which in reality may have nothing to do with what is happening now or in the near future. Although the outcome is not yet known and may be completely different, your mind creates concern and worry as if the situation has already been perceived to have turned out wrong. Stress is created when the mind tries to take the body somewhere it can't go, such as backwards to a past event or forwards to a future event that has yet to occur.

This mind stress puts your body into the fight and flight response and is greatly damaging to your body. For instance if something doesn't go the way we plan, such as running late for a meeting, worrying about an impending rent increase or a relationship argument, the initial response creates tension in the body in readiness to either run from the problem or stay and work it through. It is like being on the run for twenty four hours a day and is exhausting for your body.

Sometimes just thinking about what might have happened is enough to trigger the response. When this response is triggered we look for everything that could possibly go wrong. It is natural to look for the negative rather than the positive. We look for connecting incidents that caused similar responses in order to validate what we are feeling. The fight and flight mechanism gets stronger the more we seek the negative response. All the resources of the body are set into specific actions so it becomes a self-sabotaging or self-fulfilling prophecy.

Because our lifestyles invariably place us in the situation of stress, the fight and flight mechanism is continually activated. Maintaining this response is exhausting for your body and uses a tremendous amount of nutrients.

Your body thus becomes susceptible to disease because the immune system is depleted, and digestion is impaired because blood is drawn away from the digestive system. Over time this causes imbalances resulting in a lack of nutrient absorption and eventually Gut Dysbiosis (an over-growth of unwanted bacteria and gut toxins). Emergency chemicals are released, but not used. These break down into toxic substances that need to be excreted, placing a heavy workload on your liver.

This downward mind/body spiral cannot continue indefinitely without taking its toll on your body, and may eventually lead to depression and fatigue.

The Telltale Signs Of Stress
Tightness in the throat or chest

- dry mouth
- nagging pain in the stomach
- loss of concentration, erratic mood swings
- loneliness
- loss of memory
- restlessness
- fear of silence
- loss of appetite
- impatience
- palpitations
- sleeplessness
- obsessive behaviour
- sharp anger
- insecurity
- not socialising
- not answering the phone
- compulsive behaviour
- fatigue

People with a higher level of stress in their life are prone to illness and body imbalance more frequently than those less stressed. Stress perpetuates stress, as the cells become accustomed to stressful behaviour and replicate the metabolism accordingly.

Healthiness reflects order and unification of the spirit, mind and body. A happy, well person is likely to be radiant, full of life, energetic and clear minded. Their cellular structure radiates health because they are producing natural opiates such as oxytocin and endorphins. Their body is in unison with their mind and spirit. Inner harmony is possibly the greatest treasure that most would seek.

Anxiety

Anxiety is a state or feeling of apprehension, uneasiness, agitation, uncertainty and fear resulting from the anticipation of threat or danger. Characteristics may be subjective or objective.

- objective characteristics include cardiovascular excitation, vasoconstriction, pupil dilation, restlessness, insomnia, trembling and increased perspiration

- subjective characteristics include increased tension, apprehension, increased helplessness, fear, distress, worry and feelings of over-excitement.

In pregnancy this can prelude Antenatal Depression or lead to Postnatal Depression.

Ways to deal with Anxiety and Fears

See fear as a natural safety mechanism. Fear assists you to judge a situation and escape if you need to for your health and wellbeing. Too much fear can be harmful as may prevent you from taking positive risks and opportunities, doing what you want and being the best you can be.

It is okay to be fearful as long as it is manageable. If you have issues dealing with your fears and anxiety, here are the some strategies to incorporate in your daily life.

1. **Positive thinking.** Changing your thoughts changes your behaviour. It takes practice, but becoming aware of what you are thinking then choosing to switch your thought to a positive one can make a huge difference. Looking at the glass as half full instead of half empty. **You** are in charge of what goes on in your mind, the choice is yours to decide what you want to think about. Remember, your thoughts fuel your actions!

2. **Accept the fact that you have fears.** Fear is a normal part of life, it is important to express how you feel, accept it. Being positive is not denying how you feel, it is understanding that you feel this way then choosing to let it go. Take time to feel sad, worried, fearful, or anxious. The more you push these feelings away, the more they will be stored in your body, creating dis-ease.

3. **Be your best friend.** The first person to understand you should be you. Look in the mirror and speak kindly to you. Acknowledge all the great things you have done in your life. Pamper yourself so that you feel loved and appreciated by you. Spend time with

yourself doing things that relax you. Learn to hang out with you, it can be such great fun.

4. **Seek out a therapist.** Find ways to understand and let go of your fears and anxieties. Seeing a professional therapist can assist you to remove the neuro emotional charge, the triggers that create the stress. They can also help you formulate strategies to observe your behaviour so you can better understand why you react the way you do and how you can change it.

5. **Practice deep breathing.** When you breathe your mind is occupied with focusing on breathing. Your body is able to relax, receive oxygen and nutrients as well as clear the charge that is causing the reaction. Breath breaks the emotional reaction cycle. See Psychosomatic Breathing.

6. **Hang out with positive people.** Choose positive relationships, even if that means removing yourself from your family for a while. Sometimes we need space to create new habitual behaviour with constructive, supportive people.

7. **Be mind aware.** Amidst your busy schedule, take a few minutes to relax and de-stress your mind and body. While on a bus for instance, just close your eyes and visualise yourself being in a peaceful, tranquil place. Slowly drop your worries and anxieties, and feel your heartbeat slowing down. Self awareness meditation is one proven strategy to manage fears and anxiety.

8. **Gratitude.** Practice gratitude meditation. Recite in your mind all the things you are blessed with - for example running water, food, comfortable bed, a roof over your head, a body that is functional and healthy. When you awaken say thank you to your pillow and bed. Expect to feel refreshed and optimistic! Make this a daily habit and you will see how it can greatly improve your quality of life.

9. **Choose life.** Your daily routine affects how you think. Get up and exercise! Attend a yoga class, eat healthy, sleep on time, avoid alcohol and cigarettes and de-stress regularly! Try out different activities until you find what you really like doing.

10. **Focus on your most important values.** Focus your mind on the things you want rather than on what you don't want.

Dealing with Stress

There is only one kind of healing - self-healing.

Your cells are agents of renewal, enabling your body-mind to regenerate consistently and purposefully. Every atom in your body is replaced annually governed by the laws of nature. Every second millions of cells are created, of which approximately one third are abnormal and are deleted by your immune system. The efficiency of your immune system relies on the state of harmony and peace your body is in - healthy body-mind communication.

What you think and what you feel feeds negative or positive energy to your cells, creating negative or positive environments that your cells regenerate in. The choice is a conscious decision from an attitude of mind that directs the unconscious behaviour of the body.

> "The cells in your body react to everything that your mind says. Negativity brings down your immune system."
> http://rawforbeauty.com/blog/?s=The+cells+in+your+body+
> react+to+everything+that+your+mind+says.+Negativity+
> brings+down+your+immune+system.

Harmony and calmness are absolutely vital in pregnancy. Continuity of care during pregnancy and birth is very important. I thoroughly recommend that you find yourself a midwife who is prepared to spend time with you during your pregnancy to clear any fears or concerns you may have and is prepared to be with you for the birth and to care for you after. Support is one of the main things I am able to provide through my practice.

It is important not to struggle on alone. Seek professional help such as reflexology, breathing exercises, counselling, massage, relaxation, yoga, meditation and neuro emotional therapies. Specific herbal formulas can be very successful when given under practitioner supervision.

High quality nutrition is of utmost importance during times of stress as your body uses up vast amounts of nutrients to cope with the excessive demand for energy. Take time to feel your feelings. This new life is connected to you, the mother, and will take on your emotional baggage. Stressed mothers are far more likely to have stressed babies.

In my practice I have found FrequenSea with Marine Phytoplankton, Frankincense, Rose and Nutmeg Oil to be an exceptional food for the nervous system. The Frankincense and Rose are very calming and nurturing to the brain cells.

http://casadelsole.fgxpress.com/farmers-market/

Emotional aspects to consider here could be a very strong need to control life and the outcome of the pregnancy. There could be high expectations or a feeling of being overworked and overburdened, and over worry and concern of what being a parent may mean.

Relax in a bath of essential oils combining 10 drops Lavender, Geranium & Palma Rosa or use as a massage oil, whilst affirming and visualising:

I stay in truth, live and move in joy, I love life and allow things to flow naturally. I let go and trust.

See _Anxiety and Stress_ in the 'Complimentary Therapies For Discomforts of Pregnancy' section.

Reflexology points to work:

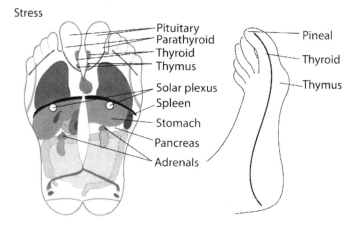

'Aim for success, not perfection.

Never give up your right to be wrong,

Or then you will lose the ability to learn new things and move forward with your life.

Remember that fear always lurks behind perfectionism.

Confronting your fears and allowing yourself the right to be human can paradoxically, make you a far happier and more productive person.'

Dr. David M. Burns

http://feelinggood.com/

Clearing Subconscious Thought Patterns

My philosophy is that whatever is created in the physical body has come from some subconscious thought or belief system. Injury and disease mostly occur if there is an imbalance in that part of the body in the first place.

For example consider two people sitting in a car at a stoplight. Unknowingly they are shunted from behind by another car. The passenger who tends to be flexible in their thinking and more relaxed will go with the impact and therefore is likely to receive less injury. The passenger who is rigid in their thoughts and actions will most likely sustain an injury in the neck and shoulders due to resistance created from the imbalances and stress.

Thus whilst people may endure the same accident the impact on their body will depend on what weaknesses and imbalances already exist.

We have three states of mind:

1. the unconscious mind
2. the sub-conscious mind
3. the conscious mind.

The Unconscious Mind

Is the one that looks after us, connected to the body and intuition. The unconscious mind contains the necessary intelligences for your survival, such as digestion, healing, movement, genetic intelligence and physical growth. In other words looks after our existence. When did you last think about breathing? The unconscious mind is the large abyss that human science has yet to explore. Only greatly disciplined Yogis have had the ability to control the unconscious mind, some to the point of hardly breathing. This takes years of disciplined training, most people have no idea what their unconscious mind is doing. Pregnancy and labour is governed by the unconscious mind.

The Sub-conscious Mind

Estimated to be eighty eight percent of our mind, this is where you hold the patterns and programs that drive your life. This is why changing behaviours and beliefs can sometimes take considerable effort. Consider that whilst you may be actively using the twelve percent provided by the logical conscious mind, the core belief stored in the subconscious mind may be quite different. Overcoming these subconscious beliefs is the challenge and where emotional release therapy truly assists.

The sub-conscious mind holds our memories and emotional attachments, the movies that we continually 're-run'. When you hear music or smell a certain perfume a memory may be triggered of a pleasant or unpleasant experience, triggering a positive or negative emotional response. The sub-conscious mind often needs tending to. Through actively making decisions regarding our thought patterns by using the conscious mind we can change the emotional response triggered by the memory.

The Conscious Mind

The conscious mind is connected to the ego and wants to be right based on previous experience, ignoring feelings and pushing the body to do. The conscious mind is the thinker, the worrier, predominantly thinking about yesterday or tomorrow, tending to waste a lot of energy because it is not thinking about the here and now. The conscious mind contains your everyday thoughts and is the decision maker, even though those decisions are often fed by the subconscious memories.

The conscious mind is estimated to hold only twelve percent of our beliefs, the majority being held in the deeper layers of the subconscious mind. Often the logical conscious mind holds a different idea to that of the belief you actually hold. This is why body testing works so effectively, as it shortcuts the conscious mind directly to the subconscious mind. Many people are surprised when they test positive to a belief that does not make sense to their logical mind. For instance, you may think you have no issue around finances, but when tested you may test positive to a deep held subconscious belief that prevents you from having abundance.

The Superconscious

There is a never-ending flood of personal power, intuition, insight, creativity and love available to you when you tap into this amazing resource within you. The superconscious is the only way through to who and what you truly are, to a permanent and higher state of consciousness.

This is where intuition, inspiration, higher intelligence, genius, psychic powers and creativity live. It is the part of your mind that integrates with the absolute consciousness or supreme intelligence of life itself. The power to make your life what you want it to be, to awaken your artistic and creative powers, to become a great spouse and parent - these things can only come from your superconscious.

The unconscious, subconscious and conscious are contained within your mind. Your superconscious has access to all aspects of higher intelligence. It is in touch with your individuality as well as the intelligence of life itself. This is why coincidences can happen. Opening to your superconscious not only allows you to awaken to your innermost nature, but it also gives you the means to create your life in whatever way you want it to be. Visualising and creating ideal labour and birth is activating the superconscious.

Affirming statements and positive visuals work at placing new behaviours and thought patterns associated with conditioning into the unconscious mind. By doing this you are erasing the sub-conscious patterns.

We have an innate ability to attach ourselves to material belongings and especially to other human beings. When we suffer the heartache attached to a loss it is lodged deeply within our sub-conscious mind as a strong feeling or emotion. Recall is triggered by a conscious thought, smell or vision, which results in the feelings being replayed.

Counselling often works at bringing these feelings to the fore, with the hope that eventually the pain associated will be less. Unfortunately this is not always successful and often just becomes a record being replayed and replayed. The attachment at the sub-conscious level has to be broken by breaking the pattern.

Emotional Release Techniques

I use several emotional release techniques in daily practice. The process of emotional release has the potential to provide profound change, assisting with the release of old behaviours, thought patterns and beliefs that may be preventing you from being or doing all that you are truly capable of.

The Process

My belief in this process has led to the development of my own emotional release process, called 'The Process'. You can visit my website for further information (www.casadelsole.com.au).

Why is emotional release so effective? Because the cells of your body hold memory. The memory is created when you have a strong emotional reaction to a situation. Peptides and hormones create a neuro

363

emotional charge (NEC) that lock onto the cell surface and create a cellular reaction. Then each time the emotional memory is triggered, the reaction occurs again, with each response becoming more embedded until the response becomes habit. This is why we often find ourselves in a similar situation over and over again wondering why we keep repeating this same behavioural pattern. Each organ and gland meridian in the body has tendencies towards certain emotions. For example the liver holds anger, resentment is stored in the gall bladder, grief in the lungs. This explored further in the Eastern Techniques.

The trained practitioner uses muscle testing to discover which meridians in your body are holding the energy and then use word association to track down the memory. Specific techniques can then be used to interrupt the pathway and delete out the data. The result is that you can still experience the memory without the emotional pain or charge.

Some of these techniques are:

- The Process
- Psychosomatic Therapy
- Neuro Emotional Technique
- EFT
- Kinesiology
- Theta Healing
- Emotional Release Therapy

Relaxation Exercises

Endorphins are hormones that occur naturally in the body. Endorphins are released in response to positive thoughts, laughter, joy, love and when we experience a sense of well-being. Endorphins are also produced in response to an injury or physical stress to reduce pain and promote a feeling of wellbeing. Morphine and related medications have a similar chemical structure to endorphins, which explains their strong pain-killing effects. In fact, 'endorphin' is made up of two words, endogenous or native to the body and morphine, an opiate-like substance.

Runners and other athletes experience a natural 'high' after about half an hour of sustained physical exertion. This is attributed to the steady release of endorphins during exercise, which reaches a threshold point within an hour, before which time their effect cannot usually be felt. This is one of the reasons exercise is such a great antidote to stress. The same occurs in labour, natural painkillers are released throughout.

The 'Gating' Effect

This pain relieving technique is very simply described using the example of stubbing your toe then rubbing it to ease the pain. Pain messages travel via the nerves to your brain, where they are interpreted and tell you that you actually feel the pain. Rubbing this same toe vigorously releases endorphins, which travel to your brain faster than the pain messages, thus reducing pain. Breathing deeply and expressing what you feel also helps.

In other words, the rubbing sensation has 'closed the gate', so painful messages cannot get through. Touch, focus and breath can activate endorphins at any time as can positive thoughts and behaviours. This is why touch, focus and breath is so commonly used in labour to distract your mind from the intensity of the experience.

The greatest thing we can do to improve the world is to change our thoughts to positive ones.

Tuning your frequency to activate endorphins rather than adrenaline is far less taxing or stressful on your body. The following simple technique has been created to help tune your thoughts to positive ones, thus helping you to produce stress reducing healing endorphins.

Exercise 1- Awareness

Our bodies produce a frequency which generates four volts or thirty eight hertz of power. This has been measured and if you sit quietly and tune into your body you will feel this energy as a sense of lightness or tingling.

Sometimes we can feel other peoples' energy, especially if they are particularly excited, happy or angry. Our energy system picks up on this frequency and depending on the message we receive, we decide if it is safe or if we need to move away from it.

Often our frequencies are emitted without us consciously being aware. For example you may think of a friend only to find that same friend telephones not long after the initial thought. How often do you hear the words 'I was just thinking about you'. Is it coincidence? Not necessarily. It is possible that our own generated power carries our thoughts by way of intent through the airwaves, especially when activated from the heart chakra. If we truly embrace and understand this fact we can intent anything and make manifest our daily happenings. Test it out for yourself and see what happens. Take notice of how you feel in different circumstances and observe the feelings and vibrations around you.

Exercise 2 - Change the Channel

It is only natural to change the channel on a radio if you do not like what you are listening to. Therefore why not choose to change the channel on what is playing in your mind if it doesn't serve you?

So why do we persist in listening to the same old songs and stories we play in our heads, songs that remind us of our traumatic experiences or stresses we have felt previously or are currently experiencing? Simply choose to change the channel and focus your mind on something that feels good. With practice this becomes a way of being.

Exercise 3 - Clock

We can change the channel of the experience or stress that's playing over and over in our head, but it must firstly be identified that it exists and is real.

Sit quietly, close your eyes and take a few moments to think of an experience that has stressed you:

- how does your body feel?
- where is it located/ where do you feel it in your body?
- what happens to your breathing?

It is quite likely that you experienced a tightening in your body, a quickening of your breath and an overall sense of tension. Give this experience a time on the clock, for example 3pm.

Now take three very deep and long breaths, exhale with a sigh. Feel your body soften and calm down as it shuts off adrenaline. Think of an experience that makes you feel happy, relaxed, fun filled or warm and fuzzy. It may be the people you love, the animals that unconditionally adore you, the places throughout your life that have captivated your soul, foods you like eating. Let your mind run wild with these wonderful thoughts. Again notice how does your body feel? It is likely that you are feeling lighter in every sense. Give this feeling a different time on the clock, for example 6pm. This number now represents the happy events. This number now becomes your key to happy energy flow in your body.

This activity generates endorphins, the happy hormones that heal and relax our body systems.

All it takes is a choice.

You may be in the middle of a stressful situation that you have no control over, such as a fight between two other people which doesn't involve you, other than being in the same vicinity. You may be instantly transported back in your mind to an experience you had earlier in your life, which can tune your channel into the stress around you and the memory of what happened to you.

The key here is to breathe, don't buy into what the other people are expressing. Change your own frequency to the number on the clock face that represents love and harmony. Your frequency will instantly be picked up by the other two people fighting and the ripple of your calming frequency will have a calming effect on them.

The only way to peaceful resolutions is to intent calmness, sometimes a real challenge but one worth considering.

Throughout the day pause and check what you are feeling, what your stress levels are, then make a conscious choice to feel at '6pm'.

Exercise 4 - Bio-Field Balance

Step 1: Scan your body - close your eyes and tune into your body. Feel if it feels even and balanced.

- scan your legs for feelings of one being longer or shorter, thicker or thinner, heavier or lighter
- scan your arms for feelings of one being longer or shorter, thicker or thinner, heavier or lighter
- scan your neck for feelings of lopsidedness, tense muscles or stiffness
- scan your spine for any discomforts or feelings of crookedness.

Step 2: Introduce the Time Line

1. imagine a silver thread coming into the centre of your forehead, going through the centre of your head and out the back of your head
2. check that this is straight. Your future lies ahead, your present is in your head, your past is behind, gone and unable to be seen.

Sometimes your time line can become off centre or even go sideways. This is a good indication that you are off your 'path' and feeling 'out of sorts'. Just recognising this and bringing your timeline back into balance will have a great beneficial effect.

Step 3: Imagine You Are Walking Barefoot Along a Lovely Soft Path Made Of Grass Or Sand (not concrete, gravel etc)

As you walk along this path ask your Higher Self which way do you need to walk to bring balance to your body.

- do you need to move forwards or backwards, to the left or right or combinations of these (eg. forward and to the right, back and to the left). Move in whatever way you would like to and as far as necessary.

- after the first move check if your legs, arms neck and spine feel more balanced
- an adjustment has most probably occurred, but if you don't' feel balanced look back at the path and make another move in any direction. You may feel like swimming, running, dancing, let your mind run wild.

DO NOT use your logic - the first thought is always the right direction.

Keep checking with your body and fine tuning it by adjusting your moves on the path. If you cannot attune your body you may need to get off the path and do something else like get on a pogo stick, bounce off onto a mountain in the distance to sit on top and admire the view, or even go for a swim in a river nearby.

You may need to strip off your clothing and wander into a beautiful pool beside the path to lie there and relax. You may need to simply sit on a log beside the path or wander off the path completely. Your first thought will always be right. Let it guide you where you need to be on the path.

Finally

If you feel still not quite balanced look at what emotion is upsetting you. Where are you feeling it in your body? Now give it a shape. Focus and watch it change shape, softening and becoming smaller until eventually it disappears. Now check how you feel. You are bound to feel better. This is a great technique to use before going to sleep. By attuning the etheric body the physical body can become balanced. Please use this and pass it on to others.

Affirmations

'The words "I am..." are potent words;
Be careful what you hitch them to.
The thing you're claiming has a way
of reaching back and claiming you.'

A. L. Kitselman, E-Therapy, Masterworks International.

Affirmations are like a blatant lie to the sub-conscious mind, told over and over again. Consciously saying the affirmations every day and visualising the desired outcome tricks the mind into believing it is true. This eventually creates reality and over time becomes a new behaviour.

Two basketball teams of equal talent were used in an experiment. One team spent an hour every day visualising and constructing his or her game plan and spent less time in physical practice. The other team practiced solidly every day on the court for the same amount of time. The team that used visualisations and affirmations played a strong, well-constructed game and won easily.

We can work on the physical perspective emphatically but without the conviction of the mind the result will always be substandard. Focus on the birth you would like, not on what you fear.

Fear and Love

Emotional reactions come from two basic thought processes, fear or love. Fear or love, the first emotions felt by baby in the womb, can be carried from generation to generation within the cellular structure that makes up your body. New cells replicate according to their environment, taking on a negative or a positive energy depending on the thought patterns and emotional vibrations at the time.

We all transmit invisible signals to those around us. Our belief systems send out a vibration which others are affected by. Your thoughts and emotions are powerful, others pick up and respond to your thoughts and emotional vibration. That is how we evolve as a race. When enough of us believe in something it becomes manifest. This has been discovered in many experiments and is still an enigma to many a scientist. It is often referred to as the hundred monkey syndrome.

Affirming, especially last thing at night, enables new cells to change whilst you sleep. Success depends on practice, repetition and intent. On average change will occur within 21-28 days of daily practice.

Exercise 5 - Visualing Your Birth

Begin by visualising the labour and birth that you would like. Bring detail to the vision so you can see it like a video. Re-run this video in your mind as often as you think to, at least twice a day. A meditative space does assist in a deeper memory shift. The process relies on trust. Australian Bush Flowers can certainly help shift emotional blockages as well. Watch positive birth videos and read positive birth stories. Saturate your mind with positive ideas.

Write down three words that represent how you feel at this moment. Then investigate ways to turn these feelings into affirming statements and explore alternative sub-conscious visualisations. By doing this you will be concentrating on the positive not the negative.

Socialise with positive and supportive people who have similar beliefs to you. When we are clear about what it is we desire for ourselves and the kinds of relationships we hope for with the people around us, we can begin to put out the energy necessary to make those things happen.

We do affect the world around us by our thoughts and our behaviour. Focus on what you would like to happen, rather than on what you are worried might happen, and you are more likely to set up the environment that will attract your desires. You are also more likely to be aware of options and opportunities you wouldn't otherwise allow yourself to see.

An example is when you constantly worry about something that could go wrong tomorrow, you are actually sending out a chain reaction of thought energy that programs the subconscious mind to create it. If instead you think about the outcome you desire then the subconscious mind is programmed to create that desire.

As explained in the section Fear Creates Pain, fear interferes with the birth process. It can be an exhausting experience trying to allay a woman's fears whilst helping her give birth, compared to the less energy required when she has trust in the process.

An affirmation is in the now, not in the future. If you constantly say I want then the state of being created is a state of want. Whereas saying and seeing I have then the state created is that of having.

Using the words 'I am' pulls on every bit of what you are stating to validate it. You do not have to believe your affirmation, although the stronger the intent the quicker the outcome.

Doreen Virtue recently studied the vibration of words and found that negative words have a flat vibration whereas words that are positive have a high vibration. Positive, loving words affect the cells of the body in a healing way. The most healing and powerful word is Peace. Simply stating 'I am at Peace' can have a relaxing effect.

Pregnancy Meditation

In the yogic tradition our sensual creative reproductive energy is known as kundalini shakti, seen as a coiled serpent that lies at the base of the spine and rises up through the body toward the head. As it rises it passes through the chakra energy centres. Each chakra has its own colour and sound. Meditation on the chakras arouses the kundalini energy and balances the body. For more information on the chakras see <u>The Chakra System</u>.

Yoga is an ideally designed practice to not only train your mind and body, but to access your chakras. The word yoga means yoke or union. Yoga is both energising and relaxing. In traditional practice in China and Japan pregnant women were encouraged to practice meditation daily and to communicate with their babies during pregnancy in the following way:

- Sit quietly either crossed legged (lotus positon) or on a chair with your legs uncrossed, well supported with the feet directly below on the floor so that your posture is in the upright position (your back straight and head in line with your spine, not pushing forward).

- It is better to meditate sitting rather than lying as the energy moves up the body from the earth below and you are less likely to fall asleep.
- Take a few deep breaths and allow yourself to let go, relax and become quiet, calm and centred. Bring your attention to your baby. Visualise your baby's tiny body enveloped in the warmth and safety of your nutrient rich womb.
- Take a moment to connect with your baby and allow yourself to sense what he/she may be feeling or experiencing.
- Imagine the warm amniotic fluid caressing your baby's body and what it must be like to float lightly, blissfully and fluidly without the restraints of gravity.

The psychic connection between you and your baby is established long before the birth. Your baby feels what you feel, so the more calm and relaxed you are the more your baby will be on entering the world. In the womb your baby moves while awake and also sleeps and dreams.

Alongside the physical body, emotional responses and senses such as hearing, sight, smell and touch develop. When you breathe deeply your baby's movements increase to bring attention so that you can centre your awareness on the child within. You will find the best moments in pregnancy are when you sit blissfully connected to your child.

Preparation
for Birth

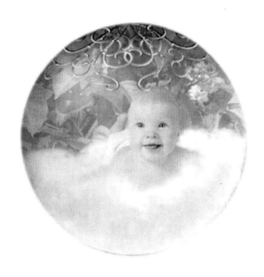

Bill Of Rights

The World Health Organisation Recommends:

- women should be able to move around during labour and choose a position for birth that best suits them
- drugs should not be routinely used for pain relief
- babies must not be separated from their mothers and breastfeeding should be promoted.

And Argues:

- electronic monitoring of the baby's heart in labour should not be routine
- induction rates should not be higher than 10 percent of pregnancies
- artificial rupture of the membranes (bag of waters) should not be routine
- episiotomies (perineal surgery) should be avoided
- the Caesarean section rate in any region should not be higher than 10 - 15 percent.   http://www.who.int/topics/pregnancy/en/

What Does 'Natural Birth' Mean?

To many it means able to give birth the way nature intended, for others it means without any medical assistance, to others it means being surrounded by the people they choose in their own environment. What it does imply is that which comes as a natural occurrence to the individual. One woman choosing to birth lying down doesn't make her birth any less natural than the one who chooses to squat. The woman who chose to lie down may have found squatting totally foreign to her natural way of being so squatting may have caused her undue stress.

Childbirth education is about helping women become attuned to their own body, to know what is right for them and know their limitations. This is often difficult for women, especially if their conditioning has been to ignore their body's signals for the sake of others. Birthing is as individual as playing sport (so to speak) some love it, others hate it. One would wonder that 'natural' birth and childbirth education are contradictory to each other. If a woman is able to give birth naturally then why does she need to be taught at all?

> "Doesn't the female body who knows how to grow a body also know how to birth it?"
>
> Elizabeth Noble, 'Channel for a New Life, The Outdoor Water Birth of Carsten Noble Sorger', 1988.

Unfortunately not all maternity units, doctors and midwives treat women as being able to do what their body is designed to do and birth naturally. When birth attendants do not have faith in women's ability to birth they may assert their own perceptions, fears and doubts onto birthing couples. If a woman was encouraged at each antenatal check to take note of her body's signals, then her attunement with her body would increase rapidly. How often do we hear from experienced midwives that the births that are best are those left to their own progress? This is not promoting irresponsible birthing but encouraging birth attendees to look to the mother for signals rather than to technology.

Why Keep Birth Natural

Michel Odent (1999) clearly expresses this concern in his well researched book, 'The Scientification of Love'. His website contains thousands of research papers that reinforce why we need to keep birth normal. The sad thing is that in order to keep things natural we have to prove why.

www.birthworks.org/primalhealth.com

Being born

> "The stress of journeying through the birth canal is not harmful to most infants. In fact, the surge of "stress" hormones it triggers can be important to the neonate's survival outside the womb."
>
> Lagercrantz & Slotkin 1986.

A 1999 survey of English female obstetricians and midwives found that one third of the obstetricians would prefer a caesarean birth, compared to ninety six percent of the 135 English midwives surveyed who stated they preferred a vaginal delivery (British Medical Journal 319, Oct. 9, 1999). Authors of the study said that female obstetricians were more likely to opt for a caesarean because they rarely attend an uncomplicated delivery, and that witnessing traumatic deliveries drives them to prefer a caesarean, regardless of the fact that it entails major abdominal surgery with a recovery period of at least two months. Midwives on the other hand are generally the primary carer for a woman following caesarean, making them aware of the difficulties a woman has nursing and caring for an infant following what amounts to major abdominal surgery. Obstetricians tend to be held in high esteem by women and therefore have immense influence on birthing women's choices worldwide. This has resulted in an increasing number of women choosing elective caesarean sections. It is predicted by some experts that by the middle of this century caesarean sections will become the norm, with most women choosing not to face what they see as the unpredictable outcomes of vaginal birth.

But in avoiding the journey of labour both mother and baby miss a vital emotional and hormonal experience imperative to life itself. The impact of this upon society could be immense. Will we breed a society void of primal urges? Looking beyond the perinatal period Michel Odent is able to express why it is so important not to disturb the natural process of birth in terms of the long-term effect on the next generation.

During birth the baby is squeezed through the birth canal for up to several hours, during which the head sustains considerable pressure. The baby is intermittently deprived of oxygen by compression of the placenta and the umbilical cord during the uterine contractions. Baby is then delivered from a warm, dark, sheltered environment to the cold bright lights of the delivery room. What a shock!

Throughout the strains of birth, hypoxia and pressure on the head the baby produces unusually high levels of the 'stress' hormones adrenaline and nor adrenaline (catecholamines, the fight and flight hormones). These catecholamine levels are higher than those produced by adults under taxing circumstances such as heart attack, the presence of these hormones would usually indicate life threatening stress. However this is not the case for the birthing baby under normal circumstances. The stress response of the baby is more limited than that of the adult. The adult, who can fight or run in response to stress, is equipped to increase the heart rate and shunt oxygen-rich blood to muscles in response to stress. The baby needs to withstand oxygen deprivation and is exquisitely equipped to do just that and little else.

Research by Hugo Lagercrantz and Theodore A. Slotkin showed that the baby is well equipped to withstand stress, even early in gestation, and that the catecholamines afford much of the protection from such adverse conditions as hypoxia. The finding was that catecholamines prepare the baby for survival outside the womb, therefore it is important for the baby to undergo stress inducing moments during birth to elicit the production of stress hormones. These hormones assist in physiological changes that clear the lungs ready for breathing, mobilise readily useable fuel to nourish cells, ensure that a rich supply of blood goes to the heart and brain and may even promote attachment between mother and baby.

Foetal monitoring often detects subtle changes in the foetal heart rate during uterine contractions. In exploring the monitoring process researchers have found that the normal birth process gives rise to a surprisingly large increase of plasma catecholamines in human infants. Even at the beginning of labour levels were found to be five times as high as the concentration in a resting adult. After birth the catecholamine levels were found to have doubled or tripled again, indicating that they surged during the next stage when the mother was pushing. Studies further revealed that those infants who were asphyxiated due to a breech position or umbilical cord involvement had catecholamine levels as high as 500 - 1000 nanomols per litre of plasma, which would cause a stroke in adults but acts to protect the baby during a stressed labour.

Research revealed that pressure to the head during second stage of delivery and a resultant hypoxia seen in all newborns also increased the secretion of catecholamines. Babies delivered by caesarean without labour had low catecholamine levels. Those delivered during labour by an emergency caesarean had a surge only slightly lower than that of vaginally delivered infants.

The role of the catecholamines is not only to protect the baby during delivery, but also to enhance the infant's ability to function effectively when separated from its mother. This includes facilitating breathing and other effects that prepare the infant to survive a lack of nourishment, oxygen deprivation or other adversities during the first few hours of birth.

Breathing is an important adaptation by the baby and catecholamines surge at delivery to facilitate this change. Infants born of elective caesareans often suffer from breathing difficulties, usually due to inadequate absorption of lung liquid at birth causing wet lungs and an inadequate production of surfactant. Both rely heavily on the sustained increase of plasma catecholamines in the hours immediately before birth. It is also crucial to lung function not only after birth but within a couple of days after birth. Studies of vaginally delivered infants compared with surgically delivered infants showed few differences immediately at birth, but within two hours of birth the vaginally delivered infants had significantly better lung compliance.

In addition to promoting normal breathing, a catecholamine surge before birth also speeds up the infant's metabolic rate at birth. This accelerates the breakdown of stored energy into forms that can nourish cells once the infant no longer receives a steady supply of nutrients from the umbilical cord. The formation of the sugar glucose, free fatty acids and glycerol all occur immediately after a normal delivery at much higher rates than those born by elective caesarean.

The third major adaptation effect of a sharp catecholamine rise during delivery is to alter blood flow. The vaginally delivered infant is born with an enhanced blood flow to vital organs, and a restricted flow to the periphery, especially enhancing the survival chances of newborn experiencing breathing difficulties. Catecholamines continue to be important to the newborn's survival during stress, just as they are for the unborn or the adult. If a newborn is starved for several days, the catecholamine response mobilises needed fuel from the liver's glycogen stores and from fat. If a baby becomes cold, stored brown fat is mobilised to produce heat.

Infants delivered by elective caesarean section are at a disadvantage. Therefore it is best to allow a mother to labour as far as possible before commencing a caesarean section. Drugs also interfere with the catecholamine production, hence the breathing difficulties of infants born to mother's drugged in labour.

It should be a comfort to parents to know that from the infants' standpoint the stress of labour during normal delivery is likely to be less unhappy and more beneficial than logic would believe. For more detailed information read the article, 'The "Stress" of Being Born', Scientific America, April 1986.

Based on this research, if you require an 'elective ceasarean' please allow yourself to labour for as long as possible before undertaking the ceasarean. Elective caesareans are generally scheduled at the doctor's convenience rather than the baby's.

> "Birth does work, almost all of the time. When we trust that it will and when we are respectful and relaxed. I remind women over and over and over again that they come from strong and proven stock, that their grandmothers had babies, and their great-grandmas, and their great-great-great grandmas—all of their ancestors since the beginning of time have birthed—and they have been designed to birth, as well! I also remind them that contrary to what we have been taught (oh Oprah, would I love a private session with you, sweet woman!) and shown on TV programs like ER, when you are respectful of the process, birth is not a disaster waiting to happen. I am extraordinarily grateful for the help that we are

given by skilled, attentive and supportive doctors when there is a situation that needs additional expertise. However, with healthy mothers it is rare to have an emergency that is not preceded by a situation, which, had it been addressed, would not have escalated into a complication or an emergency (this, too, is a subject for another day). And being in the hospital does not preclude birthing women from having problems; in fact, being there often creates the problems that are then "solved" with devices—and knives"

Nancy Wainer, Midwifery Today 2001

Is Hospital Safer?

Different care givers have differing philosophies when it comes to birth. There are two main models of care, medical and midwifery. Within these two models will fall both medical carers and midwives who cross both disciplines with their beliefs.

I have come across many midwifes who have little faith in the birthing process, believing intervention to be best. I generally term these midwives as obstetric nurses. There are also obstetricians who behave more like midwives than doctors, those people who have a strong belief in natural birth, and I have had the pleasure of working alongside one or two of them.

Woman-Centred Care

The medical model defines birth within a medical framework, assuming there are inherent risks. It manifests that all women should be treated equally, with routine medical tests and interventions to ensure a safe delivery, generally within a hospital complex near neonatal intensive care and operative theatres. This has been the dominant birthing option in our society for over fifty years. However with more research supporting natural birth as a preferred option for the better outcome for mother and baby, more mother-baby friendly options are becoming available based on woman-centred care, generally care provided by midwives.

The woman-centred model uses a more holistic approach, where the woman is treated as an individual and assessed personally, having a choice of birth environment such as home, birth- centre or hospital. Research repeatedly proves that women who birth within this model of care experience less pain due to the natural flow of endorphins. This happens because the mother is more relaxed in a trusting environment. The reduced pain means the mother is less likely to experience intervention, especially if the birth place choice is home.

Midwives or doctors who provide woman-centred care tend to be more patient, not driven by policy or procedures which put undue stress on the birthing woman. If the woman is birthing at home or in a birth centre she is more likely to have the same midwife throughout her pregnancy and birth. This brings many benefits as the midwife knows the mother and has built a relationship of trust. The midwife is also fully focused on one labour, not trying to cope with two or three at once which can occur in busy maternity delivery suites. Hospitals are notoriously understaffed and the belief they are safer begs many questions.

> "No empirical evidence supports the claim that hospital births are a safer option than planned homebirths backed by a modern hospital system for selected pregnant women."
>
> Olsen 1997

So is Hospital safer? The only certain way of answering this question would be a randomized controlled trial (RCT). This could have been done in the 1950s but such a trial of home versus hospital was not suggested. Such a trial now would require 500,000 women to answer the safety question. This is practically impossible so we make do with data that may suffer from the bias that women choosing home birth may be different from women choosing hospital, however well we may try to match them. Nevertheless, we can look at the outcomes in relation to place of birth.

One of the first to do this was Marjorie Tew, a statistician working at Nottingham Medical School. An outstanding lady, I had the great pleasure of meeting Marjorie when she came to Tasmania promoting the safety of homebirth in 1989. In her large-scale and detailed study, Marjorie analysed data from the 1970 British Births Survey and compared perinatal death rates in different places of birth (Tew, 1985).

Marjorie recognized that you would expect more 'high-risk' deliveries in hospitals than at home and attempted to control this by using both antenatal and labour prediction scores to categorize expected risk. Marjorie found that babies were more likely to survive if born in a General Practice (GP) or at home, rather than in hospital, at all levels of risk scores. Only at the very highest level of risk were the better results at home and in GP units not statistically significant. Even though Marjorie was unable to publish her results in a medical journal due to the climate of thinking at the time, it is possible that these results may show that prediction scores do not foretell problems. They were not, however, her scores, but were provided by obstetricians. Marjorie's results have not been refuted and the 1970 survey data do not support the prevailing view from the time that hospital was safer.

> "Tew has displayed great courage over the years, initially being one voice crying in the wilderness. She can now take pride in her part in getting people to question that prevailing view"
> Geoffrey N. Marsh and Mary J. Renfrew (Eds), Community-based Maternity Care, Oxford University Press, 1999).

Homebirths are no riskier than hospital births, according to the first major Canadian study to compare the two types of deliveries. The study compared 862 planned homebirths in British Columbia, with 571 midwife-attended hospital births and 743 doctor-attended hospital births between January 1998 and the end of 1999. It found no increased maternal or neonatal risk associated with planned homebirth under the care of a regulated midwife. Of the women in the homebirth group 3.6% required emergency hospital care for complications ranging from breech delivery and reduced foetal heart rate to respiratory distress, no different to what would be expected in hospital.

More intervention is often required in hospital due to the over use of routine procedures leading to complications. Researchers found that women who deliver their babies at home are less likely to undergo any of the range of medical interventions that generally accompany hospital deliveries, including epidurals, episiotomies and medically induced labour. Only 6.4% of women giving birth at home had caesarean sections, compared with 18% of those births overseen by a physician (Blais, 2002).

In her book 'Homebirth Bound, Mending the Broken Weave', New Zealand midwife Maggie Banks stated convincingly that the research and evidence indicates that homebirth is a very safe choice for birthing couples.

Maggie states:

> "The consistent evidence is that when women at low risk of complications plan to birth at home, their birthing is more likely to result in healthy outcomes for themselves and their babies than it is if they birth in an obstetric hospital using specialist services."
> "Birth takes some women to the extreme limit of sanity and they have to make their own way individually each and every time. To imply that women who literally suffer birth are in any way lacking in courage or self-control is to belittle their individuality and their birth accomplishment"
>
> Casey Makela, Midwife
> http://traditionalmidwife.com/unassistedbirth.html
>
> http://www.foodmatters.tv/articles-1/
> we-had-a-baby-and-here-is-our-unusual-story

Childbirth Education

Who needs it and why? Childbirth classes have been happening since Grantly-Dick Read first instigated their use around the 1930's. He came to see that women needed more knowledge about this aspect of life as birth became more medically orientated and women less informed. He created structured classes believing that if women were more informed they were less likely to experience fear, which would reduce the complications of long and painful labours. Although his philosophy was based in creating positive results for women, it relied on bringing women to the birth place rather than taking the place of birth to the woman. The classes involved lecturing and dictating to women about what would happen rather than what could. Over time other methods evolved such as Lamaze and the Bradley method, again promising to assist women in birth but from a medically placed way of thinking, almost teaching women to expect intervention and procedures as normal.

Traditional societies pass on their knowledge gained by observation and experience through the extended family. However, modern Western society has become far more nuclear with some women having no experience of babies before having their own.

Many books and classes have concentrated on the 'How, Where and What', rather than 'Who' is involved. From the 1980's on a new childbirth movement evolved created by radical birth doulas and midwives who desired to get real knowledge to women and allow women to make informed choices. Men were invited to take their place at the woman's side and began to attend these classes as well. Women birthing at home were observed to use a variety of ways to manage their labours successfully without pain killing drugs and interventions.

We began to understand about innate behaviours and the role of hormones in the birth process and that birth doesn't need to be managed at all. The term Active Birth became the catch cry for midwives the world over during the 80's and 90's, a philosophy that when the woman is allowed to embrace the passage of birth fully and totally a beautiful experience becomes an empowered one.

However, there is no amount of training or education that can be done to ensure the birth goes exactly to plan and the baby is as desired. New born babies are unpredictable. Some can be born from the gentlest of birth and scream their life away, others born from the most traumatic of births grow to be peacefully serene characters. So it is fair to say that the newborn brings its own characteristics and personality that does not necessarily match ours. Couples need to know that to have a child means accepting whatever this new character may bring to their home and be prepared to live with them for the next twenty years. Childbirth preparation brings an opportunity for couples to focus totally for a few hours at least on the pregnancy and imminent birth. It allows questions to be highlighted and answered as well as dispelling myths associated with local knowledge or gossip.

For midwives the biggest positive of childbirth classes is the opportunity to pass on relevant information about birth rites and the over use of procedures in hospitals, what to look for and how to diminish the risk of intervention. Effective classes help to develop your own instincts so that you believe in your own ability. Classes also provide a supportive learning environment for your partner and support people so they can truly understand the nature of birth. This way they can feel safe and confident in allowing the natural process of birth to unfold without intervention, thus supporting you well.

As expectant parents, you can only make informed decisions about procedures and whether they are right for you and your baby by knowing what procedures are and why they are given. Choose classes carefully, check the philosophy of the educator. If classes are held in a hospital, know that the educator will be bound by hospital policy, so may not explain all the choices fully.

Childbirth education is not about teaching that one method is better than another, rather that each individual birth must have the method that best suits. Often antenatal education becomes stuck on teaching about the intellectual process of labour and delivery whilst criticising current birthing trends.

Too much factual knowledge goes hand in hand with control. Expectations are set and you are left feeling inadequate if unable to meet the standard. It is better for you to awaken to your own physical and psychological changes, open to finding your own path and experience of childbirth. You need to understand that the professional has their own self-awareness, their own view on birth, their own fears and attitudes to the many facets of pregnancy and birth.

We must take responsibility for our own lives first. How far are we prepared to empower women? As professionals are we prepared to take our role into consideration, are we prepared to become superfluous?

Fathers Attending Births - Joy or Trepidation

Men present at the birth of their child is still a relatively new phenomena, only becoming a common factor over the past forty years. Some men would still prefer not to be there and many feel like a 'fish out of water'.

Just as the mother-to-be needs to be prepared so does the father. For most women pregnancy comes with a great deal of confusion, many women having had no experience of babies prior to becoming pregnant. For men it can be even more alienating. Unprepared fathers can be a huge hindrance to the birth process, rather than a support. Seeing the woman they love appear to be in intense pain can be daunting and terrifying.

It is the natural instinct of a male to protect and want to take the pain away. This is the very action that could destroy the whole experience for the woman. It is imperative for men planning to be present at the birth to be well-informed and ready to coach and support their woman through this experience. Men must trust in their partner's ability and the natural birth process. I like to think of the male partner as the 'Ugg Man', the traditional cave man who protects the lair whilst his partner births. In order for men to do this they must know what the perimeters of normality are and what could be over servicing by the maternity service being used.

Medical intervention is not a requirement during the normal healthy pregnancy and birth, but it does have its place when the need arises. Knowing when the need arises is the important role for the male, especially if he is going to be the woman's advocate as well as her support person. It is worth considering hiring a midwife or doula (a woman to assist you) to birth with you or taking a special relative or friend that you can rely on who is well informed and trusting in the natural birth process. This takes the pressure off your partner of having to be aware of all that is happening, thus allowing them to be totally absorbed in the journey. The extra person can also be a great asset of extra energy and support to the mother. Most woman need constant support and encouragement, which can be exhausting for the support team when it encompasses many hours. Support people need to be able to relieve each other and give each other a break without leaving the birthing woman alone.

Birthing was traditionally 'women's business' and if men are to take their place next to their birthing woman they must be able to understand the intensity of birth and the need for patience. During many birthing experiences, I have observed the negative effect an unsupportive partner can have on a birthing situation. I have seen women be coerced into medical intervention to speed up the process to satisfy the nervous anxiety of her partner.

When a woman is birthing she is vulnerable and easy prey to nervous behaviour and fear. She will pick up on the fear of the supporting people and begin to be fearful too, slowing labour down and increasing the pain of the contractions. A patient, experienced birth attendant understands that time has no place in a birthing situation. If mother and baby are fine then leave well enough alone. Birth does not need attending to, it needs quiet support and observation.

Recently a client expressed that she would like to have a homebirth but was concerned as her partner was less than enthusiastic. She expressed that he was under the influence of his mother and grandmother, both nurses but not midwives, who held strong opinions about homebirth. When I had the chance to speak with her partner, to discuss his fears and provide well researched information about the safety of homebirth, he changed his mind and became very enthusiastic about homebirth.

Correct information is essential to making the decision that is right for you. Many people offer unfounded advice not based in truth but distorted by their own emotions and fears. Had this couple listened to this information they would have missed out on the wonderful, life changing experience of the birth of their child at home.

When a couple work in unison, it is the most wondrous experience to observe. As a midwife I love to sit back and allow the couple to birth their baby. I'm just there for support and guidance, it is their birth not mine. Many studies have shown that when a woman is caressed, kissed and whispered sweet, loving and encouraging words throughout labour, oxytocin levels increase speeding up cervical dilation decreasing pain.

Partners - make love to your woman in this way during labour, it may be the most important role you could ever have in assisting your newborn into the world.

Preparation Exercises

Physical Exercise

Physical exercise is very important in pregnancy. The fitter and more flexible you are the better your ability to cope with labour and birth. I suggest a twenty minute walk every day with some uphill component, building to one hour.

- swimming is an excellent exercise, especially as you get bigger as the water holds your weight, enabling you to move joints move fluidly. There are many facilities providing antenatal water classes
- probably the best option is to seek out a pregnancy yoga teacher, as this provides both relaxation and resistance exercise
- it is important to avoid high-impact aerobic activity, bike riding and horse riding as these can jolt the joints, which have softened due to the hormonal changes and create an over-tight perineum.

During your pregnancy one of the most beneficial things you can do is exercise and move your body. Dancing is excellent and has been part of pregnancy and birth preparation in Eastern Countries for centuries. Belly dancing has its origins as the dance of fertility and birth. To find a 'Dancing for Birth' class in your area cock on http://www.dancingforbirth.com . Dancing helps your baby to move and find the correct position for birth.

Pilates Exercises (Julie Hills, Pilates Instructor at PilatesJ)

Pilates is the perfect partner to pregnancy. The more movement we have in our life, the stronger we are physically, mentally and emotionally. Pilates, under the guidance of a professional, fully trained instructor in an equipped studio, offers a safe environment for appropriate exercises during pregnancy.

There is no better time to discover the joy of movement than during the months that lead to the birth of a new life. Pilates practice teaches breath, body awareness, control, balance, efficiency, concentration, flow and precision. Pilates teaches you first how to focus on your breath and how to co-ordinate breath with movement from a stable centre. With a focus on recruiting inner core strength, Pilates builds a support system from within for the ever changing pregnant body.

During pregnancy, the hormone relaxin is responsible for relaxing and softening the ligaments around the pelvic joints to prepare the passage of birth. When this happens the joints become unstable and muscles have to take over the role of stabilising the pelvis.

Abdominal and gluteal muscles need to be both strong and flexible to support the growing uterus and changing posture. Abdominal muscles that are too strong or too weak can prevent the correct positioning of the baby for birth. If the abdominal muscles are too strong they can split, creating a condition called diastasis rectus. Moderation and working the abdominals in a safe and protected way, such as on the stability ball is the key. Hip circling on the ball is very beneficial as this movement encourages a correct birthing position.

The stability ball is also an excellent tool to both stretch and strengthen your pelvic floor. Mothers are rewarded with a faster delivery, less discomfort in the perineal area and a faster return to normal after the birth. Pelvic floor muscles interact with the deep abdominal and spinal muscles and the diaphragm. In the early days after birth, the pelvic floor and abdominals can be exercised and strengthened simply using breath practice to encourage recovery.

Movement is vital to giving birth. Women with practiced preparation can move their way through labour and delivery circling, rocking and swaying to a rhythm that comes from within and allows the body to open and release. Breath practice put into action provides for calm in the spaces between contractions, pain management and power when needed during labour.

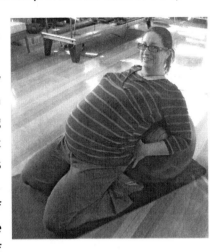

For some women, especially very fit women, there can be a problem with tight pelvic floors. Learning to relax and release your pelvic floor during pregnancy encourages a shorter pushing stage at delivery. In an upright position the action of baby's head pressing against the perineum will initiate stretching of your pelvic floor muscles, and taken slowly they will slip over the baby's head without damage. The pelvic floor is supported and maintained when the mother is allowed to take her time at the pushing stage.

Pelvic awareness and practicing pilates with neutral pelvis is excellent preparation for birthing. When the pelvis is aligned in neutral position the angle of the baby allows for a faster delivery.

If a woman is lying on her back to push, the sacrum will be restricted in its ability to open the pelvis, hindering the birthing process. It is much better to give birth in an upright or hands and knees position or even side lying. A popular tool for labour and birth is the stability ball. To feel confident using the ball during labour and delivery, it is very beneficial to have incorporated it into pilates practice during the months leading to birth.

Pilates provides support during pregnancy and mind- body training in preparation for a joyful, moving birth and the confidence and knowledge to bring your body back to optimal function as you begin to share a new life with your precious newborn.

Newborn Feeding Restriction

In some cases due to positioning through the birth passage, a newborn has difficulty turning their head in one direction, be it left or right, for feeding. This situation may be relieved by an Emmett muscle release technique of the SCM the sterno -cleido-mastoid muscle, a very simple and quick release movement which then allows freedom of the neck for feeding.

Kegal Pelvic Floor Exercises

The pelvic floor forms a base to the pelvis and consists of eight pairs of interconnected muscles, the superficial perineal muscles, fascia and the deeper levator ani and coccyges muscles, capable of a wide range of movement. It is like a pudding bowl, made from strong elastic, hanging from the pelvis.

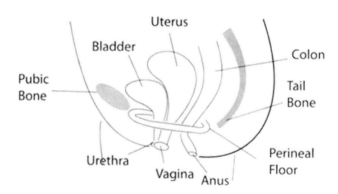

The Functions of the Pelvic Floor:

- forms a base to the outlet of the pelvis
- supports the pelvic organs
- counteracts changes in abdominal pressure caused by such actions as coughing and lifting
- assists in maintaining continence (urinary and faecal)

- produces a gutter to assist in the rotation of the foetal head during delivery
- increases sexual enjoyment during intercourse.

Signs and Symptoms of Weak Pelvic Floor Muscles:

- incontinence - leakage of urine during exertion such as jogging,coughing, laughing, sneezing or lifting
- vaginal slackness
- vaginal wall or uterine prolapse and feeling of heaviness
- passing 'wind' - gas from the bowel or trapped air from the vagina
- tampons slipping out.

Reasons for Doing Pelvic Floor Exercises

To increase muscle control and muscle tone, so that the pelvic contents (particularly the uterus) are well supported. This is particularly important during pregnancy and the postnatal period, and throughout life.

During the last three months of pregnancy the baby enlarges and presses on the bladder and pelvic floor. At the same time hormones relax the pelvic floor and pelvic ligaments in preparation for delivery. Forty two percent of women experience stress incontinence at this stage of pregnancy. Many continue to have leakage problems after the birth of their baby, one third will continue to have problems. Intensive pelvic floor exercises will help prevent this.

Daily pelvic floor exercises help to increase the ability to open up and let go during the second stage of labour, giving you more awareness and ability to push effectively, preventing tears or the need for an episiotomy. Start the exercises early in pregnancy and continue throughout and for at least three months after.

- prevention is better than cure
- the exercises need to be done four times a day
- you can fit them into your regular daily routines

- they need to be done slowly and smoothly without using unnecessary muscles
- always finish an exercise series with a tightening of the pelvic floor, to maintain good muscle tone
- do not expect too much too soon. These muscles are often weak and not accustomed to regular exercise. They fatigue easily causing more weakness.
- therefore it is important to assess how many of the exercises you can do at a time without over-fatiguing the muscles and causing more weakness.

Pelvic Floor Exercises

It important to engage your core whilst doing these exercises to ensure you are using the correct muscles.

1. Imagine trying to stop yourself passing wind. To control the wind you must contract the anal sphincter muscles around the back passage. Your buttocks and thighs should not move at all. Be aware of the skin around your anus contracting and your anus being pulled upwards away from what you are sitting on.
2. Whilst sitting, contract the muscles of the pelvic floor, those around the openings of the urethra and vagina. To help you locate the muscles concerned, imagine you are trying to stop the flow of urine. Next time you wee stop the flow and note which muscles you are using. Relax and contract, repeat six times. Feels like a wave-like motion. Practice this pattern of six contractions as often as you think of it each day, standing, sitting or at rest.
3. This exercise will help you gain further control of these muscles, which is important for the second stage of labour. Think of tightening your vaginal muscles in stages, as though you are going up in a lift - 1st floor, 2nd floor, 3rd floor, 4th floor, hold for 5 seconds. Then down again, 3rd, 2nd, 1st, ground. Now go down to

the basement and feel the vagina bulge out. Feel the whole area loose and bulging. This is what you will be doing in second stage of labour as you consciously open up to let the baby out. Repeat six times. If you are doing this exercise properly you will find that as you bulge out your perineal area you also bulge your lower abdomen (not pulling it in). Practice this several times each week. Especially good in the squat position.

4. Lying on your back on a bed with your legs bent and knees wide apart. Envisage someone trying to stick a pin into your perineum between the vagina and the anus. Put your finger on the perineum and feel it move as you contract the muscles. Concentrate. When you relax again feel the perineum fall back onto your finger.

5. In the same position, put the finger of one hand on the tail bone (the coccyx) which you will feel just behind the anus. Put a finger of the other hand on the pubic bone which you will feel in the pubic hair above the clitoris. By contracting the pelvic floor muscles, bring your two fingers closer together. You should feel a slight movement of the tail bone up towards the pubic bone as you contract the muscles. Be sure to keep your legs bent and knees apart so that you cannot cheat by using other muscles. Whilst in this position imagine you are wagging your tail side to side using the pelvic floor muscles not the buttocks.

6. Lying on your back with legs bent and knees apart, lubricate the index and middle fingers of your right hand with a crème, lotion or oil. Gently insert one then both fingers inside the vagina. Now separate the fingers as in a scissor action from the top to bottom of the vagina. With fingers held apart attempt to squeeze them together using the contraction of the vaginal muscles to do so. At first there may be little movement, especially if there has been a difficult delivery, a large baby or many prior deliveries of children. If you feel nothing, continue to concentrate and squeeze hard. The muscles need to relearn their role. Eventually with practice the fingers can be squeezed together. This exercise will enhance sexual pleasure as well.

7. Now, inserting a tampon into the vagina, pull gently on the string, contract the muscles around the vagina to retain the tampon within the vaginal cavity. If your muscles are lax you may need to dampen the tampon before inserting and then allow it to swell before beginning this exercise.

Other beneficial hints:

- decrease caffeine intake
- keep weight under control
- share heavy loads
- exercise daily - brisk walking will do. Weight bearing exercises like walking also helps to strengthen bones and so prevent osteoporosis
- ensure adequate calcium intake.

By now you should have a clear idea of which muscles to contract. You will appreciate that all the above exercises require contractions of the same group of muscles. The pelvic floor muscles and sphincter muscles work together in these exercises, closing the urethra, anus and constricting the vagina. At first a great deal of concentration is required to do these exercises. Remember which muscles you are using and the sensation you experience when you contract them.

Perineal Massage

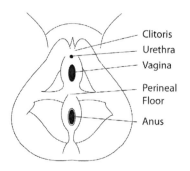

Clitoris
Urethra
Vagina
Perineal Floor
Anus

Perineal massage helps you get used to touch and pressure in a very private area.

During pushing, most mothers respond to the pressure and stretching sensations with tension and attempt to withhold the birth, rather than relax and give birth.

Women who practice regular perineal massage:

- appear to have a shorter second stage
- report less stinging and burning sensations associated with the stretching during birth
- are able to relax and let go of the perineal muscles, facilitating an intact perineum, therefore the less likelihood of episiotomy.

** **Contra-indications** do not do this massage if there is a herpes or vaginal lesions outbreak.

Perineal massage is best undertaken in conjunction with kegal pelvic floor exercises and relaxation techniques. You will be preparing yourself for a slow, controlled second stage with panting and pushing to avoid tearing. Natural positions for birth are also advocated.

Getting Ready

A warm bath or warm compress on the perineum can help relaxation before beginning. A lubricant is needed, either oil (coconut, wheat germ, sesame, almond or olive), cocoa butter, vitamin E or natural vaginal lubrication. Wash hands well. Clipping long pubic hairs makes the massage easier. Begin around the 34th week of pregnancy.

Self Massage:

Get a mirror, lean back comfortably on pillows so that you can see your perineum in the mirror. Put some lubricant on the perineal area. Massage the lubricant into the perineal area until it is worked in.

Relax and enjoy the sensation. Then add more lubricant and place your thumb shallowly inside the vagina (approx. 3-4cms, do not reach the cervix), press the perineal floor towards the rectum and to the sides. Gently stretch the opening, pressing down until you feel a slight burning sensation or tingling. At this point maintain the stretch and pressure for approximately two minutes until the area becomes somewhat numb. Then slowly and gently work the lubricant in with your thumbs, still maintaining the stretch and pressure.

Avoid the urethral area because of the risk of infection, you'll also find its uncomfortable. Massage for 3-4 minutes concentrating on any previous scar tissue which is especially non-elastic. You can pull the perineum forward a bit when massaging, which mimics the action of the baby's head as it begins to emerge.

Partner Massage:

Massage some lubricant into the perineal area until it is absorbed. Then add more lubricant and insert the two index fingers, or the index and middle finger of the one hand, shallowly into the vagina and gently press the perineum down and to the sides.

After the burning sensation diminishes, massage with the index fingers as above especially over any scar tissue. Massage in a sweeping action side to side or by separating the fingers in opposite directions. Ask your partner to acknowledge sensations and feelings whilst concentrating on relaxing.

Progression

After about one week there will be noticeable increase in flexibility and stretchiness if you have been doing the massage once a day. At the end of a few weeks the perineum is likely to stretch enough so that you can massage with two fingers of each hand inside the vagina. Once an opening of up to seven cm can be massaged without burning or tingling then massaging every other day is adequate.

The Epi-No

If you can't get the hang of perineal massage, and some women can't, try the Epi-No birthing trainer. An inflatable balloon like device that is inserted into the vagina. It helps stretch the perineum in the weeks before your due date. Feedback from this technique has been very positive.

http://www.epi-no.com.au/

Vaginal Massage

I have been teaching vaginal massage for pregnancy for the past fifteen years and the feedback has been very positive. The massage is an extension of perineal massage, taking the massage deep into the vagina and particularly focusing on the back muscles behind the cervix.

These are the muscles that must be relaxed in order to facilitate birth. Women who practice vaginal massage become familiar with their bodies and are more in tune when it comes time to birth. They also experience intact perineums even when delivering large babies.

"There is no evidence that delivery practices that avoid perineal trauma are correlated with low Apgar scores, birth trauma, or cerebral palsy. Passing through the bony pelvis might sometimes be traumatic for foetuses, but there is certainly no evidence that soft tissues of the perineum damage foetal brains. In Klein's study of restricted versus routine (median) episiotomy, sexual satisfaction in women 3 months' postpartum was best with intact perineums."

Klein et al. (1994)

Getting Baby Into the Right Position

In some ways labour can be likened to an endurance race. It can be one of the most enduring challenges you will experience as a woman, whilst also being one of the most exhilarating accomplishments. No serious athlete would turn up to the starting line for a marathon without putting in some form of preparation. The preparation you undertake during pregnancy can make a difference to your birth experience. Research suggests that although ensuring a healthy mum and new born is an important outcome of birth, just as important is how the journey or experience is perceived for both. The partnership of mother and baby is essential for a smooth labour and delivery.

Most maternity carers would agree that the best position for the baby to lie in is with your baby's back lying mainly to the front of your belly and slightly to your left side. In this position baby's head will be well flexed deep into the pelvis and face looking toward your back. When the head is flexed it creates a smaller diameter, facilitating an easier birth.

Sometimes the baby chooses to lie with its back lying mainly to your back, with its head deflexed. This results in a larger head circumference and less moulding during the labour which can lead to a slowing of the labour and more back pain involved with contractions, due to the pressure of the head on pelvic nerves. Posterior labours have an increased need for labour intervention such as epidurals, forceps and caesarean sections. But don't be over concerned if this is the case for you as many babies do turn in labour, especially if you use the positions and exercises suggested ahead.

An Anterior Position Facilitates:

- the baby's head engaging easily into the pelvis
- more effective moulding of baby's head (easier fit)
- the likelihood of spontaneous labour at term, therefore induction unlikely
- membranes less likely to rupture prematurely
- more effective and co-ordinated contractions
- less strain in labour to mother/baby
- less intervention and medical complications
- shorter and more efficient labours.

Does an Unengaged Head Impact on the Outcome of Labour?

After thirty six weeks there seems to be quite a focus on whether or not your baby should be engaged or not. Being engaged means that the baby has dropped into the pelvis and is resting at the level of the ischial spines. When measurements are done by your birth carer they are assessed according to how many fingers your baby's head is above or below the 'spines'. In the past there has been some thought that if a baby has not engaged by the time of labour that this can impact on the effectiveness of the labour. Your baby knows when it is ready to enter the world and whether it is engaged or not has little to do with how you birth. Many babies drop into the pelvis once labour starts.

According to research by Johns Hopkins University School of Medicine (1989), who undertook a retrospective study of 803 first time mothers from the database at Baltimore Maryland Hospital, only twenty nine percent of the women presented in active labour with their baby's heads engaged, and they had the lowest caesarean rate at five percent. Caesarean rate for the women with the foetal heads unengaged was fourteen percent. The study concluded that most first time mothers present with an unengaged foetal head in active labour. Despite the fact that first time mothers who present with an unengaged foetal head have a longer first and second stage of labour, the majority delivered vaginally (Obstetrics & Gynaecology, March 1999, Vol. 93, No. 33, pp. 329-331).

The most important thing to understand is that if the baby's head is not engaged and you rupture your membranes, then you must get checked out as there is a slight risk the cord could drop below baby's head. This is known as a prolapsed cord and needs immediate medical attention, however it is rare. Induction is not recommended by artificial rupture of the membranes if the baby's head is not engaged. If mother and baby are fine I tend to err on the side of leave well enough alone. If you and your baby are well then patience is the best policy as induction of mothers with a high head has a seventy to eighty percent higher risk of caesarean section.

The Role of the Pelvis

Your Pelvis Makes a Cradle for Your Baby During the Pregnancy
The pelvis is made of cartilage, not bone, and consists of three sections:

1. The brim is the top opening. Widest from side to side and usually causes little difficulty in birth.
2. The cavity is the middle or circular cavity defined at the bottom by the Ischia spines which can be the reason for birth problems

If this space is compromised by the position of the mother or sometimes physically being too small. To optimise ensure you are moving around and choosing different positions such as all fours or leaning over to assist your baby move through. Lying down decreases the space in the pelvis, thus the cavity is where the deflexed head is most likely to get stuck during birth.

3. The outlet is the bottom opening, which generally causes little problem if the mother is left to assume the position that feels right for her. Most women prefer all fours or kneeling when pushing their baby out.

In Labour

To help make this easy, nature assists in several ways:

- The pregnancy hormones help to soften ligaments around the joints in the pelvis, the pubic joint at the front and the sacroiliac joints on each side of the spine in your lower back. This helps the joints to become more flexible and supple.
- Roumuls of Michael – the pelvic ligaments relax and widen across the back of the pelvis during Second Stage, adding centimetres to the pelvic outlet. Very important that you are off your back when pushing, preferably try on all fours, kneeling or leaning over.
- The bones on baby's head are designed to over-ride each other slightly as the head is pressed down into the pelvis in labour. This makes the baby's head smaller in diameter, helping it fit more readily through the pelvis.

Gravity will assist these two procedures of moulding and opening of the pelvis. To take full advantage of gravity you need to be upright. By being upright and taking the weight on your open legs you can increase the size of the pelvic outlet by as much as thirty percent, which may mean the difference between a forceps/caesarean section or a normal delivery.

Mapping the Pelvic Outlet

Mapping the pelvic outlet allows you to become familiar with this area of your body and to gain confidence in its size and the ability of your baby to fit through. By pressing through the skin, you can feel the hard bony prominences of your pelvis.

- find the pubic arch in front (see A, diagram below). Place your thumb on this. Stretch your hand through your legs so that your middle finger is in contact with your tail bone (see B), which may be a little harder. You might find squatting or asking a partner to help makes this easier. Using a piece of string to measure may help.
- hold the stretch then mark this on a piece of paper. This gives you an idea of the distance from front to back.
- now measure the distance between the sit-bones on the backside (see C and D). To get to the sit bones, sit semi-squat so you can feel them through your buttock cheek. Mark your sit bones onto the sheet as indicated by the diagram.
- join the points together and you will have a diagram of the opening to the outlet of your pelvis.

You will be pleasantly surprised to see how large this opening is. Now you can move around with different positions to see which positions give you a greater opening. Try full squat versus semi squat, kneeling open versus one knee up. One foot on a chair, one foot on the floor then squat down. Notice the depth of the opening. This is a great exercise to do with other women or in an antenatal class as you will see that the opening is very different for each woman. Some will have a pointy pubic arch, another will be longer and squarer. Each woman is an individual.

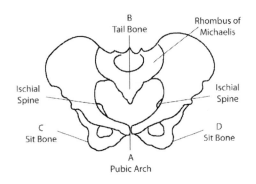

Birth Positions

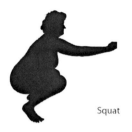

Squat

It is best to avoid the semi-lying position as the uterus and birth canal end up facing upwards. This results in the uterine muscles and baby having to work against gravity.

Though the squat position can be of great benefit, the baby has to navigate the curving and upward facing birth canal.

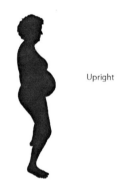

Upright

In the upright position the uterus has less resistance to work against, however the birth canal has a curve that the baby must navigate.

Ideal Birth Positions

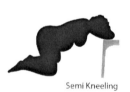

Semi Kneeling

The semi kneeling position provides least resistance to the uterine contractions, giving an almost straight line of passage through the birth canal. This results in an easy outlet of birth for baby and less pain and perineal trauma for mother.

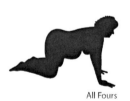

All Fours

Many mothers find all fours or kneeling most comfortable and the most effective way to give birth. It is important that you have discussed this with your birthing team before labour so they are in alignment with your wishes.

The Baby

The baby is the navigator of the birth process. Your baby is not symmetrical, thus it has to negotiate its way through the birth canal during labour. It is greatly assisted by the postions and movements you adopt. A mother birthing in tune with her body and her baby will naturally adopt positions that best facilitate baby's need to navigate the pelvis efficiently.

Your baby's:

- head is longer from front to back and the shoulders are wider from side to side
- skull is designed to mould easily when in the correct position but takes longer in other positions. If baby's head is moulded incorrectly the pressure of the uterine contraction can cause small bones and tissues to become misaligned, trapping various nerve endings and blood vessels. This may lead to settling and feeding problems. Cranial osteopathy post birth can assist if this is the case.

The Uterus

The uterus houses the powerful uterine muscles, which are specifically designed to protect the growing baby and to contract to birth your baby when the time comes.

The uterus:

- continually contracts throughout pregnancy as it grows and stretches
- forms the lower uterine segment around 32 weeks of pregnancy onward. The lower uterine segment assists the moulding of the foetal head, to allow it to fit through the pelvis.
- provides correct even pressure of the head onto the cervix, ensuring smoother dilation in less time.

Mother's Role

Aim to practice exercises and lifestyle behaviours that assist your baby into the right position, such as:

- using upright leaning forward positions that allow your pelvis to tilt forward
- 'duck waddling' and semi-squatting

- keeping the knees lower than the hips therefore maximizing the amount of room in the pelvis, especially from 34 weeks onward
- avoid sitting on couches or low settees as these tend to encourage a lowering of the pelvis
- straddling a chair backwards, leaning forward into the backrest with a pillow under buttocks for at least half an hour daily
- placing a cushion under the buttocks when driving to keep the pelvis tilted
- lying on the left side for resting and sleeping
- avoiding deep squatting. Unless your bottom is at knee level the inlet space becomes constricted.

Active Labour

A labouring mother will naturally bend forward when left to assume the position that best suits her. This allows the baby to move down the birth canal in the correct position so that it will continually tuck its head into its chest, making the head smaller in diameter.

Adopting positions as your baby is pushed through the cavity that allow the ligaments to be released at the back of the pelvis (known as the Rhombus of Michaelis) allows an extra 2cm of room for the baby to fit through. This is best if you are on all fours, leaning forward in a kneeling position or semi squatting over a chair.

Posterior Presentation

A persistent posterior presenting baby will be easy to recognise. You will tend to have a flatter tummy with lots of lumps and bumps, as the back is positioned inwards with the legs and arms out front. You will likely express that you feel lots of movement across the abdomen from these active limbs. There are many

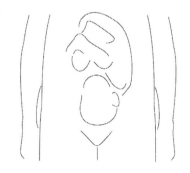

reasons why a baby will choose to lie backwards. One of these may be a tight diaphragm. The following diaphragmatic release can be very effective at releasing the tension.

Diaphragmatic Release

Lie on your back with a cushion under your left side so that the weight of the baby is not crushing your major arteries, otherwise you may feel faint. Ensure you place a small pillow or adequate support behind your lower back.

Begin with deep relaxation breathing, taking several deep breaths and holding for 5-8 seconds then releasing. Connect with your abdominal region by pulling in your navel, as though you are pulling it through to your back, whilst continuing to deep breathe. This in itself will relax the diaphragm area.

Close your eyes and become centred in your body. With the help of your partner or a friend, get him/her to stand at the top of your head. Extend your arms around their back whilst continuing to deeply breathe. They create a counter pull with their back against your arms, thus stretching the abdominal area and releasing the diaphragm. They can then gently pull up on your ribs to release around the diaphragm at the same time as you are stretching your arms and deeply breathing.

For Practitioner - Abdominal Release

If you are the practitioner stand next to the woman and place one hand horizontally under and across her lower back where the uterine ligaments attach. This is where you would usually apply lower back pressure during labour. Allow the mother's weight to apply the pressure on your hand, you do not need to press. Now place your top hand horizontally across the pubic bone with the thumb again upward without pressure. Now just wait. I generally enhance the movement with Reiki.

In time I usually feel a wave like movement under my top hand and the sense of a contraction taking place with my bottom hand. As you allow this to build it will begin to feel like the movement is flowing backward and forward from your bottom hand to the top in a circular motion. Continue to allow the release to happen for as long as is necessary usually about 20-30mins. This action allows the muscles to relax and the baby is more encouraged to turn into the correct position. The mother may or may not express emotion as the issues in the tissues are released. Our muscles habitually learn how to contract and shorten, and need to be encouraged to relax and lengthen. Often it can be related to an incident where the mother's abdominal muscles were twisted, for example where there has been a car accident and the seat belt held one shoulder down, whilst the other went forward.

Psychosomatically it could be because of long held repressed anger, where there is the sense of wanting to hit out but can't. This gets locked up in the tissues creating tension.

The process may need to be repeated over several visits. This exercise also works well for turning breech babies.

The Lunge

The lunge is a great way to turn a baby, or to assist a posterior presentation by giving baby more room to move. Stand face forward with a chair beside you. Place one foot on the chair seat, with knee and foot pointing to the side. Remaining upright, slowly 'lunge' or lean sideways, toward the chair so that the leg on the chair bends. You should feel a stretch on the insides of both thighs. Stay in the lunge for a slow count of five then return to upright. Repeat during or between contractions.

If you know your baby's position lunge toward the side where his or her back is. If you don't know the position try lunging in each direction to find the one that is most comfortable. Also lean, with your feet wide apart. In this leaning-wide position sway, dance, stomp, lean on your partner's or doula's back.

Asynclitism

Asynclitism is the term used to describe when the suture lines of the baby's skull are not felt to be aligned exactly halfway between the symphysis pubis and the sacrum. If the baby's head is tilted up toward the pubic bone, it is called anterior asynclitism. If tilted toward the sacrum it is a posterior asynclitism. If the baby is not deeply engaged in the pelvis, the head may be adjusted by your midwife manually lifting the baby's head upward if posterior or moving it downward if anterior. Climbing up and down a flight of stairs sideways may correct the asynclitism.

If no stairs are available duck walk while being supported. Bend your knees, broaden your stance and walk, swaying from side to side, rotating your hips out and forward. Also use the lunge position described above or place one foot on an elevated surface (eg chair or table), with the lifted foot higher than the other knee. This position is held for several contractions and then the alternate leg is elevated.

Visualisation Exercise

Following is a simple visualisation I have used to clear emotional blocks that may be preventing a baby getting into the right position.

- relax, breathe, close your eyes
- imagine you are sitting by a stream
- watch the stream's flow
- are the banks clear or full of reeds and trees?
- notice how the river runs. Is it gentle and easy or turbulent and tumbling over rocks?
- does it make you feel at peace or anxious and nervous?
- notice what rocks and boulders are in the river, look closely at them, are they large or small? Do they look like they could be easily moved or do they look huge and impossible to move? Ask to be shown what each rock stands for. Relax, don't try too hard, in time you may see words written on them. These words may represent what fears or emotions are coming up for you.
- now visualise these rocks being lifted out of the water onto the bank. Use whatever means you need to remove them such as cranes or big angels lifting them out, or see them as styrene foam making them light to lift.

- once they are out of the water notice now how the stream flows. Continue to go back and move any blocks from the stream until you feel a sense of calmness.

Placing earphones over your abdomen during pregnancy has been found to be very beneficial in relaxing the baby. Many studies have found that after birth babies respond to the same music that was played during pregnancy. When mothers played the same music in the humidicribs in neonatal intensive care, the neonatal staff noted how relaxed and happy the babies were in comparison to those without music. This is a great way to help move a baby, it relaxes them and they become more aware of their surrounds, moving themselves into the correct position for birth. Studies have shown that babies have a definite predisposition to the music of Bach.

Tips for Obstructed Labour

An obstructed labour occurs mainly when the baby is in the wrong position. The head can press onto the cervix, causing it to become swollen and less able to dilate. This occurs around 9cm dilated and is referred to as a 'cervical lip'. The majority of the cervix has gone but a small part remains, blocking progress. Sometimes if it is soft enough it can be pushed over the baby's head during a contraction.

Some midwives are experimenting with Homeopathic Arnica tablets dissolved in sterile water and applied to the oedematous cervix of the swollen anterior lip. The recommended use is either two tablets at 30x in 5-7cc of sterile water or three tablets at 30x in 10 cc of sterile water when a cervix is completely oedematous. Generally, within five minutes the woman no longer has swelling and delivers shortly after.

Tips When There is Mal-positioning.
In early labour walk up some stairs, stepping sideways bringing your second leg up beside the first on each step. Step toward the way you would like the baby to rotate.

- rock from side to side rotating the hips the way you want the baby to rotate
- later in labour march on the spot with high legs or alternatively lift one foot after the other onto a small stool, sideways again
- rotating the leg high over the hip is of great benefit
- sitting on the toilet can often be of great benefit as it tends to be a good position and allows the perineum to be free
- if confined to bed (unsatisfactory and most difficult birthing) try side lying with a pillow or two under the uterus in order to lift it to the midline. Then the upper hip can be moved independently, gravity is not so important it is better to concentrate on encouraging the baby's head to turn and align.
- if possible change position as often as possible to cover all opportunities
- if there is a hand presentation, the midwife may ask you to lift one or the other hip to allow the head to slip past the hand. Whilst standing, bring the hips forward by swinging your body to one side whilst bending your knees and rising up on your toes. This rocks the baby's head and can assist in moving the obstacle. Also the midwife might touch the hand on vaginal examination which may encourage the baby to pull its hand up out of the way.

Normal birth means an active mother involved in the process of labour with her baby, adopting positions that free and release the pelvis and pelvic floor (Scott & Sutton, 1995).

Breech Babies

Around four percent of babies are breech (bottom against the cervix) at term. About twenty percent of babies at 28 weeks will be breech with fifteen percent remaining in breech by 32 weeks. Breech presentation is more common before 37 weeks of pregnancy as often these babies have not settled into position yet and the chances are high that the baby will turn into the correct position. Some babies do turn by themselves after this time, but it is less likely and measures are usually taken to assist them to turn or discussion about delivery options needs to take place. About ten to fifteen percent of breech babies are discovered for the first time late in labour.

Preterm Breech

If a woman goes into labour before 37 weeks with a baby in breech position, frequently a caesarean section will be advised, particularly if the baby is between 27-30 weeks as there is the fear of risking damage to the baby's undeveloped brain. Some obstetricians advise a vaginal delivery if there are no other problems.

Term Breech

This is where a baby is found to be breech at 36 weeks. Mode of delivery will depend on the obstetrician's beliefs. Some may feel confident to deliver naturally others will insist on a caesarean. A scan will be done to check for the position of the baby's head as this will give an indication as to whether it can be delivered safely vaginally as well as check for the position of the placenta. A low lying placenta (praevia) can lead to breech presentation, and one third of women with a praevia do not have any bleeding, which would normally alert to this problem. Placenta praevia is usually ruled out by the scan at around 18-20 weeks.

Positions of Breech Babies

A. Extended or frank breech - hips flexed, with the thighs against the chest, and feet up by their ears, best for vaginal delivery.
B. Flexed breech - hips flexed with thighs against the chest, but knees also flexed with the calves against the back of the thigh and feet just above the bottom.
C. Footling breech - as above, but hips not flexed so much, and the feet lying below the bottom, less advisable for vaginal birth.

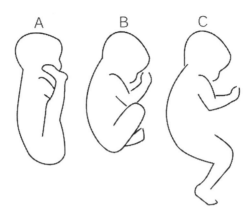

What You Can do to Encourage Your Baby to Turn

I suggest:

- spending fifteen minutes every two hours of the waking day lying on your back in the knee-chest position will help the baby to turn (Elkin's manoeuvre). I have certainly had great results with this technique accompanied with <u>reflexology</u> and Moxa (<u>Su-Jok</u>)
- hypnotherapy may be useful
- acupuncture/acupressure, use the reproductive points outlined
- Pulsatilla homoeopathic - use a maximum of one dose three times to assist a baby turn. Take a warm bath to relax muscles and then take pulsatilla 200, two doses two days apart. After taking the pulsatilla do the knee-chest position for twenty minutes and repeat the exercise again that day. This is best done around thirty five weeks or after.
- moxibustion burned near the outside of the small toe. Two hundred and sixty primigravidas with breech presentations at 32 weeks were randomized to the moxibustion group or to be given no treatment. By the end of two weeks of either daily treatment or twice daily treatment for fifteen minutes on each side, 72.4 percent of the women in the daily treatment group and 81.4 percent in the twice a day treatment group had vertex babies. There were 47.7 percent vertex presentations in the control group

(Women's Hospital in Jiangxi Province and Jiujiang Women's and Children's Hospital in the People's Republic of China JAMA Nov. 11, 1998).

- chiropractic – Webster technique
- place a flat board (a folded ironing board can be ideal) on a couch so that when you lie on the board your pelvis is higher than your head. You must be accompanied by another person when doing this exercise to ensure the board is secure. Use pillows to raise your pelvis if needed. Do this throughout the day for twenty minutes at a time. This encourages baby out of the pelvis to give it space to turn.
- yoga cat moves, rocking pelvis
- cold peas, ice on top of the uterus to make baby uncomfortable
- sitting backwards on a chair can create discomfort for baby, encouraging baby to turn
- gentle massage of baby in the direction you want
- soft, relaxing music into pubic bone/lower abdominal area.

In my experience breech often occurs when there has been an emotional problem with a relationship. It is associated with fear and lack of trust. The baby turns itself upside down because the mother is feeling 'topsy turvy'. One situation involved a 38 week pregnant mum with a breech presentation. When I asked her what she was not happy about she expressed her concern that the baby's nursery was not complete.

This may seem trivial, but to her it was a real concern. After she had expressed this to her partner, he promised to complete the project that weekend. Whilst we were talking the baby began to turn. When I saw her the following week the nursery was completed and her baby was now lying in the correct position.

Melissa's Story

Melissa came to see me at 37 weeks with a breech presentation, very stressed and worried that she would have to undertake a caesarean, something she so didn't want. On palpation I found the uterus to be very relaxed with plenty of room and the baby quite movable.

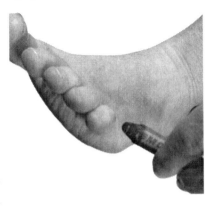

I heated up the TCM and Su-jok points with moxa (outlined in the natural therapy section), plus worked specific reflexology points. I paid particular attention to burning moxa next to the small toe, the UB67 point as shown in the picture. I also gave her some to burn at home between visits. I then gave her a relaxing reflexology session whilst gently and energetically stimulating the uterus point in order to create energy to the area.

We discussed her stresses and concerns. Melissa had moved from the outback town in Western Australia she had been living as there was no maternity support there and was now living at her parents' home. Melissa was very keen to birth naturally, she expressed that her partner was not very supportive and had remained in WA planning to return closer to the time of the birth, but she felt there were relationship issues that were not being resolved. All of this was impacting on her emotional state and therefore the emotional state of her baby.

After completing the reflexology session I took her through a deep relaxing visualisation and emotional release technique, where she was able to clear some of the subconscious baggage. Whilst she was in the deep relaxed state I was able to connect to the baby through Reiki with my hands using gentle pressure to encourage the baby to move around the uterus. Slowly the baby began to move of its own accord. The movement also triggered a Braxton Hick contraction which assisted the baby to move. Melissa expressed that she could feel the baby moving in a positive way. We continued to work like this for about thirty minutes.

By the end of the session the baby had turned into the head down position. I checked the heart rate and Melissa expressed feeling great. When Melissa got up and stood she felt a strong contraction with the need to go to the toilet quickly and the sense of the baby moving down into the pelvis. I again checked the foetal heart and all was good. Melissa came to see me twice a week until 42 weeks when she delivered her beautiful son during a straight forward three hour birth.

Labour of Term Breech Babies

Generally there is little difference in the labour of a head down presentation and a breech. Some doctors advise an epidural for a breech birth, but this is not necessary and may cause more problems as it is widely understood that a woman needs to be able to assist the delivery by feeling the urge to push.

There is some evidence that epidurals increase the risk of a caesarean section. Labour is not normally excessively long and continuous monitoring of the baby's heart rate is advised. When it comes to the actual birth, some doctors use forceps to control the delivery of the baby's head, others prefer to just assist with their hands.

Some will insist on an episiotomy (perineal cut) for first-time mothers, but it really depends on how well the skin stretches, the progress at the time of delivery, the size of the baby and the skill of the delivery attendant. A paediatrician will usually be present at the birth to check the baby over, but there is no reason why the baby shouldn't have skin to skin contact with the mother immediately after the birth. Congenital hip problems are more common in breech babies and this explains why some are breech in the first place. Congenital hip is treatable after birth.

In 2000 the Term Breech Trial (Hannah et al., 2000) became the single research project that almost halted vaginal breech deliveries across most of the developed countries, leaving women with few choices because most obstetricians have not had the opportunity to deliver breeches vaginally. Recently a new consumer driven advocacy group has been formed called the Coalition For Breech Birth (CBB). CBB advocates for the renormalisation of vaginal breech birth. CBB provide information, networking and support to women and their families as they prepare for the birth of their breech babies. CBB also facilitates training and networking opportunities for care providers who wish to support informed choice in breech birth. In July 2008 CCB submitted a petition to the Society of Obstetricians and Gynaecologists of Canada (SOGC) for a change in breech delivery guidelines. In June 2009 the SOGC released the new guidelines, which encourages the practice of vaginal breech birth and initiatives to restore the teaching of vaginal breech teaching to Canadian medical schools is now underway.

http://www.breechbirth.ca/Welcome.html
http://www.facebook.com/groups/breech/

Summary

There is rarely a straightforward way to advise on what is the best option if you find your baby to be breech toward the end of pregnancy.

The most important thing is that you have considered all the options available and reach a decision that is right for you. Many women feel strongly that a caesarean section is the only acceptable option for them, and few obstetricians would deny them this.

Others are very keen to avoid surgery and consider a breech birth just a variation of normal. An excellent book to read is 'Breech Birth, Woman-wise' by Maggie Banks, published by Birthspirit books, Hamilton, New Zealand.

Labour and Birth

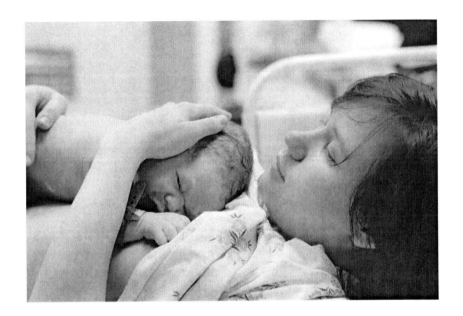

Natural Birth Is a Birthright

> A birthright is a right, privilege or possession to
> which a person is entitled by birth.

Human Right—from the Universal Declaration of Human Rights
http://www.un.org/en/documents/udhr/

Article 1: All human beings are born free and equal in dignity and rights. They are endowed with reason and conscience and should act towards one another in a spirit of brotherhood.

Article 2: Everyone has the right to life, liberty and security of person.

Article 5: No one shall be subjected to torture or cruel, inhuman or degrading treatment or punishment.

Sarah Buckley (MD, birth activist) talks about physiological birth as 'Mother Nature's blueprint' for all births (2000):

"Birth is the beginning of so many things besides the condition of a right bearer and it can be viewed from very different angles. For one it is a moment in a mother's life that requires the respect of her rights, as a woman, to make choices and to have them respected, and as a birthing woman, to have access to proper care during her pregnancy and her birth. On the other hand the baby has the right to be born with and into his rights including security of person. Both child and mother have a right to come from the birth with life and health but also in well-being and optimal beginnings, with the best start possible as bio-psycho-emotional being. Bonding, bio-neurological neonatal adaptation, and optimal jumpstart of the immune system are some of the documented differences between just birth and optimal birth. Birth is a sensuous experience, it is natural, and not a catastrophe."

Since the late 1940s the management of birth has become industrialised. The business side of birth has become the focus and hospitals and medical centres are hubs of economic turnover. The use of technology and the ability to interfere in the natural process of birth has been created through the illusion of safety. We have, as a civilization, succeeded in transforming natural birth into a medical pathology or condition and a natural abnormality.

> "So most people now profoundly believe that this is the way of giving birth and they have not yet understood how much has been lost in the process."
>
> Elena Piantino, Midwifery Today, 9:3, 2009.

This medicalisation of birth poses the great risk that we are losing our way back to nature, back to the innate knowledge of natural birth. Most doctors and midwives are now being taught more about technology and pharmaceuticals than developing an understanding of the basic physiology of birth.

We need to turn the tide and head back to the innate knowledge of what it is to be human, the knowledge that we once honoured. All individuals have the right to be born in an optimal way and given the best opportunity to do so. If interventions become necessary they should only be instigated as a result of clear, valid evidence-based research.

Fear Creates Pain

Giving birth is one of the most powerful experiences you will have in your life. In order for you to give over to the forces of nature and let go, enabling you to give birth freely and easily, you must understand and accept the functions of your unique body. You must take responsibility for your pregnancy and your birth experience.

You cannot expect to hand over this responsibility to the midwife or the obstetrician. For taking on this responsibility you will receive the greatest of rewards. It can be the most awe inspiring, uplifting experience and discovery of one's self to be able to master labour and the birth of your child through your own efforts, not to mention the safest way to give birth.

Pain is generally the body's indicator that something is not quite right, it is the warning bell. In labour it is not pain but an intense emotional experience created for a specific purpose. It is unlike any other experience and cannot be described as pain. Giving birth is not a dangerous event. It is a natural event requiring little intervention.

If a woman is led to expect pain then she will be in a state of tension in anticipation of labour. Her body is on alert. The 'fight and flight' mechanism has gone into action and she will experience unnecessary pain due to muscle and ligament tension.

Fear can become so strong as to change the pattern of the labour, interrupting the natural progress. When you go into labour your body is 'on alert', super sensitive to outside stimuli in order to ensure a safe and quiet environment for you to birth in. If you are experiencing fear your body becomes tense, creating greater discomfort. This creates a state of 'high alert' with adrenalin pumping throughout your body. The message your body hears is that it is not safe for you to give birth to this baby in this environment.

If this occurs during the first stage of labour it can slow labour down. The round muscles of the cervix resist dilating and opening in reaction to this 'fight and flight' mechanism in order to protect your baby from the perceived danger. However the longitudinal muscles of the uterus will continue to contract, with contractions often getting stronger and stronger but without effect. The adrenalin produced also inhibits the production of natural endorphins which help to relax you. This creates conflict within the body. Even though you seem to be labouring well there is little progress. Sometimes this is termed 'failure to progress' and can result in a caesarean section if the fear is not addressed. If however this occurs during second stage (the pushing stage) of labour, when your cervix is already open, then there may be a huge rush of adrenaline giving you the strength to push your baby out so that you can pick your baby up and protect it.

When drugs are used in labour they inhibit the natural production of endorphins (the bodies natural pain killers) as the body tends to stop creating endorphins once the synthetic drug has been introduced. Drugs change the delicate balance of the body, which can cause the birthing woman to become disorientated and not as centred or able to believe in her ability to birth without further interventions.

> 'A woman has an absolute need to drop her mask
> to stop being a person. In privacy and with humility,
> the labouring woman accepts her mammalian condition.
> She needs to bend forward. Praying and giving birth are presented
> as intensely private events which effectively keep the human
> community at a distance.'
>
> Michel Odent (1999).

Therefore it stands to reason to aim to create as relaxing an environment both internally and externally to facilitate an optimal birth experience.

Ways of Checking Dilation

During years of birthing with women I have come to understand the one thing that a birthing women is focused on, and that is how dilated she is. Dilation lets her know where she is at right now regardless of what has gone before. The progress of labour is very important to the mental and emotional state of the mother. How she is informed of her dilation can have a great impact on the outcome of her labour. Being told she is 'only' 1-2cm dilated after several hours of early labour can shatter her self confidence.

Then on the other hand telling a mother she is 7cms with not long to go, after only a short time of labour, can be very presumptive and lead to a state of impatience if the labour then continues for several more hours.

So the question is what is good information and the right time to impart it? For the majority of people the first thought is vaginal examination. However there are many other signs that indicate progress other than putting hands into your vagina. Vaginal checks come with risks such as accidental rupture of the membranes and the risk of infection.

Some studies have indicated that vaginal examination may not be as accurate as first thought with accuracy measured at around 48-56% (Phelps et al., 1995). This figure worsens when more people's assessments are added into the equation, as assessment techniques may vary and all rely on individual interpretation. For example, you may be examined by the midwife looking after you. The midwife may then get a second opinion from another more experienced midwife, who then may seek further assessment from the doctor in charge. All three may provide a different result, so who is correct?

I do however recommend a vaginal examination to ensure there is full dilation before allowing mum to push, to ensure the cervix is completely out of the way. Pushing on a cervix that may not be completely dilated can obstruct the progress of labour. This is especially important for first time mothers.

Other Signs

The birthing woman not lying down in labour, being ambulant and using different positions allows the birth attendant to view other signs of progress.

There is a dark line which can sometimes look quite purple that presents along the line between the buttocks. When a women is on all fours, kneeling or bending over it is easy to see. It begins close to the anus, which becomes distended by the birthing baby during birth. As labour progresses it moves up the line of division between each cheek. Once it has reached the top generally it indicates full dilation (10cm). The cervix is now out of the way and you are ready to push. A good thing to do is to get your midwife or birth attendant to check out this line before you birth so that the changes that are occurring as you labour are easily visible.

BMC Pregnancy & Childbirth published a study in 2010 (Shepherd et al.) indicating the existence and accuracy of this delineation line for most women. Seventy six percent of the women studied presented with the line at the same stage of labour. It was more likely to be present in women who commenced labour naturally than those who were induced. The line became more notable from around 4-5cm, becoming the most visible around 7-8cm then fading away closer to full dilation. This is where you may feel distension as the baby begins to move down, indicating pushing is imminent and full dilation has generally occurred. Lancet (1990) also published a study discussing the existence and accuracy of the line. This study noticed a significant correlation between the station of the baby's head and the length of the line.

Communication During Labour
There are emotional signposts along the labour trail.

Early labour (0-4cm) you may feel excited and probably quite chatty but as the labour progresses you will go inward and begin to draw on your internal energy.

Active labour (4-6 or 7 cm) you will begin to use your breath, deeply breathing through the contraction. You may even begin vocalizing, moaning, humming or even chanting. Generally conversation becomes minimal with one or two word statements during contractions. Resting between contractions will become a priority.

Transition (7-9cm) you may find you become quite noisy using guttural primal sounds. There is a to and fro of needs. Becoming hot and cold. Often changing position. You may have a great need for support by the birth helpers here too. Then you may also become snappy, tired and impatient. Many women state 'I want to go home' or 'I can't do this' at this stage.

By full dilation you may well retreat within and become quiet, not wanting to speak at all. There is often the calm before the storm. This is a time of energy gaining, resting in preparation for the pushing phase. It is important to stop and rest here.

Early pushing sounds, little grunts during the contraction, are often the first signs of full dilation. A holding of the breath and bearing down. The sounds become strong and very deep. Low and open sounds are very beneficial. Keeping the jaw relaxed without clenching helps the pelvic area to open.

Smell & Intuition

When you have been birthing with women for some time you begin to recognise smells and intuitive senses. Just before the start of transition, there is an earthy and very 'birthy' smell. Musky and deep, it speaks to some inner part of our being and psyche. There is a sense of knowing.

Fundal Height

At full term the fundal (top of the uterus) height is normally 5 finger-breadths below the breast bone. Once labour begins and the cervix begins to open, the baby starts to move down into the pelvis and the uterus pulls up from the cervix, becoming shorter. As dilation progresses, the finger-breadths between the fundus and the breast bone becomes smaller and smaller. By full dilation, there is no longer a gap between the two. This measurement must be done at the height of the contraction, and while mother is on her back.

Doptone Position

You can also check progression via the doptone. In early labour the baby is lying higher so the heartbeat will be found around to the side and higher up from the pubic bone. As labour progresses the baby moves around and down so the heart beat can be tracked down until it will be found almost directly above the pubic bone, indicating it is getting closer to birth.

Bloody Show

A bloody show often indicates that labour is imminent. There is also another bloody show and release of fluids that can occur around 7-8cm dilation as the cervix begins to open up wider.

All of these signs can be used to indicate the progress of labour without the need for vaginal examination. I recommend using vaginal examination only if it is absolutely necessary in order to make a decision about the next step in the labour journey.

The Muscles of Labour

There are three layers of uterine muscle fibres involved in birth.

- spiral or oblique fibres begin at the cervix and run in all directions around the uterus. Their major role is to take up, shorten and dilate the cervix until it is wide enough to allow the baby to pass through. These fibres also assist with contracting the uterus to prevent blood loss after the placenta is delivered.
- longitudinal fibres run from the cervix, or neck of the uterus, up to the fundus and down the other side. On contraction they shorten the uterus and are used mainly in the expulsion of the baby during second stage.
- circular fibres pass in a horizontal manner around the lower part of the uterus. When these contract they close the cervix and inhibit activity of the lower part of the uterus.

The uterus appears to be supplied with nerves from the autonomic nervous system. In a smoothly coordinated labour the longitudinal and spiral muscles contract and start to open the cervix and the circular fibres around the cervix stay relaxed to allow this to happen. This unopposed muscle contraction does not in itself produce pain.

The only pain receptors are those which detect excessive stress, tension or tearing of tissues. The intestines and uterus can be burnt, handled or moved without any sensation of pain but if they are stretched or torn considerable pain and shock results. Therefore it appears the pain in labour must be due to one or other of these two stimuli. So by encouraging relaxed muscles less pain is then experienced.

Grantly Dick Read in his book 'Childbirth Without Fear' discusses the issue of how a women's attitude to her sexuality can have strong bearing on her ability to understand the flow of nature in labour and birth. If the mother has a negative attitude to her monthly menses, believing this to be uncomfortable, tiresome and a nuisance, often experiencing Pre-Menstrual Tension and severe period pain, then labour will likely be perceived in the same way. What can then follow is a mind-body entanglement that results in strong, difficult and ineffective contractions.

What Creates the Intensity of Labour?

Whenever we experience any form of stress and trauma during life, we are often able to look back and see the personal growth that was achieved by this experience. The intensity of labour provides positive feedback to the birthing woman so as to direct her attention inwards to focus on the job at hand. This is an important right of passage from pregnancy to taking on the responsibility of motherhood. It never ceases to amaze me the incredible personal growth that women attain through pregnancy, labour and birth.

Physiologists have found that when a woman is labouring she uses the primitive part of the brain, that completely instinctive side we share with all mammals. It has been my experience that when women experience a natural birth they rarely complain about the pain of labour but invariably relish in the achievement of giving birth the way nature intended. The intensity of labour is positive with a positive end - your baby. It is not the same kind of pain that suggests illness or problems. The intensity of each contraction is different, each one a step nearer to birth. Contractions build gradually and allow the body's natural endorphins to reach their peak, allowing your mind to accept the intensity as it increases

The intensity changes with each stage of birth. The first stage of labor is passive as you focus inward and allow your body to do what it needs to do. In the second stage there is less intensity and more activity. You wake up and become alert in order to birth your baby. When the head crowns the intensity is there to tell you to take it slowly, to gently birth your baby, to allow the perineum to stretch.

The third stage of labour is the delivery of the placenta. Here you will receive more signals letting you know when it is time to push the placenta out. Allowing yourself to relax and believing in your ability to birth gives you a greater ability to accept and allow the intensity.

The intensity of labour is there for a reason. We need to understand it and accept it, and not be afraid of it.

Where women and their partners are well educated in the benefits of actively working with their body, more effective and shorter labours with less pain and far less intervention are likely, with successful outcomes for mother and baby. Women don't necessarily know what to do in labour or how to work with contractions. This needs to be taught through effective antenatal classes that concentrate on empowering them and their support people to fully understand their options and how to use 'The System' most effectively.

A study on expectations of labour pain included postpartum women who had delivered single infants at term in one of two hospitals, one in the Netherlands and one in Iowa. Within fourty eight hours of delivery they were asked about their prenatal expectations of pain in labour and measures available for pain relief, and then about their memory of labour pain and whether or not they had received pain medication. The Iowa women were significantly younger than the Dutch women (mean age 24.7 as compared to 28.9 years). The number of primiparas (first time mothers) in each population was similar (52.2% of the Iowa group and 45.5% of the Dutch).

Of both groups twelve to thirteen percent had had their labour induced and neonatal data was similar. The Iowa women in general expected labour to be more painful than did the Dutch women and anticipated more often that they would receive medication for labour pain. In virtually the same proportion as anticipated, the Iowa women did receive analgesia. By contrast, the Dutch women did not expect labour to be painful, tended not to anticipate receiving analgesia, and usually did not receive any. When asked retrospectively to assess the painfulness of labour, both groups gave similar responses, divided roughly equally among the choices "more painful, less painful, and about as expected" (Obstetrics and Gynaecology, April 1988).

Around the turn of the twentieth century, many of the early feminists believed the pain and problems in labour were a direct result of the commonly held belief that the female body was inherently inferior to that of the male. They heard about Indian women who were giving birth painlessly and easily and believed that with the proper mindset, they could do the same. So childbirth became a way for women to prove to themselves and others that women were strong and capable of determining their own fates. Elizabeth Cady Stanton wrote:

> "My girlhood was spent mostly in the open air. I early imbibed the idea that a girl is just as good as a boy, and I carried it out. I would walk five miles before breakfast, or ride 10 on horseback ... I wore my clothing sensibly. ... I never compressed my body. ... When my first four children were born, I suffered very little. I then made up my mind that it was totally unnecessary for me to suffer at all; so I dressed lightly, walked every day ... And took proper care of myself. I walked three miles. The child was born without a particle of pain."
>
> Laura Kaplan Shanley, Love is the Heart of Labour,
> Midwifery Today Issue 24

No honest doctor would ever suggest that drugs given for pain are without risks. But in their pursuit of relieving a labouring mother's pain, doctors inevitably resort to prescribing drugs when, in fact, there are many non-pharmacological ways to relieve pain. For example, scientific research has proven a number of drug-free techniques to be effective in relieving the pain of normal labour, including:

- the continuous presence during labour of a midwife, a doula or a loved one
- sitting in a tub of warm water or standing in a shower

- freedom to move about and assume any position
- massage
- acupuncture
- reflexology.

None of these techniques involve any risk to the woman or her baby and are often promoted by midwives but rarely promoted by doctors (Wagner, 2000).

Many studies have been conducted on labour, birth and pain. Grantly-Dick Read, the founder of Antenatal classes as far back as the early 1930's, challenged obstetric carers on these grounds. He noted:

- that no other animal appeared to struggle with the birth process except when complications arose
- many primitive cultures where birth was embraced and looked forward to with joy and anticipation appeared to have little signs of suffering through childbirth unless complications arose
- that pain receptors are not present as such in the uterus or birth canal and that the physiological process of pain in our body is related to fear and tension
- experience shows that if the woman is prepared spiritually and psychologically for the birth then there is little or minimal suffering in labour
- the pain associated with labour is directly linked to the amount of fear and tension present in the body.

Most women who have experienced a natural birth are overwhelmed by their feelings of achievement and empowerment and rarely become engrossed in describing the pain.

Assisting a Productive Labour and Birth

- Create the right support team - support must be positive, patient and encouraging, they must have faith in you to give birth naturally.
- If possible woman-centred care ensures you know who will be with you during the birth and you can build a strong working relationship with one midwife. Express and clear feelings and fears with your birth carer.
- Use affirmations, visualizations, yoga and relaxation during your pregnancy and birth.
- Attend effective Antenatal Classes, read natural birth books, spend time with Natural Birth Midwives and doulas.
- Write a birth plan, clearly stating what your wants and desires are.
- Choose a birth place that feels safe, comfortable and non-threatening. Seek out the options in your area and visit Delivery Suites, Birth Centres and talk to Homebirth Midwives. Become familiar with the environment that is going to be your place of birth.
- Set the environment of your birth. Place bean bags on the floor with mattresses, take in your favourite coloured materials, music, photos, aromatherapy.
- Become very informed so that you are able to make informed decisions without fear attached, therefore avoiding unnecessary interventions which often cause more problems once they are introduced.
- Have a regular massage, learn what feels good and what you dislike. This allows you to know what sort of massage works best for you so that you can indicate this to your support people. The more familiar you are with touch the better.
- Practice different positions with your partner/support people for first and second stages of labour.
- Women who begin labour at peak fitness are able to cope better. Begin walking every day, building up to an hour of fast walking or swimming by late pregnancy.

- Movement is essential in labour and a woman who is fit and flexible will be able to take full advantage of different positions to assist.
- Have regular Reflexology sessions throughout pregnancy and labour, this has been proven to significantly reduce labour pain and time.
- Relaxation and breathing exercises need to be practiced regularly to become habitual. Being able to totally let go and relax between contractions can be the greatest asset in labour. Hypnotherapy has becoming a popular form of deep relaxation for labour. Therapists are available in some states.
- Use water in labour as this can significantly reduce labour pain and time. Showers, baths or water tanks and pools can be of great assistance.
- Explore complimentary therapies, such as those discussed in this book. Body therapies greatly enhance your birth experience.

Ways of Diminishing the Intensity

I believe that mastering the pain of labour and giving birth can provide you with incredible personal growth that spans your whole life. Men have no assimilating experience in their life yet it is often men who dictate how a woman will act or what care she will receive in labour.

The life force of labour need not be feared but understood for the beauty it really is, I give thanks for being able to continually experience the energy of love and power that is created by labour.

The most common reason for long painful labours is the posterior presentation of the baby. It is important to work towards the right position. Keep the pelvis tilted forward and higher than the knees. Don't slouch. Practice hands and knees (all fours) exercises, semi-squats and sit backwards on a chair daily (see Getting Baby Into the Right Position).

Address as many fears as possible through re-birthing, maternity reflexology, hypno-birthing and counselling. Even though you may feel you have no fears, fears may be carried from your own mothers' pregnancies and lay dormant deep within your cellular structure.

Also consider:

- keep upright throughout labour as much as possible. Gravity is a great assistant to the baby. Walk around, rock, squat and lean forward.
- hot packs and towels locally applied to tense areas relieve discomfort. Heat and cold applied especially to the lower back and front of the pubic bone can be a great relief. Most women find really hot packs to be the best. This can be one of the main roles for the support person, holding a pack on the front and back during a contraction.
- change position as soon as contractions become uncomfortable. This may be difficult at times, but the discomfort is nature's way of telling you to move to allow the baby to negotiate its way through the pelvis.
- a TENS (Transcutaneous Electrical Nerve Stimulation) is a battery operated device with wires that are attached to your body by adhesive pads. It sends a small electrical current through the skin to the muscle, which interrupts the pain signal being sent to the brain as well as stimulating the natural production of endorphins. It allows the user to move around and control the level of impulse being sent. Most sets need to be hired by the user.
- listen intuitively to your body and push when it feels right to do so.

Baby Josef (pictured below) was a large baby at 4.4kilos. Josef was born vaginally and his mother, Eleanor, maintained an intact perineum. Eleanor credits the lack of trauma from perineal tearing or need for episiotomy to her ability to trust her intuition. Whilst her midwife kept telling her to push, Eleanor said 'No, it's not ready', pushing instead when her intuition told her it was time.

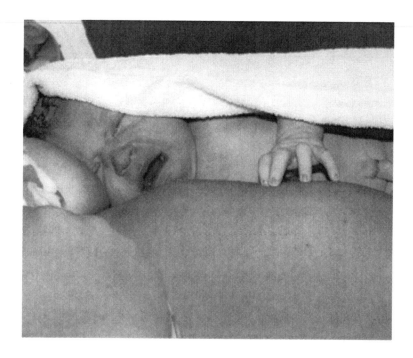

Visualisation Exercise for Labour

This is a good exercise to practice before labour with your partner or support person. The aim of this exercise is to bring your focus inside and to distract the mind during contractions. If possible have someone guide you through each step and give your guide verbal feedback after each step.

1. Scan the body for a sensation, pressure, pain or tightness (contraction).
2. Where is it? In relation to the other parts of the body?
3. If you could give it a score out of 10, with 10 being the most painful and 1 for no pain, what number would you give it?
4. If it had a shape what would it be? For example round, square, triangular.
5. How big is this shape?
6. What colour and depth is it?

7. What texture is it? For example soft, hard, metallic, wool.

8. What score is it now?

Continue to work through these different questions or similar until the pain has reduced. Ask questions such as what does it look like? Does it remind you of anything? Can you move it? The technique allows the body to relax as the mind is preoccupied with thinking, allowing your body to get on with labour.

As the labour progresses begin visualising your birth canal. Imagine it is like a tunnel with a light at the end. Focus on this light, seeing it become larger as if you are opening the gateway. Try not to focus on the intensity, the aim is to distract your mind. If we keep thoughts in the form of visualisations actively happening they block the pathway for the pain molecules to reach the brain.

What to Expect in Labour - a Practical Guide

Pre-Labour

What's Happening to Your Body?	What You May Feel	What You Can Do	What Support People Can Do
• Baby's head engaged in the pelvis. • Muscles begin to relax due to hormones. • Braxton-Hicks contractions. • Softening of the cervix. • Bloody Show, increased mucous discharge. • Baby less active and is settled. • Slight diarrhoea. • Pelvic pressure. • Membranes may rupture with no contractions.	• Period pain • Backache (lower back) • Tired sore legs. • Waves of light contractions. • Bursts of energy. • Increased bowel movements. • Nesting behaviour around the house. • Need to house clean. • Emotionally scattered, unsettled.	• Rest as needed. • Gentle exercise such as swimming or walking helps establish labour. • High energy food and drinks. • Relaxation and yoga. • Hot bath / shower. • Massage / Reflexology. • Ensure you have all you need. • Let your midwife and support people know, particularly if you are planning a homebirth so they can organise their schedules. • Remain calm, it may be a couple of days yet.	• Relax and get organised. • Reassure and clear any fears. • Reflexology for relaxation. • Massage • Spend time with mum. go for walks, exercise. • Just be there, be available, but also get on with your own life. Do not hang around as it creates a state of anticipation and impatience. • Encourage mum to be patient.

What to Expect in Labour - a Practical Guide

Labour Begins

What's Happening to Your Body?	What You May Feel	What You Can Do	What Support People Can Do
• Cervix is thinning and begins to dilate, from 0-4cm dilated. • Contractions become more rhythmic and regular, building to 5 - 20 minutes apart. • Waters may break. • This stage may last for several hours or even a couple of days.	• Stronger waves of contractions making you stop to breathe. • Pressure on the cervix. • Increase in mucous production. • Increased need to wee. • May feel like you are wetting yourself but it could be the membranes leaking. • Excited, impatient, scared. • The need to be upright.	• Eat a healthy energetic meal. • Drink frequently. • Relax. • Take baths and showers. • Rest as much as possible. • Listen to your body. • Make sure you and your support team are fully organised as labour is hotting up.	• If you haven't already, notify the midwife things are starting. • Encourage relaxation, go for walks. • Stay very calm, try not to get too excited. • Massage, Reflexology. • Keep the energy positive. • Be very patient.

What to Expect in Labour - a Practical Guide

Accelerated Phase

What's Happening to Your Body?	What You May Feel	What You Can Do	What Support People Can Do
• 4-5 cm to 7-8cm dilation. • Contractions become strong and regular, 2-5 minutes apart, lasting 60-90 seconds. • Nothing else exists except what is happening to your body. • Baby begins to move lower. • Body functions spontaneously. • You will begin to feel very earthy, making guttural sounds, deep breathing with moaning sounds. Often the birthing dance can begin to happen now.	• This is it, no going back. • Can be overwhelming. • You are preoccupied with labour, nothing else exists. • One word answers, body swaying, deep breathing, guttural sounds. • Intensity of body sensations, sometimes backache, strong pubic pressure, pelvic pressure from the baby, cold feet, most likely want your clothes off by this stage. **All that matters is healthy mum healthy baby - Time is not important.**	• Talk to your baby, breathe with each contraction. • Stay focused, try not to get into thinking mode. • Use relaxation techniques. • Switch off between contractions and rest. • Keep active, change positions. • Wee frequently. • Take showers and baths. • Express your needs clearly. • Lean on your support people.	• Stay positive. • Talk quietly. • Breathe with her. • Respond quickly to her requests. • Help her focus, use visualisations. • Massage, hot packs. • Offer frequent energetic drinks with ice. • Maintain eye contact. • Keep distractions to a minimum. • Keep environment relaxed. • Time to go to hospital if mum is planning to birth there. Do this calmly and quietly. Mum will probably be most comfortable in the back seat of the car.

What to Expect in Labour - a Practical Guide

Transition

What's Happening to Your Body?	What You May Feel	What You Can Do	What Support People Can Do
• The body is busy clearing out in preparation for pushing out the baby. • Hormones and endorphins are at their highest. • You will be receiving many mixed signals. • Contractions are strong and regular but with a deeper relaxation between. • Membranes will most likely rupture now. • There will be frequent bowel motions and weeing. • Most likely vomiting as well. • This is a great time to be in the shower, bath or water pool.	• Contractions will be strong and overwhelming, it will feel like your body is taking over and you must just follow its lead. • Your endorphins will make you feel very high, allowing you to rest and regain energy. • You may feel tense feelings between each contraction. • Do not push until your body really wants to. Listen to your midwife. • You will feel many sensations - panic, cramps, pressure, soreness, stretching, hot, sweaty, tired, exhausted, fed up. • You may fall into a deep sleep between contractions.	• Panting, blowing, shower, wee frequently, go with the flow. • Breathe deeply, focus on relaxing. • Know it is almost over, rock, dance, sing, groan, and ask for your needs to be met. • Lean on your support people, pull on their energy. • Do not push yet. • Avoid distractions, go within, focus on your baby, talk to your baby. • Use visualisations. • Focus on opening up. **The toilet is a great place now.** • Loose lips Loose Perineum.	• Eye to Eye contact, stay very positive. • This is when you will be most needed. • If you can't handle the intensity get out. • Speak positively and confidently, assure her of the progress. • Don't ever say 'you're only'. • Massage, hot packs, follow the midwives instructions. • Support the partner, they are feeling it too and may be overwhelmed. **POSITIVE, LOVING, ENCOURAGING** • Support her positions. • Take photos. • Make the experience very special. • Keep Smiling. **TRUST THE PROCESS**

What to Expect in Labour - a Practical Guide

Second Stage

What's Happening to Your Body?	What You May Feel	What You Can Do	What Support People Can Do
• The body begins to bear down with intensity, similar to pushing when having a bowel action. • Bowel and bladder will completely empty. • Lots of pressure in the pelvic region and across the pubic bone. • Your body will choose the most comfortable positions that facilitate and open the pelvis. • It can take a couple of hours to push your baby out if this is your first baby, but is generally much quicker for subsequent births.	• An unusual sensation, may feel like you are pushing your baby out of your bottom. • Mixed sensations, go with your body's direction. • Do not push unnecessarily, your baby will move down by itself. It feels good, allow your body to guide you. • You will wake up and become very active. • You will feel continual pressure between each contraction.	• Use many positions to help your baby move through the pelvis. This is the time to really work. • Don't be in a hurry let your body guide you. Talk to your baby. Listen to your midwife. • Completely let go and rest between contractions this can be hard work. • **Breathe with the contraction until you feel the need to push then take a big breath and using your abdominal muscles just like you are doing a great big POO push into your bottom. Hold the pressure there then take another breath and continue to push until the contraction has gone.**	• Support the mother through any positions she chooses, stay focused, light and positive. • Do not get over-excited, keep everything calm and quiet. • Do not over encourage pushing, allow her body to do what is best for her. • Talk positively with eye to eye contact. • Guide her pushing into the bottom so as to use contractions effectively.

What to Expect in Labour - a Practical Guide

	Crowning and Birth		
What's Happening to Your Body?	What You May Feel	What You Can Do	What The Support People Can Do
• Pelvic floor stretches and dilates. • Pelvis relaxes and opens, baby rotates. • Head is born first followed by the shoulders.	• Stretching, burning sensation, overwhelming fear, need for direction. • A very short, intense emotional time, let go and let your body do what is needed. • You may like to touch your baby's head as it is birthing. This gives great reassurance.	• Follow your midwife's instructions, pant, try to relax, keep lips loose, smile. • Push through the stretching, visualise or use a mirror. • Focus on your baby whom you will meet soon.	• Relax, smile enjoy the experience, follow, the midwives instructions. Keep everything calm, take photos. • Begin to drop back from the intensity, allowing the parents to be the focus.

445

What to Expect in Labour - a Practical Guide

Immediately Following Birth

What's Happening to Your Body?	What You May Feel	What You Can Do	What The Support People Can Do
• Baby needs to be passed immediately to mum. • Baby will usually breathe fairly soon after birth. Just needs to be held and welcomed. • Skin to skin is imperative. There is plenty of time. Do not allow anyone else to impose on your bonding time. Preferable to leave the cord uncut until after the placenta is delivered. Let your baby get the best start. **BONDING IS IMPERATIVE NOW**	• Overwhelmed by the birth. • Cold and shaky. • You may feel a bit shocked. It has been a big experience, be gentle on yourself. • It often takes time to fall in love with your baby.	• Hold your baby, take time to relax and enjoy the experience. • Make sure your baby is placed skin to skin. • Look into your baby's eyes and connect and bond. • Take the time to be together as a family.	• Drop back and quietly begin to tidy up. • Leave parents and baby together to bond. • Take photos if requested. • Have a quiet drink as you wait for the placenta, which may take a while.

What to Expect in Labour - a Practical Guide

Third Stage - Delivery of the Placenta

What's Happening to Your Body?	What You May Feel	What You Can Do	What The Support People Can Do
• A resting time takes place as the body's hormones gather and the changes occur for the delivery of the placenta. This can take an hour or so. • As long as there is no bleeding everything is fine and time is of no consequence. • The body will show signs when it's ready to birth the placenta. • There will be a strong contraction, a gush of blood and lengthening of the cord. • Your body knows how to deliver the placenta, trust in the process.	• A strong contraction and sensation to push, a gush from the vagina and movement in the cord. • You will feel like getting up and pushing the placenta out. • You may feel like breastfeeding if your baby shows interest. This can also help with the delivery of the placenta. **YOU MUST DO THIS YOURSELF to prevent risk of haemorrhage or tearing the placenta, causing a retaining of products.**	• Best if you can move into a squat position over a bowl and gently push your placenta out with the contraction. You may need to guide it by holding onto the cord. **DO NOT PULL.** • If it resists wait and push with the next contraction. Stimulating the nipples and breasts can help with a release of oxytocin.	• Assist mum to squat over a bowl. • Do what ever you can to facilitate a natural delivery of the placenta. Take time to look at this incredible organ, it has sustained the life of a child for nine months. • Ask the parents if they would like to keep it and maybe plant a tree over it for their child.

447

What to Expect in Labour - a Practical Guide

Post Birth

What's Happening to Your Body?	What You May Feel	What You Can Do	What The Support People Can Do
• The baby begins to take in its new world. Its body changes from living in the womb to living on earth. • The baby may want to feed but just as likely not. • Involution of the uterus, your uterus will contract to the size of a cricket ball. • There will be bleeding and you may have small tears and lacerations that will heal over the next few days. • You may feel quite shaky when you first walk.	• You will feel sore and tired but extremely excited and in love with your child. • This is a very special time so take as much time as you like. • You may feel like breast feeding but your baby may not be ready yet. It can take a couple of days.	• Just hold your baby and enjoy it. • Relax and be pampered. • You have just achieved the most important job in the world bringing a baby into the world. Feel very proud of yourself.	• Help clean up, make drinks, and generally just support the couple. • Celebrate with a birthday cake. • Make Nettle Tea for mum • Be a good friend and support the couple every day through meals and cleaning for a few weeks. • Often it's the next few days that is the most difficult and you will be needed the most, especially at home.

448

The Delivery of the Placenta

Many midwives have remarked that the delivery of the placenta is a natural progression, so much easier and complete when the cord remains attached to the baby. It is a time of adjustment, healing and letting go of the pregnancy. A time of acceptance of motherhood and an opportunity by nature to provide necessary nutrients and hormones to the baby as it adjusts to life outside the womb.

Throughout the first two stages of labour uterine muscles at the placenta site are protected from the contractions. This prevents the placenta from separating from the uterus and depriving your baby of oxygen. Once baby has birthed and begins to breathe for itself the cord ceases to pulsate and foetal blood no longer reaches the placental site. The placental site starts to lose its resistance to contractions and begins to separate.

The expulsion of the placenta is most likely to be accompanied by the force of gravity, with the mother in the squatting position. It has been my experience as a midwife that when a mother is assisted to gently squat and push her own placenta out there are far less complications.

Unfortunately modern birthing practices dictate the active management of the delivery of the placenta by routinely injecting an oxytocic drug to the mother shortly after the birth of the baby.

This causes a rapid contracting of the uterine wall, forcing the separation of the placenta in a short period of time. This can be a shocking experience for the woman. The placenta must be delivered quickly or the rapidly contracting uterus will cause the cervix to re-close, resulting in a retained placenta. The woman must then be taken to theatre for removal of the retained placenta. This is not a good way to begin life as a new mother. This management of third stage can cause the problems it is meant to prevent, that of post-partum haemorrhage and retained placenta.

It is far more pleasant if the mother refuses the drug and takes control by delivering her placenta herself, which will usually occur within one hour of the birth. It is my policy to strongly recommend hands off by the birth attendants and let the new mother do this herself. Mother and baby assist each other in a most essential critical way. The sucking activity of the baby not only stimulates oxytocin release, which instigates bonding and separation of the placenta, but also promotes prolactin, establishing the let-down reflex for breastfeeding.

There are many differing opinions regarding the management of the cord and placenta after birth. Shivam Rachan celebrates the placenta through the Lotus Birth:

> "Lotus Birth extends the birth time into the sacred days that follow and enables baby, mother and father and all family members to pause, reflect and engage in nature's conduct. Lotus birth is a call to return to the rhythms of nature, to witness the natural order and to the experience of not doing, just being"
>
> Shivam Rachan (2000).

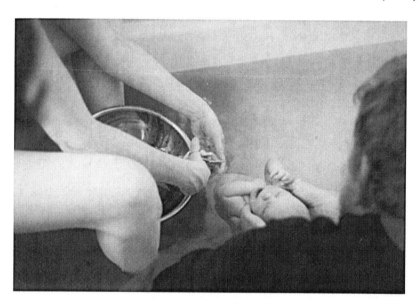

Shivam undertook extensive research into the relationship of the placenta to the baby's early postnatal period. She discovered that the earlier the cord was cut the longer the time it took for healing of the umbilical wound. When the cord was cut immediately the average time for healing is 9.56 days, 7.16 days when cut at the end of pulsating and 3.75 days when cut after the placenta was delivered from the mother. This supported the notion that the later the cord is cut the better for the baby. Her research also indicated that doctors were sixty eight percent more likely to cut the cord immediately compared to twenty two percent of midwifes.

The Royal College of Midwives (RCM) guidelines advise clamping of the cord within thirty seconds in order to reduce the risk of jaundice. The RCM is now reviewing this guideline and has indicated support for midwives not to immediately clamp cords. In August 2012 the RCM indicated they expect to change their guidelines to advise waiting three to five minutes before clamping. RCM cites research from Sweden and the USA that indicates later clamping of the cord may help protect the newborn from anaemia and iron deficiency whilst allowing the transfer of vital stem cells (RCM 2012, http:// www.rcm.org.uk/midwives/news/clamping-update-to-be-delivered/).

The time between the birth of the baby and the birth of the placenta is a period when "TIME SHOULD STAND STILL", as mother and baby get to know each other and fall deeply in love. Michel Odent (1999) refers to this time as the critical bonding time, when a mother and baby look into each others eyes and fall deeply in love, imperative for their future relationship together. He recommends that being still connected to the placenta after birth allows the baby to reconnect with its former sense of inner stability, of connection to a deep unchanging reality. The baby can remember the familiar resonance of deep unconscious knowing that still resides in the placenta. Time is of the essence so that the completion of this stage can occur. The fact that time is taken away from us may be the basis of why this world is always in such a hurry.

http://cord-clamping.com/2011/12/19/mother-baby-after-birth/

In the case of the lotus birth there is less pressure on the baby to breathe immediately, and the transition between the intrauterine environment and condition of utter dependence to the first steps of independence outside the womb is not as severe and threatening.

451

Traditional cultures are strengthened by a belief in the existence of spirit or soul that inhabits the physical body. Thus the respectful care of the placenta was often referred to as the double soul, secret helper or brother and was either buried or placed in a tree on a pole (Elizabeth Noble, 1988).

> "By respecting the placenta we respect our origin and our connection to the beyond as the inspiration for our spirit, and to the earth as the nurturer of our body."
>
> Shivam Rachan (2000).

Not cutting the cord until after delivery of the placenta allows baby to receive optimal nutrients from the placenta. I have often found that if you ask a baby if they want their cord cut or not they will let you know. Usually they crunch up if not ready, indicating a protection of the umbilical area, whereas if they are ready they will open up their arms and legs allowing access to the cord. This may sound bizarre but I have seen it too often not to take notice. Elizabeth Nobles' waterbirth video from the early nineties demonstrates this theory wonderfully (1988).

Preventing Postpartum Haemorrhage

Ordinarily the myometrial fibres of the uterus contract and retract causing kinking of the blood vessels at the placental site. The kinked vessels cease providing blood to the placental site and bleeding is controlled. Uterine atony (ineffective uterine contraction) is responsible for eighty to ninety percent of postpartum haemorrhage cases. This failure may be due to uterine dysfunction, anaesthesia, ineffective first and second stage contractions, over distension of the uterus, exhaustion due to a long labour, multiparity (many pregnancies), myomas (fibroids), operative deliveries which traumatize the uterus and mismanagement of the placental delivery stage of labour. Most of these causes can be anticipated and the appropriate management taken to lessen the risks of a haemorrhage.

By applying these keys both prenatally and in the third stage, the incidence of postpartum haemorrhage can decrease considerably.

1. Good nutrition is imperative as outlined in the Nutrition section.
2. Make a tincture of equal parts nettles, yellow dock, alfalfa and red raspberry. Take 1-2 teaspoons daily in the last few weeks of pregnancy and regularly throughout labour.
3. Take an antioxidant formula like FrequenSea and A.I.M. along with Pure.
4. Make sure your carer has a good understanding of your previous birth experiences and your emotional status.
5. Ensure you have good pathology reports and recent blood assays, including platelet counts, to ensure you have adequate clotting factors.
6. Allow the natural delivery of the placenta as outlined above. Most postpartum haemorrhages are caused by being in a hurry to deliver the placenta. In these cases, I believe haemorrhage is caused by the intervillous spaces in the uterus not having a chance to contract and help control the flow of blood. Consequently the over manipulation of the uterus to facilitate placental delivery can cause lobes to be left on the uterine wall which result in uneven contraction of the uterus. These lobes then need to be manually removed under anaesthetic to prevent postpartum infection. This is not any fun for you the mother or for the birth attendant.
    I have seen birth attendants not give the placenta time to deliver, pulling on the cord and/or massaging a uterus with an as-yet unseparated placenta attached, causing a partial separation with the resultant bleeding by vessels that still have maternal blood coursing through them.
7. Reflexology can be one of the most effective tools at this time. Vigorously work the uterine point. One study showed that vigorous reflexology resulted in spontaneous expulsion of the placenta within thirty minutes of delivery.

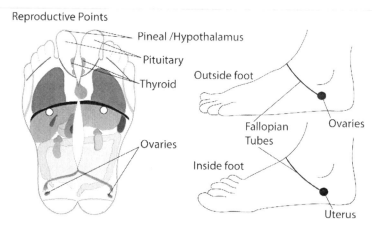

Reproductive Points

Pineal /Hypothalamus

Pituitary

Thyroid

Outside foot

Ovaries

Fallopian Tubes

Ovaries

Inside foot

Uterus

8. So a policy of hands off, unless there is due cause, is the most important key to preventing postpartum haemorrhage.

9. Shortly after delivery (while waiting for the placenta to deliver) drink a glass of very warm sweetened water with 30 drops of *blue cohosh/shepherd's purse* with ginger tincture added to it. This reduces the incidence of haemorrhage and also helps improve your condition following the birth. The hot water replaces some body heat and fluids whilst sweetening the drink makes it palatable and gives you a little energy boost.

    The blue cohosh encourages the uterus to clamp down firmly. Shepherd's purse seems to slow internal bleeding because it is a haemostatic and coagulant, whilst ginger promotes circulation and warmth in the pelvic region. Improved circulation helps the uterus do its work better (Feral, 2000).

With the introduction of FrequenSea, Pure and A.I.M. to my clients over the past few years I have not experienced any of them haemorrhaging post-birth. The phytonutrient properties of these formulas seems to provide the uterus with optimal nutrition.

The Miracle of Valentine's Birth-Day

Elizabeth came to see me when she was five months pregnant with her first child and feeling very exhausted.

Elizabeth had been diagnosed with Multiple Sclerosis, along with Glycogen storage disease type 5 (McArdle Syndrome), which meant her body was unable to transfer glycogen in the muscles to glucose for energy. Both of these conditions are very debilitating, especially the Mcardle Syndrome. Elizabeth has great difficulty getting her muscles to function normally, so therefore tends to be very slow and deliberate about her movements.

This is Elizabeth's Testimonial:

I was told years ago by my specialist that due to the major gynaecological problems I have experienced there is no way I would ever get pregnant. I have only one functioning ovary. The other has dystrophy and is not detectable on ultrasound. I only ovulate once or twice a year at the most. I accepted that my life would be childless. I was quite happy really. I had some friends at the time who had dreadfully behaved children and whenever I visited them I always counted my blessings that I didn't have to experience what they were experiencing. Subconsciously I think these thoughts were my reasoning and way of excuse to validate my barrenness of ever experiencing being a mother.

I met William in December. We started dating by mid April. Our relationship is very special and by May I found myself pregnant. What a miracle. I went to the doctor because I was feeling so ill. I was late for my period but for me that was nothing unusual, he took a pregnancy test and to my shock, horror and delight it was positive. I immediately knew that this was meant to happen, that it was a miracle. I figured out that I had fallen pregnant most likely on the first night we had made love. I had just completed a period so thought there would definitely be no risk. It is so special to know our beautiful son was conceived in such a very loving environment and special way. I was not expecting my life to change so much and was surprised at my reaction of elation when I found I was pregnant.

The pregnancy was particularly difficult because of the immense tiredness I was experiencing. I was also very cold all the time even though in pregnancy you have an incubator glowing within, growing and keeping you warm. This was not the case for me. It was a real shock to the system. I just couldn't get or keep warm. I guess the majority of my energy was going to making the baby which left little for me. I felt so ill the majority of the time no matter what I took, this lasted for months.

At six months into the pregnancy I began to get headaches. A precious friend gave me a gift voucher to visit Vicki then continued to pay for my treatments. I am so grateful for her generosity, foresight and believing that Vicki (a wonderful spiritual midwife and her assistant) would be able to assist. I took specific nutrients to relieve the incredible headaches I experienced up until Valentine was born. The last six weeks I slept, fed myself and went to the toilet. I was just a baby-making machine, which was all the energy my body could muster.

The strongest memory that changed the course of events for me was when Vicki spent extra time reassuring and going over again for me what to expect at the birth. I hadn't been able to attend the child birth class. Vicki imparted some very important information which I focused intently on. She showed me videos of natural birth. I had never seen a birth before and this profounded me. It made it real somehow. Vicki taught me how to help get the baby into the right position for birth. I expressed my concern that the pressure to have a caesarean section was on me because of my circumstances and that ideally I would love to be able to give birth naturally. She casually said I could achieve a natural birth if the baby was well and I was well then there was no reason to intervene. At the end of the day I had to sign the consent form to be operated on. She also reassured me that intervention was not an enemy either, that if it was needed then I needed to embrace the technology.

I understood from her gentle and affirming nature that it was normal to experience pain during birth. She pointed out the obvious to me that

I had endured so much during this pregnancy, why now did I doubt my ability to endure labour.

The pressure to have a caesarean section was on me from about thirty weeks of pregnancy. Every time I went for a check up at the hospital, it was reiterated to me how I could not give birth normally because of my muscle disorder and that I would need a caesarean so why not just book in for one. I kept demanding to be allowed to have a chance to have a natural birth. Especially after having read how important it is to the baby to experience labour first before birth. Every visit to my doctor was a battle of caesarean vs. vaginal birth. I armed myself for battle each time I went in to be checked. It is a wonder my blood pressure didn't go up.

I sometimes organized my appointments with Vicki to coincide prior to my checkups. The reflexology reduced my blood pressure and the positive reassurance strengthened my resolve. I had weekly reflexology and the specific supplements prescribed all helped immensely. Particularly the high energy protein drink and phytoplankton products. I don't think I would have had the energy I had in labour if it were not for these products. The staff in the hospital kept offering me sandwiches. I couldn't work out why anyone would feel like ham and processed cheese in the middle of labour. I have to say with all the care and guidance I was given by Vicki, by the time I went into labour I felt the healthiest I had felt for a very long time in spite of the headaches. I looked forward to my reflexology sessions with relish and William was very dedicated to working my feet inbetween times.

Labour

I went into labour at 6am. I woke with the contractions happening around seven minutely and noticed I was bleeding. There appeared to be quite a lot so I called the hospital and they told me to come in to be checked. It turned out to be a show. My membranes were in tact and the baby was fine.

A new intern (what felt like an inexperienced) doctor checked me to see how dilated I was. She said I was five centimetres. I thought great and it hasn't even hurt yet. She was happy to allow me to continue. Then a resident doctor came in and spoke to me and began to talk me into having a caesarean section. I refused. They had begun to scrub ready for the caesarean. Because I had experienced an infection a couple of weeks before which was now resolved, and because of my disabling condition they felt that it would be best to Caesar me anyway. They gave me again all the reasons why I would be silly to go through labour for nothing when I was most likely going to have a Caesar anyway. They explained how awful labour was going to be and why put myself through the pain for nothing. I just said, "Why am I any different to any other woman? I understand labour is painful but at least give me the opportunity to trial a labour first."

I began to cry and demanded a second opinion. Eventually they conceded after checking my notes and evaluating the situation. I had some tests done to check if the infection was still there. The results were negative. So I continued to labour on.

The midwife looking after me came into the room dressed for theatre, she was still under the impression I was going to have a caesarean section. When she realized what had changed she suggested I go home and come back later when I was in established labour. It was now 11am. I had just spent four hours negotiating my future path. I went home and rested as best I could. I was happy at home and felt no urge to return to hospital.

The afternoon midwife called at around 4.30pm and suggested it might be good if I returned to the hospital to be checked again, so I came back in at about 5pm. I was still quietly contracting every five to seven minutes without too much discomfort. Another doctor examined me this time and said I was now eight centimetres so I should stay and continue on with the labour. I thought wow eight centimetres and I am not really in any great pain yet, this is too easy. Throughout the evening I continued to drink the protein drink and the FrequenSea and again I was kindly offered the white bread processed cheese sandwiches which I politely refused. All I could see was their regurgitation and return, yuck!

By 9pm things started to get a little stronger and another doctor examined me. He said I was only four centimetres and had not progressed as well as thought. He suggested I have a drip put in with Syntocinon to move things along as things were moving too slowly. I blatantly refused and again went into battle for my labour rights.

I now know why they refer to birth as labour. My contractions were a breeze compared to the pain of labouring and battling the system. I understood at some level they were genuinely concerned for me however I knew how I felt. I had no instinctual signs or sense of urgency to head down the pathway of intervention.

I asked if they thought there was a problem with my baby.

"No".

Was there a problem with me?

"No".

Then what is the issue?

"You are taking too long".

So I said. "If I am well and the baby is well what difference does time make?"

I did not want a drip in my arm hindering my movements, besides I knew that the pressure of the drug would be too strong for my body and the baby would end up in foetal distress. The doctor began to get angry with me. He began to tell me I was risking my child's life.

I said why? Give me the research that says time has an implication for hurting my baby. The Midwife then took him aside, thank God, and spoke to him. She explained that there had been human error with the earlier examinations and in fact I probably hadn't really gone into labour until early in the evening. He agreed to let me go until 11pm and if I hadn't progressed I was to agree to a drip. The pressure was now on to perform. I settled myself and focused on the baby. I visualized myself expanding and said over and over again to my baby we can do this, just relax.

By 11pm I had progressed to five centimetres so he was happy for me to continue on until 1am when I was to be examined again. I felt like I was being watched. By 1am I was six centimetres. The pressure began again to give me a caesarean. I said, 'I have to sign to consent form don't I and I refuse to do this. I am well and my baby is well'.

I continued to sip on my nutritional formulas. The midwife was incredibly supportive and spoke to the doctor again. He again allowed me to continue until 4am when he would check me again.

Things were starting to really hot up now. I was feeling tired more from the battle and lack of sleep than from the contractions. I just kept visualizing a natural birth and continued to say to myself "I can do this". To my baby "I promise I will get you out. Hang in there we are going to do this together". Throughout all of this my wonderful partner William supported me totally. Whatever I needed he was there to get it. He never once undermined my power or my ability to give birth. I just kept saying "Trust me I'll get you out, I will, just trust me."

At 4am I was examined again and there was no doubt I was nine centimetres. I knew I could feel what was happening to my body. They decided to break my waters and wow did this swing me into those powerful contractions. The baby came down upon the cervix. I believe the nutrients I was taking throughout the pregnancy made the difference and membranes really strong, which is why they didn't break easily.

At 5am I was fully dilated, wow! It was time to push. I was feeling really overwhelmed by all the things happening in my body, but my muscles in my legs were beginning to fatigue. Knowing how it was an every day effort to walk with my muscles I still didn't question my ability. What I was questioning was how to push my baby out.

At that moment my question was answered by a wonderful midwife who just happened to be passing by on her way to the birth centre. All I can remember was she wore a beanie on her head and seeing I was lost in it all, the beanie popped its head into my ward. She spoke wisely and asked what was I feeling. I said I feel like I want to go to the toilet but scared I'd mess the bed. She said "Excellent that's what you are meant to feel. Go with it push as if you are doing the biggest poo you have ever done in your life". So I did and it felt gooood. She stayed and taught me to push.

By this stage my legs were exhausted. I could no longer stand or put any weight on them I was becoming like a rag doll. A medical student was assisting with the birth. He had to hold my legs apart whilst I actively pushed. My legs were just not strong enough to get traction against the floor, the pushing was becoming ineffective. We tried the left lateral lying position with someone holding my legs but that didn't work either.

I was getting exhausted and feeling like I was going to pass out. I hadn't given up but did concede to assistance. They put me in stirrups, pulled my bottom to the edge of the bed, and sat me up with pillows stacked all around me. It was so supportive for my legs. I suddenly found I had some more energy. I read where this wasn't the optimal birthing position however this was one birth where the stirrups were extremely beneficial. The doctor said he was going to use forceps to help the baby out. That was enough to give me the huge whoosh of adrenaline I needed to complete the journey. I said "give me one more go, one more push'. With that an almighty push came from nowhere and out popped my baby. I didn't even need stitches.

At 9:14am 14 February (Valentine's Day) my son Valentine was born. He was bright and alert. I remembered what Vicki had told me about how important it is to have skin to skin contact immediately and to have that critical time of bonding following the birth for mother and baby.

I insisted that he be laid on my bare breast skin to skin. I looked into the eyes of my son and knew we had accomplished something truly amazing. I fell in love so deeply. I agreed to a managed third stage they gave me a shot of Syntometrine in my leg and delivered my placenta shortly after. I also agreed to Valentine having Vitamin K because the labour had been fairly long and arduous for us both.

We fell asleep together and basically that is what we did for three days. Slept and fed in unison with each other. Breastfeeding was a breeze and I went home on day four when I had enough energy to do so.

I have to say thank you to the midwife with the beanie, to my angelic friend for all my reflexology and nutrients - how can I ever possibly repay you? To Vicki (the most wondrous trusting midwife) for her inspiration, divine treatments and faith in my ability to birth, for her knowledge in improving my health, especially my baby's wellbeing and for enabling me to endure my pregnancy and birth. It gave me so much wisdom, insight and sincere care. I know she was with me Spiritually even though she couldn't be there physically.

"Mothers have as powerful an influence over the welfare of future generations as all other earthly causes combined."

S. C. Abbott (1833)

Sienna's Birth

Jo Griffin

In the week leading up to Sienna's birth I had experienced mild contractions on a few occasions and she was fully engaged, so I knew it wouldn't be long until she would make her grand entrance. Excitement and anticipation was setting in! I had been seeing Vicki throughout my journey of pregnancy and had worked through a few hurdles to prepare me for this precious little person.

After a wonderful, healthy pregnancy I was feeling empowered and excited to see what my body was truly capable of. The night before my due date I went to visit a friend who had just had her baby. On the way home I had a few contractions which got us excited again but alas, they soon disappeared. I had been feeling unusually tired that day and had a sense that it could be 'the calm before the storm' so I had an early night and slept well.

I was awoken at around 4.30am with some mild cramping. It seemed to be happening at regular intervals so I decided to get up and see what happened. Not long after I got up, I had a bloody show so was fairly certain at that point that it was the real deal.

The contractions continued coming at regular intervals - some more intense than others - but I was cruising through them by focussing on my breathing and using my fit ball. My husband cooked us up a lovely breakfast and we watched some TV while timing the contractions. We were very excited and couldn't wait to meet our little girl!

The morning disappeared and by 1pm my contractions were about three minutes apart, but mostly still very mild and manageable. I decided to call the hospital and update them on my situation. The midwife I spoke to advised us to come in, which I wasn't really feeling ready for as

I was coping just fine, but we decided it wouldn't hurt to get checked. I was convinced that I would be sent home anyway! Upon arrival at the hospital I was hooked up to the monitors and it became apparent that the contractions were indeed fairly intense and there was some concern that our little girl's heart rate was dropping with each contraction. I was admitted, which I wasn't expecting, but was happy enough.

It turned out that it was probably quite timely as not long after being admitted my contractions really ramped up! I was managing the pain by using a TENS machine, breathing, movement and making plenty of noise! I was determined to avoid any form of intervention as I wanted a drug-free natural birth. I trusted that my body was doing what it needed to do and I went within. Time became irrelevant and I was completely focussed on riding the wave of contractions and resting inbetween. On the peak of the most painful contraction I experienced my waters broke. They were meconium stained but I sensed no real panic about this so chose to ignore this and continue to focus on the job at hand!

The contractions at this point were very intense and I asked the midwife how much longer I was going to have to endure this! Upon checking she announced, much to my surprise, that I was fully dilated and could start pushing if I liked! This was at around 5pm, so it had all happened fairly quickly which I wasn't really anticipating as I knew first babies could take a while to deliver. The urge to push took over. The contractions slowed down a little and I focussed on figuring out how to push this baby out. My pushing efforts were a little slack to start with as I was fairly tired. Eventually I decided to give it all I had and made some progress. My husband was by my side encouraging me and letting me squeeze his hands with all my might! I found his presence very calming and encouraging throughout the labour. He was my rock!

Eventually she began crowning and I reached down to touch her squishy, wet head. She started squawking before she even came out which was the strangest feeling! She wanted out! Another couple of almighty pushes and out she came. A beautiful, pink, screaming healthy baby! It was 5.52pm. She was placed straight onto my chest and looked me right in the eyes. It was the most surreal moment. Pure love.

I delivered the placenta naturally after the cord had stopped pulsating, as I had requested. Unfortunately I hadn't contracted properly and the doctor wanted to administer Syntocinon. I agreed to this as I was thrilled to have delivered without any intervention to that point and understood the need.

I was so elated and proud of my body for labouring so beautifully. I was holding my beautiful daughter, Sienna, and experiencing the biggest high of my life!

I truly believe that simply trusting my body's ability to birth Sienna helped me to have the wonderful birth experience I had. Vicki had been instrumental in bringing me to this point. I had been bombarded with horror birth stories from the moment I announced my pregnancy but allowed them to wash over me without worry as I knew that their experience was theirs as mine would be mine. No two births are the same. I also took the supplements that Vicki had recommended throughout my pregnancy and had regular reflexology treatments. I am sure that these things helped my body to be in the best possible condition to birth Sienna so beautifully.

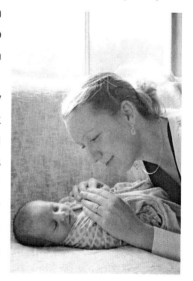

I relive my birth experience regularly and love telling my story to others. It is nice to have a positive story to tell. I visited Vicki a few weeks after Sienna was born and said jokingly "Is it weird that I want to do it all again?". It was truly the most awe-inspiring day of my life which I will always remember fondly. I can't wait to do it again!

Birth Plan Example

The following is an example of a very comprehensive birth plan prepared by a client. I'm not recommending that you need to undertake this type of plan, I have included it so that it may give you ideas or trigger the need to find out more information when making up your own birth plan.

Personal Statement:

We understand that birth can be unpredictable but come into this event with as much pre-evaluated knowledge as possible. We are presenting this birth plan to encourage dialogue and to help us achieve a safe, natural and satisfying birth and for hospital staff to be open to our beliefs and techniques.

Our baby's health and well being, now and what may impact on its future, is of utmost importance to us. We look forward to working with you, and appreciate your cooperation in helping our family to achieve our personal birthing goals.

Before Labour Begins:

- *I expect, and trust, that my practitioner will seek my opinion and that of my partner on all issues that may affect my birth experience or that deviate from this plan, whether they are mandatory, routine or otherwise.*
- *If the baby and I are fine, and if I go past my estimated due date, I would like to try natural remedies and to wait. If my water breaks at the onset of labour and there are no signs of infection, I would ideally like to wait as long as possible before induction and attempt the use of more natural induction methods.*

  o *Reflexology*
  o *Breast stimulation*
  o *Aromatherapy*
  o *Chiropractic*
  o *Acupuncture*
  o *Homeopathy*

I am more than happy to be checked daily if needed, unless there are signs of distress.

Labour

- *I would like my environment to:*

    o *have dimmed lights*
    o *to have voices respectfully lowered*
    o *include music I provide*
    o *have other devices (bean bag, fit ball, bath, aromatherapy diffuser, birthing chair or bars)*

- *I would like the to wear my own clothing.*
- *Any discussion of interventions is to be done with my partner and myself.*

First Stage, Phase II: Active Labour - Fully Dilated

- *I would like to keep internal vaginal exams to a minimum.*
- *I understand that I will be working REALLY hard. Therefore: I would like no restrictions on food or drink.*
- *I feel comfortable with very limited intermittent foetal monitoring, using External Electronic Monitor preferably a Doptone and not a Cardio Tocograph.*
- *My birth partner and I would like to take a few moments to privately discuss my pain-relief options before a decision is made.*

    o *Ideally, I'd like a drug-free birth. Only offer medications if I ask. Only use small IV amounts no bolus doses if this occurs.*

- *I would like the opportunity to try non-medical, non-invasive pain-relief methods. Some therapies I feel would be useful for me include:*

o   *Maternity Reflexology*

o   *Massage with aromatherapy*

o   *Guided relaxation*

o   *Water (shower/bath)*

o   *If bath or shower, I would like my partner to join me.*

o   *Change in position*

o   *Hot/cold therapy*

o   *Acupressure*

o   *TENS machine*

- *Ideally, I would like to be allowed freedom of movement, to walk, rock, use the bathroom and move as my body dictates.*
- *Time is not a factor as long as I am well and my baby is well there should be no reason to hurry things along.*
- *I am interested in having access to certain birthing equipment. If available, I would like to use:*

o   *Fit ball*

o   *Beanbag*

o   *Birthing Stool*

Second stage of Childbirth: Pushing and Delivery

Pushing:

When I am fully dilated, I will also trust my body's instincts to push my baby out naturally without pressure. Please encourage me to move and try different positions for pushing, for example:

- *Squatting*
- *Hands and knees on floor*
- *Kneeling, resting arms on bed/chair/fit ball*
- *Whatever feels right in the moment*

Vaginal Delivery:

- *Please do not use antiseptic wash downs that interfere with the normal vaginal flora as these are important to my baby's immune system.*
- *Ideally, I would like to avoid an episiotomy.*
- *I prefer the use of vacuum extraction without episiotomy if possible rather than forceps.*
- *I would like for my baby to hear our voices first.*
- *I prefer to be naked at birth and for my baby to be placed on my abdomen immediately following the birth.*
- *If warming is necessary, please allow baby to be warmed on my breast, covered by blankets.*

Third Stage of Childbirth: Delivery of Placenta or Afterbirth

- *Ideally, I would like to deliver the placenta unassisted - without Pitocin, uterine massage or cord traction. I would like to be given plenty of time for this to occur, at least an hour. If a procedure is necessary, please explain it to me.*
- *I understand that the placenta has been my baby's life support system, providing him or her with daily nutrients, warmth and eliminating his or her wastes. I would like to keep the placenta to take home.*
- *I would like my partner to deliver in tandem with the midwife.*

If Complications Lead to a Caesarean Delivery:

- *Please keep communication open. If, at all possible, please wait for my express consent, or that of my partner, before initiating any procedure.*
- *It is important to me that my partner(s) be present with me at all times during the birth.*

- *Ideally, I would like to remain awake and aware, avoiding general anaesthesia if possible.*
- *Please leave the screen down so I can see the birth.*
- *Please leave at least one of my hands free so I may touch my baby when he or she is born.*
- *Assuming the baby is well, I would like to hold my baby on my chest and/or nurse my baby as soon as possible whilst they stitch up.*
- *Please discuss options for postpartum medication, if needed, with me.*
- *Please provide me with the opportunity to consume nutritious food and drink as soon as possible.*

Immediate Newborn Care:

Suction and Cord Care:

- *I would like my baby not to be suctioned unless medically necessary.*
- *In my ideal world, my healthy baby will be immediately placed on my chest. If this is the case, he or she will be above the placenta and I would therefore like to wait until after the placenta is delivered before the cord is clamped and cut.*
- *I would like the opportunity to have my partner cut the baby's umbilical cord.*

Eyedrops, Vitamin K and other Procedures:

- *I would like to postpone any immunizations until a later time.*
- *I understand that it is routine to administer vitamin K through injection or oral drops in the event that internal haemorrhaging occurs in baby. Having researched this area well I prefer not have my baby undergo this treatment at all as there is clearly not enough research to support this procedure.*

Rooming-In and Feeding:

- *My preference for in-hospital infant care is:*

  o *Full rooming in - no separation.*

- *Please do not offer my baby the following:*

  o *Formula*
  o *Sugar water*
  o *Pacifiers*
  o *Artificial nipples*

- *My feeding preference is:*

  o *to be offered guidance on this issue.*

- *I would like the assistance of a lactation consultant to help me with nursing.*

Sick Baby and Postpartum Care:

- *If my baby is not well, I would like to:*

  o *accompany my baby, or have my partner accompany the baby if transported to another facility.*
  o *breastfeed, or provide my expressed milk for my baby.*
  o *have unlimited visitation for my partner and myself.*
  o *hold, rock and care for my baby, if possible.*

- *I opt for kangaroo care if possible.*

Medical Procedures

Induction

An induction is when labour is instigated via artificial means.There are many ways to induce labour, some closer to nature than others as will be discussed ahead. Induction is undertaken when there is a perceived fear that the baby may be endangered if it stays in the womb too long. The World Health Organisation states that the induction level should never be more than ten percent. However the rates in many maternity units are as high as twenty eight to thirty percent. Statistics world wide indicate that those women whose primary carer is a midwife have induction levels around two percent of cases, compared with some maternity units with obstetricians in charge having stats as high as thirty to fourty percent.

A woman who goes beyond one week of the expected due date may find herself pressured by her maternity carers to undergo an induction. However some due dates may not be correct and may possibly be up to three weeks inaccurate, especially if conception has taken place on a 'blue moon', meaning a second ovulation in a month. Even though early scans are accurate, there is still much discrepancy about what is the normal length of pregnancy. Induction will be encouraged if:

- you go over 42 weeks pregnancy
- your waters have broken but labour hasn't started within 24 hours
- at 38 weeks if you have diabetes due to possible risks and potentially larger size of baby
- if you have pre-eclamptic symptoms such as high blood pressure, oedema or kidney abnormalities.

Remember that many of these conditions can be assisted naturally. There are many natural ways of encouraging a mother to get started once the pregnancy has gone past 41 weeks. Devoe and Sholl (1983) found that thirty percent of babies testing normal prior to a medically induced labour then required caesareans for foetal distress, leading them to ascertain that the method of delivery is more of a problem than the risk of being post-dates.

Medical induction should be a last resort with the woman monitored daily and encouraged to use natural methods to encourage labour. I have a policy of checking Mum and baby daily once a mum is two weeks over. I can honestly say women in my care are rarely induced. Using the techniques in this book can reduce the need for induction.

Induction is far more stressful to the mother and the baby than the gentle natural progression of spontaneous labour.

Natural Techniques for Assisting the Onset of Labour

- vigorous and frequent reflexology to specific <u>reproductive points</u>
- <u>acupressure</u>/acupuncture
- nipple stimulation, expressing colostrum releases oxytocin which naturally creates contractions
- sexual intercourse can help release prostaglandins, which soften the cervix to start labour
- homoeopathic Caulophyllum 30c or herbal tinctures of blue and black cohosh can stimulate contractions and soften the cervix
- explore through visualisation if there are any emotional blocks (see <u>River Visualisation</u>)
- one dose of Pulsatilla can be effective if the baby appears to be in a wrong position. The dose can be repeated three times in twelve hour intervals.
- specific exercises that move the baby into the best position can help, as well as stepping up and down the stairs side ways, with high hip movements over two to three steps. See <u>'Getting Baby Into the Right Position'</u>.
- Bush Flowers and Rescue Remedy can also help
- cumin tea with a small wedge of potato in it is an old American Parterres Indian tradition
- two parts partridgeberry, one part black and blue cohosh, half a part Homeopathic Helonias. Take half a teaspoon twice a day and

one teaspoon before bed. Then increase the dose to one teaspoon three times a day.

- a spot of evening primrose oil on the cervix has been known to kick-start labour
- Su-Jok point work to the reproductive areas
- moxa to acupressure points <u>Spleen 6</u> (inner ankle) and <u>LI 4</u> (large intestine).
- most of all, patience and time as some babies just need the extra growing time.

Massage the following Reflexology points frequently:

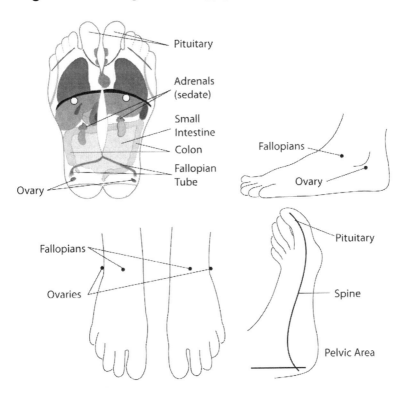

What's the Emotional Block?

Investigate with your midwife or partner in a visualisation what may be causing the delay. Sometimes there can be issues of fear that you have not dealt with, or there may be relationship problems. I have witnessed this many times. One couple rang two weeks overdue with their doctor suggesting induction the next day. After working the reproductive reflex points, mum burst into tears expressing a fear of mothering. I explored this fear and its foundations using techniques of emotional release and forgiveness and worked the Emotional Anatomy points on her hands and feet (see chart). Following a two hour session in which several strong contractions were felt, mum and partner left feeling very confident and ready for birth. Her membranes ruptured walking down the drive and she gave birth three hours later.

My sister was due with her third child. I had helped deliver the other two with ease and was expected to be very involved in this birth. With her first two labours her membranes ruptured first with labour beginning a day later. This time the membranes ruptured but unlike the other two births two days had gone by without a sign of labour and she was one week over due. The pressure was on to get things happening. I used all the techniques I usually used to no avail. On checking on her fear level there were no fears lurking.

After visiting her to do some more reflexology, I discussed the situation with another reflexology colleague who suggested taking me through a couple of visualisations to see how I was feeling. My colleague suggested that as I hadn't assisted a delivery for a couple of years it may be that I had some issues to clear. The visualisations revealed my own fear of failure. I doubted my own ability as a midwife. Once aware I was able to work through the fear with my own techniques. Within half an hour of me feeling I had cleared the fears, the phone rang, my sister calling to say her contractions had started. She gave birth within three hours and I had the privilege of catching daughter number three confidently. This was a huge learning experience for me, emphasising how fears held by others can impact on the mother's progress.

If your membranes rupture on their own prior to labour, you must believe that this is exactly the way your body needs to start this particular labour. Accept it as a sign that labour will begin sometime within the next few hours or at the least a couple of days. Stay close to home, relax, eat well, and increase your vitamin C and fluid intake. Before agreeing to be induced, you can try several natural induction suggestions: visualization, herbs or evening primrose oil (under the direction of a qualified midwife). Lovemaking and orgasm without penetration/sexual intercourse as ruptured membranes mean there is a risk of infection, may encourage labour to begin.

Many physicians worry that an infection will begin now that the protection around the infant is gone. Some prescribe antibiotics prophylactically. Others ask you to take your temperature and report any rise. Some take blood tests to check your white blood cell count. Most tell you that if you haven't had the baby in twelve to twenty four hours an induction will be scheduled. Recent research shows that the risk of infection is minimal up to five days, especially if the mother stays at home rather than entering hospital. The risk of infection increases once in hospital (in a single year 1.5 million patients were victims of hospital-acquired infections, Wainer Cohen & Estner, 1983, 'Silent Knife').

Suggested Labour Prep Tincture at 36 Weeks

An evaluation of research by Maryl Smith (1999) revealed that most studies seem to show that the group of primary concern is women with correct dates who do not enter labour spontaneously and eventually must be induced. Comparable studies of medically managed births versus natural births do not provide enough empirical evidence to support routine induction for a healthy post-date pregnancy. All studies indicated an increase in caesarean section rate due to foetal distress in the group who were medically managed using induction. The outcome for post-date mothers and babies who were allowed to go into spontaneous labour was generally good and the mortality rate was similar to the actively managed group. The conclusion was that client satisfaction is the most important factor and indicator of management style.

Emotional factors must be taken into account in prolonged pregnancy. It is important that pregnant women become familiar with the concept that their pregnancy may last as much as fourty three weeks and anything prior is a bonus. Only fourty percent of mothers deliver within five days of their due date. As long as mother and baby are well then active management is not indicated, rather patience is required (Midwifery Today, Dec. 17, 1999).

Ideas to Help a Mother Cope With a Prolonged Pregnancy:

- remind mum it is common to go past the due date, she is sixty percent more likely to go at least one week past
- reassure her all is okay, encourage her to rest in preparation for the business of being a new mother
- how has she been sleeping? Address any issues here, increase reflexology sessions and ensure adequate nutrient intake.
- reassure family and friends, encourage them to provide positive input and feedback
- allow her to express and release emotions of tiredness
- listen frequently to the baby if this reassures the mother
- research and try natural methods of induction such as those suggested in this section
- encourage her to talk to her baby
- discuss induction and encourage her to release the fears, let her know her options.

Medical Induction Techniques

Membrane Sweeps

A vaginal examination is required for this form of induction, performed by your doctor or midwife in order to gently separate the membranes from the cervix. This leads to the release of prostaglandins and hormones which set labour into motion. The success rate will be higher if your body is ready and your cervix is ripe and softened. The process can feel a little uncomfortable and may take three or four attempts before labour commences. For greater success combine with the natural techniques already mentioned here.

Prostaglandins

A synthetic form of prostaglandin, generally a tablet or pessary, is inserted in the vagina close to the cervix. Often the prostaglandin is inserted in the evening, with a second administered the next morning if there are no signs of labour commencing. Generally successful within 24 hours, depending on the body's readiness to birth. Approximately 15% of unripe cervix inductions fail.

Artificial Rupture of Membranes (ARM)

This procedure is not generally used for induction anymore as it is better for the membranes to remain intact for as long as possible during labour. If your membranes have already ruptured there may be a small tear at the top of the amniotic sac which often creates a trickle. This may be too slow and ARM may be needed to break the fore waters and speed up labour. Sometimes it has the effect of bringing the baby down into the pelvis and onto the pelvic floor, triggering natural hormone production which in turn speeds up labour. Once the membranes are ruptured there is a greater risk of infection.

Syntocinon

A synthetic form of oxytocin, the hormone that creates contractions during labour. Syntocinon is not used as frequently these days as it has many disadvantages. Syntocinon tends to create strong contractions which can be difficult to cope with for both mother and baby. Many women report greater pain with syntocinon. Certainly I can vouch for this. I could not believe the difference between natural contractions compared to the induced contractions of my first birth. Syntocinon induction poses higher risk of epidural, foetal distress, forceps delivery and caesarean so is best avoided if you can.

Electronic-Foetal Monitoring vs. Doptone

Electronic Foetal Monitoring (EFM) is a routine procedure undertaken by birth attendants in most delivery suites. It is an ultrasonic recording of the baby's heart rate, which can be heard and recorded on a written tracing. Generally there are two components, one assessing contractions the other assessing the heart rate.

The main disadvantages are that usually the mother is required to be stationary whilst the test is done and the effectiveness of the read out is still open to debate amongst researchers.

In contrast, the midwife listens to the baby's heart beat through a portable Doptone, which can be used with the mother in any position, is less invasive and can be done without disturbing mum. Experienced birth attendants can assess the baby's well being by the sound and speed of the heartbeat.

There is no scientific evidence that routine EFM during labour improves the condition of the baby at birth or reduces the possibility of brain damage (Wagner, 1994).

> "The need for universal EFM legitimates so many other contentious decisions on the place, style and management of labour that it will not be discarded in favour of [auscultation] but only displaced when another new, equally unevaluated procedure arrives on the obstetric scene". This would explain why only one study has looked at whether auscultation was feasible in a big, busy unit - finding, by the way, that it was"
>
> Sandmire, Henci Goer, Obstetric Myths Versus
> Research Realities, Bergin & Garvey, 1995.

If recent studies do not support the routine use of EFM, why is it still so widely used?

First - because many nurses and physicians have not been trained in intermittent auscultation (listening to the heartbeat).

Second- some believe that EFM might still be a valuable assessment tool with better guidelines for interpreting tracings and making management decisions, even though studies comparing the ability of experts to agree on the interpretation of an EFM tracing have shown poor interpreter reliability.

Third - physicians may fear that they will be vulnerable to malpractice lawsuits if they do not use EFM. The impact of changing to intermittent monitoring on malpractice claims is unknown.

Fourth - many hospitals are not adequately staffed to do intermittent auscultation. In one study, a university hospital centre attempted to use intermittent auscultation as the primary method of monitoring without increasing the number of staff. Auscultation was only successfully completed in 31 of 862 patients in labour with viable babies (Sweha, Hacker & Nuovo, 1999).

Dr John Ott, author of the book 'Health and Light' (1990), shed some light on non-advancing labour where the mother and/or baby is hooked up to a monitor. Dr Ott's research in the colour spectrum wavelengths led to a curiosity about the effects of electrical fields on the human body. His work led to the first commercially available full-spectrum shielded fluorescent lighting. He stated that susceptible persons are greatly weakened by artificial energy fields. Dr Ott predicted that the number of caesareans would increase in hospitals using foetal monitors. But his reasons were different than most would think. Dr Ott claimed that when a maternal or foetal monitor is hooked up, its energy field makes muscles weak for both baby and mother. And of course, the uterus is a muscle. Add to this all the electronic equipment in the typical delivery room, plus all the voltage-carrying conduits in the hospital (Judy Ritchie, The Birthkit No. 23, Autumn 1999).

My recommendation is to request foetal monitoring with a doptone where possible and use EFM only when necessary. At least now in most maternity units monitors are portable so mother can move around.

Drugs in Labour

In an article for Midwifery Today, Beverley Lawrence Beech (1999) discussed the effects of maternal drugs on the developing baby and child. Beech looked at the work of British psychiatrist, Desmond Bardon, who investigated the long term effects on neurological development on infants who had been subjected to prolonged maternal exposure to drugs. Bardon's study discussed the intricate biochemical changes such exposure precipitates within the foetal brain, and created the analogy of the building of the brain as complex circuitry, which appears to work properly but has some malfunctions due to maternal drug exposure.

Beech also considered the work of Yvonne Brackbrill, who suggested the effect of drugs in labour may stretch well beyond birth, as far as four and a half years, as the growth of one part of the human brain, hippocampus, continues until that age. Thus it is possible that drugs administered in labour have the potential to alter not only the proliferation of new brain cells, but the ability of the new cells to migrate to their correct position and then link up with other cells (Brackbrill, 1979).

An important question raised by Beech is whether or not such disruption to this process of cell migration contributes to cognitive issues such as dyslexia. This has yet to be determined, but more importantly raises the question of how much of narcotic drugs such as pethidine and morphine, and of drugs used in epidurals, passes through to the baby.

Sometimes it is necessary to use drugs in labour, and if this is your choice then I recommend asking for smaller intravenous doses of pethidine that are quick acting but have a short life rather than larger intramuscular doses that can last for hours and can take a baby days to remove from their system.

It is well known that babies subjected to drugs in labour invariably have feeding problems. An excellent study called 'Self Attachment' clearly shows video footage of babies crawling to the breast to self attach after natural births. Even those babies born by caesarean where no drugs were involved crawled to the breast and self-attached. Those born following the use of drugs did not move and were lethargic without the instinctual ability to crawl to the breast.

A trial sought to determine whether injecting sterile water subcutaneously produced less pain during labour (Bahasadri et al. 2006). Ninety-nine pregnant women at term who required relief of severe low back pain during the first stage of labour were randomly allocated to receive four injections of 0.1 ml of water subcutaneously or placebo injections in the area of the Michaelis rhomboid in the lower lumbosacral area. The placebo treatment was subcutaneous injections of normal saline.

Both groups of women receiving intra-cutaneous or subcutaneous sterile water had significant reductions in pain scores after fourty five minutes compared with the placebo group. No difference occurred in the women's experience of pain during the injections. When surveyed after birth, however, twice as many women receiving subcutaneous sterile water said they would not be willing to try this method in a future labour and birth, compared with those women receiving intra-cutaneous water.

Researchers at the University of Minnesota Medical School reported that the use of intrathecal (spinal) narcotics to manage labour-related pain may significantly prolong second stage of labour and double the need for oxytocin (Fontaine & Adam, 2000). This contradicts findings from several prior studies that support the overall safety of intrathecal narcotics compared with other analgesic options during labour. Researchers retrospectively compared the labour and delivery outcomes of one hundred women who had received intrathecal narcotics and one hundred who received intravenous narcotics or no analgesia during labour. Women given the narcotics had significantly longer second-stage labours than the other women, averaging seventy three minutes and fourty minutes respectively. Women who received intrathecal narcotics were also twice as likely as the others to use oxytocin, and had higher rates of urinary catheterization and pruritus. Intrathecal narcotic use was associated with a higher risk of caesarean delivery, but this association was not significant. On the other hand, the overall duration of active labour and neonatal outcomes were similar in the two groups of women.

In the rush to speed up labour, a woman's distress at the increased pain of induction or acceleration is often dealt with by giving a pethidine injection. Ironically, research by Thomson and Hillier (1994) revealed that unmedicated mothers had a first stage of labour whose mean length was 7.7 hours, compared with 11.7 hours in those who received pethidine (Demerol). Furthermore, an incidental finding in Rajan's research (1994) revealed that when the second stage of labour was longer than an hour there was no difference between those who received pethidine and those who did not, but in the group of women who had second stages lasting less than an hour there were many more women who did not have pethidine (436 vs 2770).

Pethidine readily crosses the placenta. The baby may have greater sensitivity to the drug because of the immaturity of the blood-brain barrier and the circulatory bypass of the liver. Research shows that pethidine is most likely to have a depressant effect on the foetal respiratory system if the dose is administered two or three hours before birth, with the higher the dose to the mother the greater the effect on the baby (Yerby, 1996). As the baby's liver is immature, it takes a great deal longer to eliminate the drug from its system, eighteen to twenty three hours, although ninety five percent of the drug is excreted in two to three days (Beverley Beech, AIMS Journal Vol 10 No. 1, 1998).

Research by Jacobsen (1987), Raine (1994) and Michel Odent (1999), among others, suggest that contemporary tragedies such as suicide, drug addiction and violent criminal acts by teenagers may be linked to the perinatal period such as exposure to drugs, birth complications and separation from or rejection by the mother. The more you can do to reduce the need for intervention the greater the long term benefits for you and your baby.

Assisted Birth

Hopefully with the suggestions presented in this book you will avoid the need for an assisted birth. However the nature of birth is that it can be unpredictable, the most prepared of mothers occasionally requires assistance. Assisted birth is required when the birth of a baby is not progressing as would be expected once the baby has reached the perineum and the top of the head is on view. On average about one in nine births in Australia require assistance. The instruments used are generally Ventouse and less often forceps.

There are many reasons why a baby may not travel through the birth canal under the propulsion of the mother's contractions:

- the baby's head is deflexed, resulting in the circumference of the head being larger, resulting in less room
- the baby's head has become malpositioned, creating less room in the birth canal
- if there is foetal distress, requiring the birth to be sped up
- if the contractions are ineffectual, particularly if the labour has been long and the mother is tired. This often happens when a baby has turned posterior or there is a medical reason such as high blood pressure preventing the mother from pushing.

The best way to prevent the need for assisted birth is to follow the suggestions on getting your baby into the right position and taking phytonutrients and minerals to ensure a strong healthy uterus that is more likely to labour effectively. It is important to let nature take its course, allow labour to commence when your body is ready and avoid induction as there is a higher chance of intervention with induction.

Be active and well supported throughout your labour and do your best to avoid an epidural. If however you do end up with an epidural ask that the dose is lighter so you can still feel the contractions. Also allow the epidural to wear off when you are fully dilated so that you have the sensation to push, which helps you work with your body more effectively.

Ventouse
Ventouse works on the principle of creating a vacuum that assists the baby to move down whilst the mother pushes. A small cup is placed over

the baby's head with one end attached to a monitored vacuum pump. In Australia soft plastic cups are most often used, most doctors prefer them because they tend to be less painful for the mother.

Ventouse extraction is less likely to damage the pelvic floor and the perineum, generally can be done without an episiotomy and there is less risk of perineal tearing. If there is no progress after two to three pushing contractions most doctors will choose to do a caesarean rather than forceps to prevent damage to mother and baby. Forceps are being used less and less.

Forceps

Because forceps take up room there is often a perceived need to do an episiotomy to allow more room around the perineum.

This is a contentious issue, as episiotomy is perineal surgery with inherent post birth problems such as pain and delayed healing. It also creates scarring that can impact on your next birth, so best avoided if you can. If you are able, discuss with the obstetrician the option of using a Ventouse, and if that fails at least try without an episiotomy.

Unless your baby is close to delivery and only requires one or two pulls with the forceps, I personally would recommend a caesarean rather than a forceps delivery. Forceps do have a slightly higher success rate than the use of Ventouse but are more likely to damage the perineum and pelvic floor. Research has shown that it is far better to undergo a caesarean than have a damaged perineum or damaged baby.

Most women go on to experience a normal birth the next time following a forceps delivery. Forceps can be an emotional experience and it is recommended that following the birth you have the opportunity to debrief with the attending midwife as soon as possible.

Episiotomy

I refer to episiotomy as perineal surgery. A cut is made with very sharp surgical scissors in the perineum at the time of delivery to speed up the birth of the baby's head. Usually the cut is made through all tissue including muscle. This causes more damage to the pelvic floor than a natural perineal tear which tends to only break through stretched thinned out tissue, so less likely to involve muscle tissue. Episiotomy can take weeks to heal and is often very painful whilst healing, whereas a perineal tear may only take days and is far less imposing on the mother.

Scientific evidence shows that having an episiotomy means more bleeding, more pain, and more permanent deformity of the vagina. Women's rights activists worldwide are rightly concerned about the practice of female genital mutilation in parts of Africa. They need to be equally concerned about the millions of women worldwide who have suffered unnecessary perineal damage during birth. A good birth attendant is patient and will allow time to prevent the need for an episiotomy. Statistically midwives are more likely to avoid episiotomy where possible.

A worthwhile read on this subject is 'Episiotomy, Challenging Obstetric Interventions' by Ian D Graham (1997) who challenged the liberal use of episiotomy by gathering research from many areas. While midwives trust women's bodies, use low technical assistance such as the skilled use of their hands, and understand the importance of preserving normalcy, some doctors do not share this faith and optimism. Lack of trust in the birth process and the medical focus on abnormality can lead to greater trust in and use of drugs, machines and high levels of technical assistance.

When deciding on your primary maternity care provider, it is important to ask midwives or doctors about their practices. Find out if they prefer to put you on your back during birth, how often they do episiotomy, forceps or vacuum extraction and caesarean section. If they don't know their rates of surgical interventions or refuse to tell you what their rates are, look out! Beware of any tendency to patronize you, to suggest that you cannot possibly understand all this technical stuff, or that you should just 'trust me, I'm the doctor' (Wagner, 2000).

Women who have previously had episiotomies should be warned that they will feel considerably more stretching and burning when no episiotomy is performed. During pushing, unprepared women are often alarmed by these sensations, insisting that something is wrong. It is important to explain the benefits of an intact birth and what to expect. Prenatal stretching will help them immensely (Frye, 1995). See 'Vaginal Massage' in the section 'Preparation for Birth'.

Epidural

An epidural anaesthetic numbs from the waist down. It is used when:

- labour progression is slow
- the mother being too stressed and not coping well
- the mother requests pain relief
- there is high blood pressure
- there are signs of foetal distress

An epidural is often used for a caesarean although the choice is usually a spinal block, which is a deeper anaesthetic placed into the spinal cord and more effective for surgery.

Possible disadvantages with an epidural:

- loss of sensation can mean you can't feel when you need to wee, so may need a catheter inserted, which can pose an infection risk
- an epidural causes a loss of fluid from the spinal area so an intravenous drip is inserted to hydrate the woman to prevent shock
- although this is rare, there is the risk of spinal cord damage
- research indicates the baby is affected by the drugs used in an epidural which can lead to difficulties with breastfeeding
- because you can't feel from the waist down you may have difficulty moving, therefore be unable to assist your body to adopt positions that help your baby move through. This creates a higher risk of your baby getting stuck, resulting in a caesarean.

- a lack of sensation during second stage can lead to ineffectual pushing, which may result in the need for forceps and episiotomy.
- the caesarean rate increases markedly with the use of epidurals. The Term Breech Trial steering committee (Hannah & Ross in MacColl, 2009: 120) reported that a woman who plans to birth vaginally but has an epidural is three times more likely to have a caesarean than a woman who does not have an epidural.

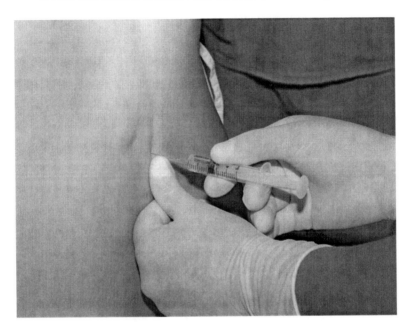

There are lighter epidurals now being used in some units which allow a mother to still feel contractions without the intensity. It may be worthwhile investigating if this is available where you choose to birth.

"It's not the interventions that save lives that are the problem. It's the interventions that are not needed and not wanted."

MacColl, M. (2009) *The Birth Wars.*
University of Queensland Press

Caesarean Birth

A caesarean section (c-section) is a surgical procedure in which a baby is born through an incision (cut) made in the mother's abdominal wall and the wall of the uterus (womb). There are two types of incisions in the uterus that can be used when having a caesarean section:

1. **A lower uterine segment incision (LUSC)** - will be used wherever possible. This is a horizontal cut through the lower abdomen just above the pubic bone and a horizontal cut through the lower part of the uterus, sometimes known as a 'bikini line' incision. These cuts heal better, are less visible and are less likely to cause problems in future pregnancies.

2. **A classical incision** - refers to a vertical incision on the uterus. The incision on the abdomen may be horizontal or vertical. These days this incision is rare and only for extreme emergencies or in specific situations, such as if the placenta is lying very low, if the baby is lying sideways or if the baby is very small. The chance of problems is greater in subsequent pregnancies when this kind of incision is used.

A baby may need to be born by caesarean section if there are serious problems that prevent the baby being born by a normal vaginal birth.

Caesarean section can be:

- Elective - a caesarean section is called 'elective' if the doctor decides it is necessary before labour begins.
- Emergency - a caesarean section is called 'emergency' if the doctor decides it is necessary after labour has begun. The term emergency is used loosely because in reality it is not an emergency. There are always warning signs and it takes fifteen to thirty minutes to prepare a mother for theatre.

490

A normal vaginal birth is the safest way for your baby to be born if both you and your baby are healthy during pregnancy and labour. There is no doubt that a caesarean birth has saved many a mother and baby's life, but as with many medical interventions they tend to be over used. Unfortunately the number of caesareans being performed is way above what the World Health Organisation states it should be. In Australia during 2006 more than thirty percent of births were by caesarean, the fastest increasing rate in the OECD and ranking Australia fifth highest among OECD nations (MacColl, 2009: 126). This is due to the growing trend of caesareans being undertaken without labour. An elective caesarean deprives both mother and baby of the experience of labour, which is so important (read 'Being Born'). It is a false belief that having a caesarean is easier than giving birth by vaginal delivery. It is major abdominal surgery and as such comes with many risk factors.

Pat Brodie, President of the Australian College of Midwives also sees fear as a major driving force in increasing caesarean rates. According to Brodie, women may choose the medical model of epidural and caesarean as it provides certainty, and this way they don't have to address their fears regarding their ability to give birth (MacColl, 2009: 135). The midwifery model works with mothers to address their fears and build confidence, reducing the perceived need for caesarean, whilst the medical model provides what may seem like an easier option.

If there are no serious problems indicating the need for a caesarean delivery but you are considering caesarean, please read the section 'Why Keep Birth Natural'. Also have a look at the website:

http://evidencebasedbirth.com/friedmans-curve-and-failure-to-progress-a-leading-cause-of-unplanned-c-sections/

When is a Caesarean Birth Necessary?

- the baby is presenting as a footling breech or is laying sideways (transverse) and is not able to be turned
- if labour is not progressing after a reasonable time and medical efforts

- during second stage if the baby does not appear to sink down or 'fit' through the pelvis after strong pushing efforts
- the baby shows serious signs of distress during labour
- the cervix (opening to the womb) is blocked by the placenta (placenta praevia)
- the umbilical cord, which provides important nutrients and oxygenated blood to the baby, has prolapsed (fallen down) through the cervix and into the vagina when the membranes have ruptured
- there is a serious health problem such as high blood pressure or pre-eclampsia.

Risks and Possible Complications

Because caesarean section has become a relatively common operation it is often perceived as a very safe procedure, which leads many women to be quite complacent about it. However, as with all surgical procedures, there are risks for both mother and baby. Some of these risks and possible complications include:

- post operative infection
- damage to the mother's bladder, other internal organs and blood vessels
- damage to the baby inflicted by surgical instruments
- research shows that babies born through elective caesarean may be up to six times more likely to experience respiratory distress.
- increased time in hospital, increased abdominal (tummy) pain
- longer post-delivery recovery period
- increased risk of blood clots
- increased risk in future pregnancies of the placenta growing or implanting too low in the uterus or through the uterus (buried in scar tissue)
- increased risk of having a caesarean section with future pregnancies
- when stitching a caesarean cut many doctors are now using a short cut method, where instead of suturing in layers they are now suturing one whole layer. This lessens the healing ability of

the muscles and viscera, increasing risks next time round (Nancy Wainer, Midwifery Today 2001).
- fertility problems have been linked to previous caesarean section
- increased complications with breastfeeding.

Some women develop serious problems after a caesarean section, which may include:

- increased pain
- pain passing urine
- leaking urine
- increased vaginal blood loss or offensive smelling discharge from the vagina
- coughing or shortness of breath
- swelling or pain in your calf (lower leg).

A caesarean section means a stay in hospital of around four to seven days, a more prolonged recovery of over two months for most women, not being able to drive for at least six weeks and implications for future pregnancies or operations. It is important to understand that there are inherent health risks, including infection, haemorrhage and that scar tissue formed during the healing can lead to pain and make future operations more difficult.

http://www.who.int/healthsystems/topics/
financing/healthreport/30C-sectioncosts.pdf

Types of Anaesthetic

There are three types of anaesthetic used during a caesarean section.

Epidural anaesthetic - a needle is inserted into the epidural space around the lining outside the spinal cord in the back, and local anaesthetic drugs are given to 'numb' or remove sensation from the waist down. The mother is still conscious and will be able to breathe normally. This is often used if an epidural is already inserted to provide pain relief during labour.

Spinal anaesthetic – this is a deeper block than an epidural where the anaesthetic is inserted directly into the spinal fluid. This anaesthetic requires the mother to lie flat for a few hours after delivery to prevent the risk of headaches.

General anaesthetic – the mother is not conscious during the baby's birth. This may be necessary if the baby must be born quickly or if insertion of the epidural or spinal anaesthetic has failed for some reason. It is not ideal as it is preferred for mother to be awake to witness the birth of her baby.

In the operating theatre - if you require a caesarean your partner or support person is able to accompany you into the operating theatre unless you require a general anaesthetic due to complications. It is important that you and your partner are fully informed of all procedures and that you ensure all your questions are answered.

** If you have chosen not to know the sex of your baby prior to birth, make sure you tell your delivery team that you want to discover the sex of your baby first, not to be told by the team.

Once the anaesthetic has been activated and the surgical team are happy with the level of the block you will be made comfortable on the table. Generally a screen is put of across your chest to prevent you from seeing the procedure. However, you are quite within your rights to ask for the screen to be lowered so that you can witness the immediate delivery of your baby. I would encourage you to do this and to have your baby lay naked on your chest as soon as possible to encourage early bonding. Your partner or support person might like to cut the cord. If your baby is alert, you might like to try breastfeeding while you are being sutured.

Usually your baby stay's tucked in bed with you, but if baby needs to go to neonatal intensive care please ensure your partner or support person goes with baby.

Because Pip chose to have the screen down I was able to snap this picture of the moment Anneliese was being born (see image below) and Pip was able to witness the birth and feel present, rather than be separated by the screen. Pip then breastfed Anneliese whilst being sutured.

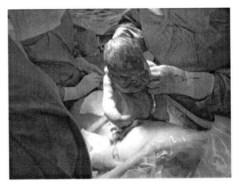

Suggestions for the Mother on Returning Home

- get as much rest as you can. Ask family or friends to help out or organise paid help if possible. Check with the local council - they may be able to provide some assistance in certain circumstances (for example, if there are twins).
- take a gentle walk every day. This can have physical and emotional health benefits.
- eat a healthy diet and drink plenty of water every day
- good nutrition is essential for preventing Postnatal Depression
- use warmth on the wound (such as a heating pad) for a soothing effect
- take painkillers regularly to begin with. If breastfeeding, check that the medication is safe for baby too. Taking codeine painkillers can create constipation and upset your gut. It may be worthwhile trying some of the suggestions in the Complimentary Pregnancy Therapies and Remedies section or Kaprex from Healthworld.
- wear loose cotton clothing and keep the wound clean and dry. Look for signs of infection (such as redness, pain and swelling) every day.
- seek professional assistance if you are feeling more anxious than usual, have guilt feelings about your baby's birth, feel sad most of the time or are not sleeping

- taking FrequenSea, Pure and A.I.M. will help you bounce back more quickly.

Vaginal Birth After Caesarean

It is a great joy to experience the birth of a baby via a vaginal birth after caesarean (VBAC). It is a huge healing experience for mother and partner. In Australia caesarean is seen as such a normality that in some birthing units women book in for the caesarean birth when they book into the hospital. Most states in Australia have a C-Section rate of twenty five percent or more with some areas as high as sixty percent. It seems that many doctors are not supportive of women who would like to try for a VBAC.

Ted Weaver, President of the Royal Australian and New Zealand College of Obstetricians and Gynaecologists, is referred to in 'The Birth Wars' (MacColl, 2009: 139) as having stated that if more women attempted VBAC there would be a reduction in the caesarean rate. However, Weaver strongly supported VBAC occurring only in hospital settings, where access to caesarean is close by. Obstetrician Mark Keirse, who worked on South Australia's guidelines for homebirth, does not rule out VBAC homebirth after a caesarean (MacColl, 2009: 139).

Pat Brodie, President of the Australian College of Midwives, also suggested that home births should not be ruled out for VBAC, rather that the reasons for the initial caesarean should be considered when considering hospital or home birth for VBAC (MacColl, 2009, 139).

Every single birth is different, every baby is different. No woman deserves to be judged on her previous birth experience. Her current experience is the only one that matters. When a woman experiences a VBAC she celebrates her achievement. The women I have helped all say similar things that they wish they could describe how they feel, what a difference my trust, confidence and belief in them made. Even those women who undertake a trial that ends in caesarean are elated at the experience.

We have to thank wonderful people like Nancy Wainer, a midwife, childbirth educator and an internationally known childbirth writer and speaker. She coined the term VBAC (vaginal birth after caesarean) and is the co-author of 'Silent Knife: Caesarean Prevention and Vaginal Birth After Caesarean', and the author of 'Open Season: A Survival Guide for Natural Childbirth and VBAC' along with hundreds of strong midwives the world over who have stood by the rights of women against all odds to help them achieve the ultimate.

The ridiculous thing is that the research supports VBAC, stating very clearly that there is less risk of uterine rupture than with a first time pregnancy. The risk of the scar tearing is extremely low because of the sheer nature of scar tissue, it is stronger than the original tissue. So many of the routine procedures used during a VBAC create more risks. Leave women alone and let them get on with what they know they can do naturally. Many of these women have to counteract the fear of untrusting birth attendants as well.

I cared for a woman choosing a VBAC with her fourth child, who with her previous child had been convinced by her doctor that a caesarean birth would be the best options as the baby was going to be too big. She had given birth vaginally to two previous healthy babies without any problems but suddenly her body was incapable, according to the obstetrician, even though there was no evidence to support this. The emotional pressure was too much for her so she agreed. When the baby was born by elective caesarean at term this baby was actually smaller than the other two. Her anger, sadness and feelings of betrayal were immense. It marred the joy of having a new baby, not to mention the pain of dealing with a caesarean scar for weeks later. So for her fourth baby she was not taking any chances and enlisted the assistance of carers who trusted in her ability to birth and to act as support and guidance for this birth. Of course she birthed easily without complication.

> "If women knew the real truth about birth, obstetrics as we know it would be vastly different—this may be a threatening thought to those who have been indoctrinated to believe that machines,

technology and computers always make things better...after almost 30 years of researching, writing, counselling and teaching caesarean prevention and VBAC, I know that most women can have safe, gentle, sacred, delicious VBAC births, and that they are safer than repeat caesareans. It is a travesty that the majority of sections and repeat sections are unnecessary. It is a tremendous sadness when women have been so indoctrinated with fear about birth that they choose numbness and technology to "get the baby out" rather than their own power and efforts. We must continue our efforts to stop the alarming number of primary caesareans and to increase the VBAC rate for those who have been cut. Spiritually conscious women want to feel the full scope of their feminine experience. They do not want to be ripped open. VBAC makes an immense difference in their lives, and it makes a positive and impressive difference in the lives of all those who are witness to that experience, as well"

Nancy Wainer, 'A Butcher's Dozen', Midwifery Today 2001.

Hints for Birth Helpers

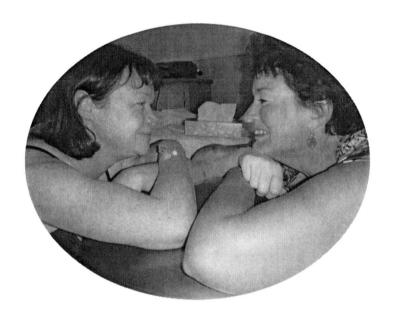

Listen to me!

- When I ask you to listen to me and you start giving advice, you have not done as I asked.
- When I ask you to listen to me and you begin to tell me why I shouldn't feel that way you are trampling on my feelings.
- When I ask you to listen to me and you feel you have to do something to solve my problem, you have failed me, strange as that may seem.

Listen! All I ask is that you listen. Not talk or do, just hear me.

> "The thing that helps more than anything, and I'm speaking as somebody who has given birth both in a hospital situation and at home, is that the person who's helping you, loves you"
>
> Ina May Gaskin, 1979

Being a Support Person

Knowing how important the process of giving birth is in a woman's life and how vulnerable she is to the people and energies around her at this time, it is important to find out what it means to be a 'good' support person. Simply having experienced birth does not necessarily qualify you, as when giving birth yourself you are far too self absorbed in the process of birthing to take particular notice of what everyone else is doing! Here are some ideas I have come across.

As a support person, knowing all about the process of childbirth is not as important as actually believing in a woman's ability to birth naturally. Helping is based on a relationship of mutual trust, honest communication and sensitivity to the woman's needs. Birth is an opportunity for personal growth for all who are present.

If you are planning to be a support person you must be prepared to go along with an open heart and mind with whatever happens, whatever choices the birthing woman makes.

Preparing for the Birth

It is important to find out what expectations the mother/couple has of you at the time of birth, whether it is providing emotional support and massage, or more general help such as food preparation, childcare, or a record of the birth (camera or video). Asking for a birth plan and familiarizing yourself with it helps to define a clear role.

Practical Preparations Near the Due Date May Include:

- light, comfortable clothing
- childcare availability
- car filled with petrol
- a bag packed ready with change of clothes, snacks and toothbrush
- ensure your families needs are met, organise childcare and meals.

If possible, get to know the midwife who will be working at the birth so that you feel comfortable around her. Attend childbirth classes with the couple and attend antenatal visits if possible.

Familiarise Yourself With:

The stages of labour, the 'Labour and Birth' chapter earlier gives short descriptions to help you know what to expect at each stage.

The couples breathing and relaxation techniques for coping with labour. Be aware of your own and the birthing family's emotional responses to labour.

Familiarise yourself with the home situation:

- how to get there, particularly useful if you are called at night
- where items needed for the birth are kept
- where food and utensils are kept, where the phone is, how to use the washing machine. I can assure you as a support person you will be invariably required to do the washing after.
- what the birthing woman will want you to do, such as prepare food, massage her back, thighs, shoulders, help her concentrate on breathing, provide an emotional support, place hot towels on her back, abdomen, thighs, help to change her position for comfort
- the help she may require before and after the birth. Enlist the help of others where necessary to provide adequate care for this period.

At the time of the birth a helper must have positive energy. Don't bring worries or ego with you. Don't chat on, even if you are excited at the prospect of the birth. Move quietly around the birth room. Maintain cheerful non-verbal support.

Present yourself well, this will boost the birthing woman's confidence. Take the time to think about what YOU might need during a long labour. Prepare yourself physically (eg. take a shower), eat a high energy meal and mentally calm your mind, try to get in tune with the birthing woman. Ensure you have good body and oral hygiene, a birthing mum has heightened senses and doesn't need to be challenged by body odour or bad breath.

Remember it is the woman's birth experience, not yours. Listen to her. If in doubt, ask her if she wants something, such as a drink, massage, or a change in position. In intense labour ask her questions that are simple and need only yes/no answers or a shake or nod of the head. Remember, you are their guest. Above all relax, enjoy peacefully, you may not be required to do anything except just be there and be available to support and hold her.

Ensure:

- a loving environment for the baby
- you are tactful, sensitive with all concerned
- a positive attitude to home birth
- be alert and aware of the signs of a quick birth. The midwife could need the help of the support person, especially if at home.

As women approach term, it is important they know to eat in labour. Some women will avoid eating for fear foods will make them nauseous. Tell them on the contrary, not eating will result in hypoglycaemia and increase their chances of nausea.

Since most first-time mothers have no idea what they are in for with their first labour, it is best if they expect labour to be at least twenty four hours of early labour and twelve hours of more active labour.

Prepare their nutrition accordingly. I encourage drinking high energy nutritional formulas such as ForeverGreen's AZUL and FrequenSea. Avoid using sugar drinks, the body needs electrolytes more to avoid dehydration.

Labour Support

Most people who ask a support person to be present are striving for a natural childbirth, so the role of all helpers is to assist this. Whether at home or in a hospital situation, you will likely be called to assist at home in early labour and be there for the transfer to the place of birth. In the hospital situation you may be required to act as the couples advocate, as a natural birth takes a little more effort in a place set up with the medical model of care. So the more informed you are the better.

Why Take a Support Person

Quite often a woman comes into the labour ward with her partner. While the partner may be well prepared and wonderfully supportive, they are also very emotionally involved. When labour becomes intense partners can become stressed and overwhelmed. This is where the wonderful support of another is great.

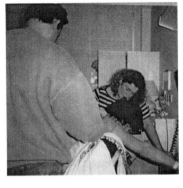

The midwife working in the labour ward is often very busy and may not be able to provide enough support. By taking another midwife or doula the pressure is off. I've seen this quite a few times, where the couple feel so confident but when it comes to the crunch neither are truly prepared for what is about to happen. Midwives and doulas are experienced, full of knowledge and skills to make this experience an amazing time. We are able to help the couple work together, connect and birth brilliantly together.

Giving direct labour support through massage and other pain relief techniques is a way in which a helper can assist. It is important you are comfortable touching and caressing the body.

Massage

May be easier with oil or talc, use long, strong downward strokes.

- effleurage - some women find that a light circular stroking of the abdomen with the finger tips gives relief during contractions.
- counter pressure - as labour progresses, the baby's head moves lower down, sometimes causing back pain due to pressure on the spine. Apply counter pressure by pressing your thumbs, knuckles or heels of your hands into the 'dimples' either side of her sacrum. Trial and error will find the right place. As the baby moves further down, you will need to apply counter pressure progressively lower.
- sacral pressure using the heel of the hand, either in a circular motion or alternative pressure and release
- back and buttock massage - with thumbs on the hip, move fingers firmly in and out from the spine to the hip. When used on one side, the effect is referred to the other.

- if it is necessary to lie on back, place fists, tennis balls or rolled towel under lower back as a counter pressure

Touch Relaxation

Practice ways to touch the expectant mum. Noticing areas of tension in the mother, shape your hand to the shape of that part of the body you are going to massage. With your hand thus shaped and relaxed, apply firm but gentle strokes to the tense area. Use continuous movements and maintain contact and pressure until the contraction is completed. If using two hands, keep one hand in contact while removing the other.

Touch relaxation is so powerful because the mother releases towards the hand that is touching her. By practicing before labour the mother learns that touch is a signal for her to relax towards that touch. Thus when the technique is used in labour mum will relax more readily, having an immediate relaxation effect.

Touch Relaxation Exercises

Mother - contracts the muscles of her scalp and raises her eyebrows.

- Support person - rest a hand either side of the scalp.
  Mother – relax, then frown.
- Support person - strokes the brow out towards the temples as she relaxes.

Continue in this manner moving through out the body. The mother tightens or squeezes muscles and the support person strokes and gently relaxes the area.

As a woman's labour increases in intensity, more will be required of helpers. The woman's ability to converse and express her needs may decrease, she will drop to using single words to convey her needs. As a helper you may need to anticipate needs and respond accordingly.

Non verbal communication may be most appropriate, such as a stroke, a smile, relaxation through touch. Good carers spend a lot of time touching in a calming and gentle way.

Helping Mum Choose Positions:

- choose positions that keep pressure off the back and tip the uterus forward
- use hot packs and towels to support the uterus. I spend many hours of labour with my arms wrapped around the birthing mum with a hot towel supporting the weight of the tummy and the other hand with a hot pack supporting the back.
- keep upright and moving as much as possible
- stand leaning against a wall, or lean on a bench or table
- sit backwards on a chair, head resting on a pillow
- kneel on the floor, arms on a chair, head resting on arms
- supported squatting such as between your partners legs with your arms over their legs. They can take your weight, allowing you to totally rest.
- side lying - relaxation position with pillows tucked around for comfort and support
- on all fours.

For acute back pain, use an ice pack at the site of pain, anywhere between the site of pain and the brain, or on the side opposite the pain. Because of the gating mechanism in the central nervous system, intense cold at any of these locations may beat a pain message to the brain. An ice pack may even be applied to the back of the woman's neck for the duration of a contraction (Lieberman, 1992).

The role of the support team is to share love, confidence and guidance.

During the Birth

Speak softly. Encourage her to listen to the person catching the baby as they will guide the birth.

Offer a mirror, this may help mum be more involved and focused on the birth. Encourage her to touch her baby's head as it is crowning, help her find the right position that works for her.

Be sensitive - remember this is not your journey. Calm your excitement.

Encourage mum to be the first to hold her baby as pictured. I assisted the birth of this baby gently and quietly while assisting mum to be fully present and catch her baby as soon as physically possible. Mum guided the birth of her baby herself, being the first to touch and hold her child. Just be silently available with love and support

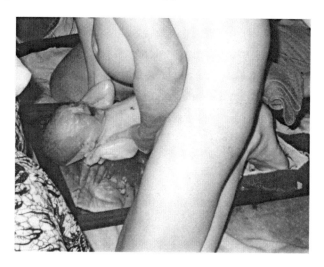

After the Birth

As soon as the baby is born the support person needs to retreat quietly after ensuring mum is comfortable in holding her baby. There is plenty of time to wait for the arrival of the placenta. Facilitate the bonding of the family unit as much as possible by doing all the fetching and carrying, allowing the new parents and siblings to 'sit' peacefully with their newborn and not be distracted or separated unnecessarily.

Mum may need some assistance in moving after the birth, and emotional support if her perineum is to be stitched, but this can wait as long as there is no excessive blood loss. The placenta usually will deliver within one to two hours and mum may need assistance with this.

When birthing at home I encourage mum to have a bath with her baby. Babies love warm water and it is a lovely relaxing space for mum to immerse herself into with her new baby.

Around three to five hours after the birth is the usual amount of time support people may be needed for cleaning up, food preparation and celebration. Use your discretion as to when it is appropriate to leave.

Whatever else you do after the birth, remember it is preferable not to judge your performance after the event. The memories of birth are precious and are better not analysed too thoroughly. Maintain a sense of humour.

Children at The Birth

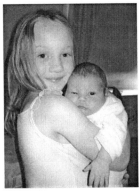

At first suggestion the thought of having a child at the birth of a new addition to the family may feel strange to some. Birth is a natural part of family life. What better way to show children that they are a valued member of the family than to allow them to be involved in the arrival of a new sibling, an event that will affect them profoundly whether they are involved in the birth process or not.

Seeing and helping when a new baby is born must surely create a bond between the siblings, whilst also giving them a valuable and healthy insight into the natural wonders of being human. I have experienced and heard many stories of children giving their mothers love and support during the birth, stories of children's wonder and excitement as they watched the baby's head emerge, stories of children revealing new aspects to their personality through the emotional high that birth creates. The most lasting impression I have gained from these experiences and shared stories is that children are not afraid of birth, they are fascinated, excited, awestruck and sometimes indifferent, but if they have been told about the reality of birth they seem to take it in their stride as a normal family happening.

It is very important that children have a caretaker to look after them during the birth that is not the mother or father but is in tune with the needs and desires of the family unit. Children are prone to getting bored during a birth and need to be entertained. Have a special present for them to receive after the baby is born as a celebration of the arrival of their brother or sister. Involve them in every aspect if this feels right for you.

Much of the information you need to divulge to a child is of course dependent upon their age and ability to understand. There are many books available such as "Mom and Dad and I are having a Baby" by Maryann P. Malecki, an excellent source of information for children and parents preparing for birth together. The book is in story format written from the child's point of view. It may also help to look at chidlbirth movies on YouTube.

What Children Need to Know:

- that giving birth can take a long time
- that baby comes out of the vagina, not the stomach. It is suggested that if the mother feels comfortable she could show the child her vagina prior to the birth.
- there will be blood, and that this blood is normal, healthy and 'natural'
- the baby may be an unusual colour when first born
- mother will be having an intense experience and may make a lot of noise, but this is natural
- some babies don't cry straight away
- mother may change her mind and not want you at the birth
- things can change and, if birthing at home, mum may need to go to hospital. If at hospital, children may have to leave the room if mum needs medical assistance.
- children don't need to know the technical jargon or about medical interventions, keep it simple. Children have the capacity to deal with the situation as it arises.
- children should be given the option of not attending or being able to leave at any time.

Don't forget the child after the baby is born, include them in the bonding process.

After the Birth

Afterbirth Pains

Women following a second or subsequent pregnancy will experience contraction like pain as the uterus involutes. It is thought this is a result of scar tissue from the placental site of the previous pregnancy combined with the placental site remaining from this pregnancy. You are likely to experience strong contractions when breastfeeding due to the increased oxytocin released causing the uterus to contract. You may also feel a gush of blood from the vagina, this is normal. The more you breastfeed the faster your uterus will involute and the more rapidly the pain will subside.

- if the pain is unbearable pressing on the uterine point on the foot can sedate the uterus
- a few mls of Pure can calm things down
- Motherwort tincture can be taken, use 1-2 droppers full in water or recharge every four hours or so. Motherwort also helps with milk production, menstrual cramps and hormone balance in general.
- lavender, tiger balm or Green oil can be applied to hips, neck and lower back whenever needed
- drink nettle tea, chamomile and rapsberry leaf teas.

Homeopathic Remedies for Post-Partum Healing

Caulophyllum 30c assists contractions to expel the placenta as well as good to take over the first few days every three - four hours to help the uterus return to its pre-pregnant state. Very good to assist with after pains.

Angelica Tincture (Dong Quai) can be used after birth to help release the placenta, 30-50 drops under tongue, combine with Caulophyllum and Witch hazel bark. Use repeatedly to control the bleeding until the placenta has been delivered.

Witch hazel bark (Hamamelis virginiana) a safe and effective astringent with additional benefits as an antiseptic.

Sabina 30c is a useful remedy for haemorrhage when there is retained placenta. Give the remedy every 10 mins for 4 doses.

Secale 30c is indicated when the contractions are not effective enough to expel the placenta. Give one dose every 10 mins.

Sepia 30c useful for retained placenta or situations where there is back pain, which is better when hard pressure is applied to the small of the back. Only repeat the dose if the pain persists or returns.

Chamomile and Arnica are excellent for afterpains and to help reduce perineal bruising. The results are almost immediate. It is also useful for cranky babies.

    ** Caution - don't use chamomile too soon after birth as it relaxes the uterus and can cause an increase in bleeding. Usually don't give mothers chamomile until about 8 to 12 hours after the birth, depending on need and bleeding.

Staphisagria combined with Arnica and Witch Hazel to help reduce haemorrhoids, varicose veins.

Calendula tincture is excellent for bathing a perineal tear.

The Newborn

The birth of a baby brings great changes for all members of the family. Birth marks the end of pregnancy and the beginning of parenthood.

    Three hormones play a key role in the immediate postnatal period.

Oxytocin (described earlier in this book) assists in the bonding between you and your baby, contracts the uterus, closes the cervix and instigates breast-feeding.

Endorphins are natural opiates that create a state of euphoria, calmness and pain relief so that you may enjoy the rewards of your hard work by being alert and able to experience and look after your baby.

Adrenaline and nor-adrenaline create the fight and flight response which enable a burst of energy for both baby and you to facilitate the final stages of birth and be awake for the initial moments after birth, then subside to create the warm fuzzy loving atmosphere necessary for bonding.

(Refer to 'Why Keep Birth Natural').

Contact Between Mother and Baby is Imperative.

"Separation will prevent the activation of specific brain functions that is nature's blueprint at this time. The separation of mother and baby after birth is 'the most devastating event of life, which leaves us emotionally and psychologically crippled."

Joseph Chilton Pearce 1992.

Immediately following birth is the critical bonding time for mother, partner and baby. It is now that the birth support team need to step back and provide a quiet serene space. As soon as the baby slips from the body, if the mother does not have hold at this time, then as soon as is possible baby should be passed to the mother's arms and be held close to the mother's skin.

At the moment of birth enormous changes occur in the baby's circulation, breathing, nerve and muscle function. With uterine contractions and the beginning of the separation of the placenta, the baby's oxygen supply diminishes. This low level of oxygen in the baby's blood stimulates the brain which in turn stimulates muscle contraction in the body. The muscles in the artery walls contract, causing changes in blood pressure, which changes the functioning of the heart. For the first time blood starts to flow through the arteries and capillaries supplying the lungs, which until now have not been used. The muscles involved with breathing (the diaphragm and intercostal muscles) also contract causing the chest cavity to enlarge and air enters the lungs - the first breath.

Adaptation to life outside the womb is a major physiological task for the baby immediately following the birth. Skin to skin contact is essential as the mother is the best incubator for her baby (and the softest). The first sounds a baby should hear are the welcoming tones of the parents. Encourage parents to welcome their baby. If the baby is a little slow waking to the world ask mum to run her fingers along the baby's spinal column from the base to the head. This stimulates the neural pathways, awakening the baby's nervous system. All parents should discover the sex of their baby. This fourty five minutes is probably the most precious time in this child's life.

'If ever there was a key trauma with lifelong consequences it is the separation of the newborn from its mother right after birth. As if the long birth struggle had not been enough, as if the harsh delivery room conditions had not been enough, the infant is then actually taken away from the one person who has been its entire source of comfort, its entire world. No wonder so many neurotics cannot be alone. Their initial entry into this world was marked by that catastrophic aloneness just after birth, when they were placed in a container, alone and uncomforted, if anything, the newborn needs to be held, comforted and touched more now than any other time in his life.'

Janov.

Leboyer (Birth without Violence, 1975) developed methods which allow the baby continuity from womb to belly by being put on the mother's belly directly after birth. Leboyer babies are reported to be healthier, rarely cry, are bright, alert and curious from early on.

Chamberlain (1989) describes the trauma and stress that babies go through today in Western hospitals, with bright lights, noise, cold rooms, instruments, rough contact with their sensitive skin and injections. Particularly traumatic is the cutting of the cord. The sad fact is that many birth assistants do not believe that babies are born with consciousness of what is going on around them, let alone that they are conscious whilst in utero. Thankfully this belief is changing. Rebirthing and primal therapy opens the doorway to understanding what a person feels or experiences through the birth process.

Re-birthing gives many indications of how people react to the modernisation of the birthing process. The child is thrown into a state of struggle to survive with intense fear when it is separated from its mother. The Western world is at risk of becoming pathologically cold and detached, materialistic and lacking in spirituality. I recently heard an interesting interview with a renowned medic who questioned whether the high state of depression was due to lack of spirituality, lack of a sense of belonging and lack of connection to fellow humans in our society today.

Rebirthing Experience

My personal experience with re-birthing was incredibly profound. As a midwife for many years I found myself unable to deal with women who chose not to breastfeed. I was fanatical about breastfeeding and it was becoming a problem with my relationships with women on the maternity floor. A friend suggested that I book in for a re-birthing session to find out why I held this view as it was obviously tied up with my own personal breastfeeding experience. So off I went to the local therapist with a very open mind.

Through a series of breathing techniques I was slowly taken deep into my inner self and then guided back to my time in the uterus. It was amazing. I could explain how I was feeling, what I was thinking and experiencing inside my mother's womb, along with what she was feeling!

I was the fifth child after four boys so my mother was very desirous of me being a girl. I felt this strongly and was very happy that I was fulfilling her dream but I was also acutely aware of the stress my mother was under, and her difficulties with coping with four boys under the age of nine years whilst preparing for another birth.

The therapist moved me through to the time of birth. I was born quickly at 12.05 am on my brother's ninth birthday. My mother had held off going to hospital in order to ensure I was born after midnight to fulfil his wish of a baby sister for his birthday. I began to crown in the lift of the hospital, which shows how quickly I came into the world. During the re-birthing session I was able to immediately experience my feelings on entering the world. It was incredibly cold, the lights hurt my eyes and I felt shocked and a great desire to be held by my mother. I felt dry scratchy cloths rubbed on my wet body and then felt myself being wrapped in layers of cloth, feeling restricted.

I was not handed to my mother immediately and felt a great sense of abandonment and a sense of not being wanted. These feelings of loneliness and abandonment have plagued my personal relationships all my life. I lay in the cot looking through metal bars at my parents. I felt my father pick me up and look at me with great love but my mother was very detached. I felt very distressed that I was not in her arms. Then I felt hungry and tried to wriggle my hand out of the cloths to suckle my fingers but to no avail. I wanted my mother to breast feed me but it never happened. My mother had breast abscesses drained two weeks before I was born and was told that she could not feed me, which unfortunately was the medical direction of the time in 1961.

As the breath therapy continued the therapist kept encouraging me to explore my cellular memories. I found myself becoming very angry and resentful that my mother did not feed me. I had made a pact with myself that it was not a nice place here and that the least painful place to be is asleep. Then the midwives tried to make me suck on a horrible tasting rubber teat with liquid that I knew was not my mothers. I stubbornly refused to drink. Talking to my mother after the session revealed how accurate my cellular memory was. She told me I slept most of the time so that she and her mother used to have to wake me up to feed, and then it was a battle to actually make me feed. I had made a decision I did not want to be here. Throughout the healing session I explored these feelings more deeply until finally I really began to understand how much my earliest experiences had impacted on my own life.

It took many weeks for me to process the feelings that came up for me during this session and to forgive my mother for not feeding me. I eventually was able to let go with a deeper understanding of what babies experience at birth. I am able to now work more fully with all women, understanding their desires and needs with less judgement, although I still am a strong advocate for the rights of the unborn child. Imagine if every birth attendant was to undergo re-birthing, wow, what a difference this would make to the way we see the unborn child and pregnant woman.

A review of seventeen controlled studies conducted between 1975 and 1985 compared newborn infants in the hospital who had routine contact with their mothers with those receiving additional contact. In thirteen studies the additional contact occurred only during the first hour of life. Nine of these noted significant positive differences in the later behaviour of the mothers toward their infants. In the four studies in which the extra contact extended through the first three days of life, the mother-child relationship was measurably better in quality for the extra contact infants, than for the control infants at one month, one year and two years of age (Midwifery Today 2000). Increased contact at any time during the first three days after birth (when the mother and baby spend this time in the hospital) produces a long-term improvement in the quality of the relationship between mother and child. Increased contact may, in part, make up for the marked deprivation that is a part of current routines in modern hospitals.

Researchers at the University College London have discovered that infants have a unique nervous system that makes them respond differently to pain than adults. By studying sensory nerve cells in infants, the scientists discovered that infants' reflex to pain or harm is greater and more prolonged than that of adults. The sensory nerve cells are also linked to larger areas of skin, which means they feel pain over a greater area of their body. In a commentary on the findings, a professor of neurobiology said that because the spinal sensory nerve cells work differently in babies, even a simple skin wound at birth could lead to the area becoming hypersensitive to touch long after the wound had healed (London Sunday Telegraph, August 2, 1998).

Do Fragile Babies Need Incubators at All?

If a baby is particularly drowsy (from drugs or other reasons) there may be too few brain signals to initiate breathing. Mouth to mouth resuscitation, gentle pressure on the baby's chest or administration of oxygen can be used until the baby's own breathing takes over. Sometimes mucous blocks the airway, and if the baby's own breathing movements are not strong enough to clear the airway, this can be cleared with gentle suction or a controlled suction pump.

A baby who has had breathing difficulties is often put into a humidicrib for a while so that temperature and oxygen levels can be controlled and he can be closely monitored.

A Swedish study investigated the potential benefits of skin to skin contact versus incubator treatment for hypothermic newborns (The Lancet, 1998, 352: 1115). Of eighty hypothermic newborns, fourty were placed in incubators while fourty received skin to skin contact. Almost ninety percent of the newborns who received skin to skin contact reached normal body temperature within four hours, compared to only sixty percent of the newborns placed in incubators. The Swedish study also found that within twenty four hours the babies placed in incubators tended to have a higher body temperature than the babies who were held skin to skin, which may make the incubated newborns vulnerable to heat stress. The researchers claimed that holding newborns skin to skin also stabilised heart and respiratory functions.

One doctor in an African hospital where there were no incubators found the best incubator to be the mother. The mother is the correct temperature, is soft and has food on tap. This particular doctor saved ninety percent of premature babies, some as small as four pounds. Compare this to the well-established research finding that mothers of babies spending time in neonatal care units find it more difficult to bond with their babies, suffer more postnatal depression, are talking less to their babies a year later as well as having a higher risk of child abuse.

Unfortunately, many babies end up in neonatal units due to interventions in the birth process. Babies suffer complications from inductions, drugs, forceps delivery and caesarean sections. These babies often miss out on the B-endorphin hormone essential for bonding with their mother. Keeping birth normal is more important for the future psychological development of the baby than we give credence (Jowitt, 1993).

Researchers provided about one hundred premature babies with a fifteen minute massage three times a day. An equal number of premature babies were given the exact same number of calories and other care as the massage group but no massage (Field, 2001). The result of this study, conducted in collaboration with the University of Miami Medical School, showed that the massaged babies gained fifty percent more weight each day and were ready to leave the hospital six days earlier than the control group. The massaged infants were also found to have substantial differences in motor skills and cognitive functioning compared with the control group.

How Does the Baby Change?

At birth the baby may not be all pink and cuddly. Your baby has been through a very dramatic experience and will have their own story to tell. As well as being covered with blood and vernix they may be bruised and marked from the birth. The skin can be quite bluish dark in the first minutes after birth but usually they pink up within one minute. It is not unusual for a small baby to have small pimples on his nose and chin, and red blotches on the eyelids, which soon disappear.

The head may be a little mishaped from pressure in the birth canal (moulding), and sometimes there is a large blister-like protuberance on the head (called a caput) which may look alarming but soon disappears. The genitals appear large in relation to the rest of the body, and the breasts may be a little swollen. Baby girls may have vaginal discharge as a result of the hormones created during the birth process.

The skin is usually covered in a white greasy texture called vernix which is a natural protection preventing the skin from drying out. It is good to rub this into the skin, don't be in a hurry to wash your baby. An interesting article in an old British obstetrics and gynaecology journal titled 'Forget the newborn bath!' indicated vernix should be left on a newborn rather than washed off because it helps the infant maintain body temperature (Austin, 1999).

Some babies have a lot of fine downy hair called Lanugo, which generally rubs off in a few days. The newborn baby has blue eyes at birth, which will usually take on their own unique colouring by three months. They can see and will follow a moving object and they can look cross eyed at times. However their eyes are unaccustomed to bright lights and they have no experience with focusing or fixing on objects so vision may not be clear.

In the uterus the baby has been curled up and therefore continues this position when lying down for some time afterwards. Straight after birth they are capable of creeping up the abdomen as the video 'Self-Attachment' demonstrates http://www.geddesproduction.com/breast-feeding-delivery-selfattachment.php. This is a wonderful record of how a baby when left on the mother's abdomen following birth crawls to the breast and self attaches to the breast. This later becomes crawling and if put on their stomach babies will quickly make their way to the end of the cot.

A new baby does not like to be suddenly lowered and shows the startle reflex if lowered quickly, or almost dropped. If held upright, under the arms, with feet touching a flat surface, they will make stepping movements. There is usually a strong sucking reflex and the baby may suck their fingers or fist. If not too drowsy they will probably suck strongly on the nipple.

A newborn is startled by sudden loud noises, but seems to enjoy continuous rhythmical sounds such as music, voices, washing machines and so on. Your baby enjoys and is comforted by rocking movements, and by movements such as those they feel in a car or a rocking cradle. They are comforted by being held closely and hearing the body sounds of the person holding them, and by deep bathing, provided the water is the right temperature.

Naming Your Baby

Naming your baby will be one of the greatest joys but can also be a tough decision. There are so many choices. There are also many different cultural practices related to naming baby.

It has been my experience that most babies appear to name themselves. I have witnessed many parents choose a name only to change it during the last weeks of pregnancy, during labour or even when it comes time to fill out the birth certificate. Often it is a sudden intuitive feeling that their child needs to be called a certain name. Some may say that their child has named themselves. If we look at the numerological significance this could be quite true, as each letter holds a number frequency which then relates to the personality type. I'd rather not go into an in-depth discussion about numerology at this point as it is a whole book in its own right, you can however find the basic principles online to assist in guiding you. Needless to say the date and time of birth is very significant and even more so in relation to the name. I use numerology a great deal in my life.

My suggestion is that through meditation, going inwards and connecting with your child you may receive a strong message in regards to the name of your child. Some people know this from the moment of pregnancy and are already referring to their baby in utero by its name. My personal experience of this was that I knew many years before my daughter was born that I was going to have a Vanessa. When I was pregnant with my third child my eldest son Justin, then aged four, told many people that his sister Vanessa would be born on the 25th August at 2am. True to form Vanessa was born at that time at home. Justin, who at the time was asleep in his room, walked out within minutes of her birth. Greeting his sister with a kiss he stated 'Hi Vanessa, about time your got here', kissed me and promptly went back to bed. We hadn't actually formally named her at that time. Quite uncanny!

There is no need to rush the naming of your child. You have up to six weeks under Australian law to legally name your child. Have fun.

Babies Immune System

Enhancing Your Child's Immunity

Children are one of the most important, if not the greatest, assets and joys in life, and to see them suffer during illness cuts to the core of every parent. As a parent you are in a privileged position to enable your child to reach their full potential through correct implementation of diet and lifestyle.

Research indicates failure to provide infants with the correct nutritional requirements early in life is likely to increase their susceptibility to immune dysfunction (allergies and infections) and behavioural disorders (anxiety, insomnia, ADD and ADHD).

Boosting a child's immune system naturally can provide long-term health benefits. Unfortunately our environment is such that it does not support this process. Over-use of chemicals, antiseptics and cleaning agents does not allow the natural development of the immune system. Children need to be exposed to every day bugs in order for their immune system to build a defence against them. Many studies have shown that children born and bred on farms where they are associating with animals on a regular basis have stronger immunity than those born and bred in clean modern home environments.

Further evidence suggests that environmental changes and over-sanitation has led to decreased intestinal flora, even if natural birth and breastfeeding have taken place. Also due to environmental toxins there have been reports of too much dioxin in breast milk. Vaccination, stress, changes in water treatment and weaning too early may all have an impact on baby's digestive system, increasing the risk of low immune systems.

Immune System Priming

Our immune systems rely on a balance of T Lymphocytes. These T Helper (TH) cells are the primary regulators of the immune system. They present in three ways:

TH1 cells regulate responses to bacteria, viruses, fungi and metastatic cells and are the dominant type of lymphocyte in tissue-specific autoimmunity conditions.

TH2 cells promote responses against allergens and parasites, and are particularly involved in stimulating the production of antibodies. They are elevated in allergic diseases and systemic autoimmune conditions.

TH3 cells regulate the activity of TH1 and TH2 if one or other becomes dominant then TH3 is activated in the gut to assist bringing immune balance back. This indicates very clearly why the gut is so important in immunity health.

A mother must become TH2 dominant in pregnancy in order to prevent her body from aborting the baby, so children are born in a TH2 dominant state and are dependant on immune challenges and TH3-type immunity to induce and maintain balance within the immune system. The micro-environment of the gut is critical in determining the normal development of immune function. Without normal gastrointestinal function children may develop much immune pathology.

The gastro-intestinal tract not only maintains digestion and absorption of nutrients required for the growth and development of infants, but also programs and develops many other systems of the body, such as the immune and neuroendocrine systems, for life. Seventy percent of the body's immunity is localized in the gastrointestinal tract. Beneficial gut flora is essential for digestion and absorption of nutrients which the whole body is reliant on. Dysbiosis, an over-growth of unwanted bacteria, leads to poor digestion which then manifests as gastrointestinal symptoms such as flatulence, bloating, diarrhoea, vomiting, colic, reflux and failure to thrive.

The mother influences the development and maturation of the gastrointestinal tract of the infant while in-utero. Stress, infection, poor micro flora status and dietary habits of the mother during pregnancy may all lead to dysbiosis in the infant post-partum. The gastrointestinal tract of new-borns is inoculated primarily by organisms originating from the mother's vagina, faeces and the environment. Infants delivered by c-section have far fewer lactobacilli in the early stages of life than those delivered vaginally, and the hygiene conditions of hospitals may prevent the full transfer of micro-organisms to abdominally delivered new-borns. The faecal colonisation of infants born by caesarean delivery is delayed, and the primary gut flora in infants born by caesarean may be disturbed for up to six months after the birth, compared with vaginally delivered infants. Latest studies indicate these infants may take up to six months to colonize their gut with beneficial flora, running a greater risk of compromised immunity (Jakobsson et al., 2014). This is further compounded if infants are bottle fed.

Many studies, including recent research by Vanderbilt University (2013) have shown that microbes play a very important role to play in the body's genetic information. Beneficial bacteria essential to healthy immune function dominate the micro flora of breast fed infants. A lack of beneficial microbes can contribute to many adult health issues. Recurrent infections treated by antibiotics also lead to the disruption of normal gut flora. It is important to note that a child's immune system must be in optimum function if you choose to immunize your child to prevent long term adverse effects.

Solution - boost your child's immune system through the gut by ensuring they have adequate levels of beneficial bacteria, either through breastfeeding or using specific supplementation under the guidance of a natural therapist. Research indicates that if mother and baby take therapeutic probiotic bacteria and colostrums during the first six months following birth, immune imbalances are hugely assisted, helping with the prevention of colic and other gastro-intestinal upsets. It is also important to ensure solids are not introduced until after six months of age, avoid processed refined food, feed children small frequent meals rather than three large meals and avoid cold drinks with meals as this decreases the digestive process.

Prevention

Pregnant mothers need to be encouraged to:

- take probiotics and gut flora throughout pregnancy
- avoid antibiotic therapy if possible, or if unavoidable take higher doses of probiotics two hours after the antibiotic
- aim for vaginal birth as naturally as possible
- do not allow the washing down of the vaginal area prior to birth with antiseptic solutions as this kills essential microorganisms
- skin-skin contact immediately following birth
- avoid suctioning at birth
- breast feed as soon as possible
- continue to take probiotics whilst breastfeeding.

Vaccination

How do you decide whether or not to vaccinate your child? It can be a difficult and emotional decision for many parents. With a background in paediatric nursing and as a natural therapist I have experienced personal stories from both sides of the story. Currently approximately 53% of Australians have concerns around vaccination. Communication with honesty must be made available for parents so that they can have real and valid information to make the right decision for them.

What is Vaccination and How Does it Work?

Vaccination is the deliberate introduction to the human immune system of minute particles of a disease (pathogen). The aim is that the vaccine is so minimal as to create a positive effect on the immune system by creating long term immunity without running too high a risk of reaction. Of course there are always risks as every person is individual and reactions are possible.

Vaccination is believed to have begun at least one thousand years ago, with people understanding that if they were exposed to a light infection of the disease, although they got sick, they were then protected for the rest of their life. In 1976 Edward Genner was the first man to create a vaccination, giving a deliberate infection of smallpox. Smallpox had been a devastating disease with a high death rate, but the introduction and widespread use of the vaccine in the years that followed saw the disease all but disappear.

What are Parents' Concerns?

There are many reasons why parents choose not to vaccinate. Their fears and concerns are valid as there are many factors involved and each case needs individual consideration. There is concern that the carrier for vaccines may be the reason that some children have a sinister reaction, leading some parents to be more afraid of the vaccine than the diseases the vaccines prevent and raising a number of questions:

- what has the vaccination been created from and how do these constituents affect the brain and the body?
- what does the carrier do once it is in the body? Is it eliminated or is it stored in the brain or the body's fat tissue?

It is a fact that viruses and germs that can harm or kill exist on our planet. I have seen the struggle to stay alive that a tiny baby, only a few weeks old, can go through when afflicted with croup and Ptussis (whooping cough). No parent wishes to endure this terrifying experience with their child. However I have also witnessed the death of a baby from encephalitis as a reaction to immunisation. So what is the logical path to take?

Do Your Research

Before you make a decision about vaccination, explore the wealth of information available. The internet is a fabulous source of information, but understand it may also be passing on misinformation. Vaccination is tied to an economic value, with pharmaceutical companies making a lot of money from the creation and sale of vaccinations.

The movie 'For the Greater Good' directs the conversation to the idea that a vaccine can be pushed through quickly and sent out to the community too fast, before good research has been conducted to eliminate the side effects or other variables, thus putting people at risk.

I suggest watching the video 'Jabbed, Love, Fear and Vaccines' broadcast by the SBS television as it provides information and insight from the more pro-vaccine perspective. Much research is occurring now into Genomics that is shedding some light on the reactions that those rare children have had in regards to immunisation. It appears that these children may carry a gene that heightens the risk of them reacting to certain triggers. These triggers may be in vaccines but also in many other areas of life, begging the idea that the child is likely to react at some point anyway. So was it the vaccination or did the vaccination trigger something that was likely to trigger anyway? Professor Ingrid Scheffer (Melbourne Brain Center, University of Melbourne) has discovered that the histories and symptoms matched a rare form of epilepsy often not occurring until one to two years of life, caused from a gene mutation (http://www.sbs.com.au/shows/jabbed) . Professor Scheffer's research suggests the vaccination triggered rather than caused the seizures, which were inevitable and would have occurred regardless.

It may also be important to take into account the health and wellbeing of society in general. Lifestyles and behaviours appear to be lowering our overall immune systems as superbugs take hold and antibiotics have less beneficial effect. There also appears to be a reoccurrence of those diseases we felt had been eliminated through vaccination. Is this a result of parents not vaccinating or a natural evolution of the virus and bacteria?

The majority of adults who contract diseases such as measles have not been vaccinated. Yet there is research that seems to imply that when vaccination has taken place there is a greater outbreak in that disease, although often mild, and that perhaps this is a natural community immunisation taking place.

Unarguably immunisation has saved the lives of many, many millions of people, particularly children. Though it would seem that immunisation is without doubt a warranted practice, the question is asked - have we gone too far and are we over vaccinating, with some children now receiving up to 17 vaccinations in one year. Does this overtax the immature immune system? From my point of view I feel that balance is required. Spread the vaccinations over a period of time, ensure your child is very well and healthy when receiving vaccination and boost your child's immune system by giving probiotics for children. Visit a naturopath or homeopath and follow some of the suggestions I have provided in this book for building your immune system whilst pregnant. Obviously building your own immune system is the best way to support your body and prevent yourself from getting sick.

Some diseases such as measles are particularly fast at replicating and can be spread widely before the carrier is even aware they are the carrier. The risk here is that as more people choose not to immunise the risk becomes greater of the disease spreading faster and infecting those that are more vulnerable. Level of immunity and immune system strength varies from person to person and there will always be those who are more vulnerable than others. Often those who choose not to immunise tend to lead healthy lives and are greatly motivated to support their immune systems through better lifestyle choices. The problem is that if their child does contract a disease although they may be lightly affected, they can become a live carrier without symptoms and can spread the disease to others who are more vulnerable to a greater reaction. This is why when a break out occurs those children who are not immunised are required to be kept away from school and confined to their homes.

Maybe our children are vulnerable if we don't vaccinate and then again vulnerable to some extent if we do vaccinate but to a much lesser extent. Life is not without its risks. Perhaps we are too quick to aim for perfection. It is a reality that a small number of children will run a higher risk of a complication from vaccination, but when we look at the number of children vaccinated every year this risk seems quite tiny by comparison.

I guess a fatalist may say that we are destined to experience life personally prescribed for each individual. This may feel a cold comfort for those who have fallen victim to life's greater challenges. We need to remember how far we have come. Looking back to the 1940s and 1950s when so many were afflicted by polio without treatment available, and now due to vaccination Polio is almost non-existent, although there are claims that the disease may be returning.

Whatever your decision I ask that you do your research, get the facts and make your decision based on what feels right for you. Make sure you explore any aspect you have fears about and check the data and the research to ensure you have the facts. A lot of information available on the world wide web is emotionally driven and may not be a beneficial source of information.

Jaundice

A yellow discolouration of the skin (jaundice) occurs in most newborn babies, some becoming more jaundiced (yellow) than others. It is usually caused by the breakdown of red blood cells the baby no longer needs. When these cells are broken down bilirubin is produced, which is usually eliminated by the kidneys and liver. Babies are not ill but often become very sleepy and may be difficult to feed. This is quite normal. It is very important to feed your baby frequently to help remove any excess bilirubin.

If the baby becomes very yellow (jaundiced), it is an indication that there is too much bilirubin for the baby's body to manage. The excess bilirubin deposits in the skin and sclera of the eyes. If your baby is becoming yellow, placing baby in the warmth of the sun is an excellent way to help the body break down the excess bilirubin. If the yellowing is become excessive a blood test will need to be done and the baby may need specific help by being placed in a cot (humidicrib) under ultra-violet lights. The lights help to break down the extra bilirubin in the skin. They are put in the humidicrib to keep them warm, as they need to be naked for the lights to affect the skin. They are usually only under lights for two to three days and it is very important to feed frequently to help the elimination process. If you are at home sometimes lights and a humidicrib can be organised for home. Excessively high bilirubin may require a blood transfusion or it could lead to brain damage, though this is very rare.

Vitamin K

One of the first decisions parents are faced with is whether to give their baby vitamin K. Vitamin K assists our body to manufacture clotting factors that prevent us from bleeding. Even though these factors are available at birth there is a need for vitamin K to activate the process. Babies tend to be born with low levels of vitamin K which generally don't reach adult levels until around six months of age. It is believed there are two reasons for this:

- very little vitamin K crosses the placenta to the baby
- babies are born with low levels of the intestinal bacteria necessary for the clotting process.

Vitamin K Deficiency Bleeding (VKDB)

A rare condition, VKDB affects between one and two in every ten thousand babies born, depending on where they are born in the world. A baby who does not have enough vitamin K can start to bleed suddenly, without warning, any time up to several weeks after birth. VKDB seems to occur in exclusively breastfed babies for reasons mostly unknown. Vitamin K supplementation was developed to counteract the risk of this haemorrhagic disease of the newborn. Research suggests that supply of Vitamin K from breast milk is not the issue, as breast milk generally has adequate vitamin K within a few days of birth. Babies presenting with VKDB almost exclusively are breastfed and when tested their mother's breast milk did contain adequate levels of vitamin K. So it would appear that the VKDB was due to either babies having difficulty absorbing vitamin K or not having enough bacteria in their gut to activate vitamin K. VKDB can also occur in babies that have an underlying health problem such as gallbladder disease, cystic fibrosis or medication side effects and again those affected are exclusively breast fed babies.

Professor Golding (1992) wrote:

> 'It has always seemed physiologically perverse that evolution should have permitted the development of what is termed vitamin K deficiency in normal term infants. If this is the case how did we come to be here at all?'
>
> Golding, J, Greenwood,R, Birmingham, K & Mott, M
> (1992) http://www.ncbi.nlm.nih.gov/pubmed/1392886

Any decision regarding a child's health is bound to be emotional. It also depends on what philosophy you come from and the choices you make and why. For me personally I tend to agree with Professor Golding. The discussion needs to be put into perspective and all sides taken into consideration.

There are many reasons why parents choose not to give their babies vitamin K at birth, one being that it is administered as an injection and feels like an intervention, especially if they are aiming for an intervention free birth. To some it would seem perverse to achieve a wonderful, calm birthing experience to then give their baby a painful injection, particularly with the knowledge that babies are hypersensitive to pain after birth.

Possible reactions to vitamin K injection include:

- mild reaction at the injection site
- haemolytic anaemia
- jaundice or rash.

If any of these issues concern you then oral vitamin K may be a better choice for you. It is available and certainly worth your while asking for it or searching it out before you give birth. You must be aware of the guidelines for its effectiveness. When administered orally vitamin K is best given a few days after birth as bile salts that are not present at birth are required for absorption (Sandra Stine, MD, Midwifery Today, 1999).

"One reason that other countries may use the oral version Vitamin K is that mothers and infants either have prolonged hospital stays after birth, or they have nurses come to the home. This does not occur in the U.S. nor often in Australia. Therefore if the oral version is used, the parents need a reminder to administer the follow-up doses, and someone needs to monitor that the infant does not spit it up. When oral Vitamin K is used it usually requires 3 doses (birth, 1 week, and 6 weeks), and the breakthrough cases of Vitamin K deficiency bleeding are often related to missing the final dose"

Samuel Busfield et al., 2013

- When infants do not receive any Vitamin K at birth, statistics from Europe show that 4.4 to 10.5 infants out of 100,000 will develop late VKDB. Rates are higher in Asian countries (1 out of every 6,000 infants).
- When infants receive oral Vitamin K at least three times during infancy (typically at birth, one week, and four weeks), anywhere from 1.4 to 6.4 infants out of 100,000 will develop late VKDB.
- When infants receive the Vitamin K shot at birth, there are virtually no cases of late VKDB.

Shearer, M J (2009)

Some parents fear that vitamin K is linked with childhood cancer and Leukaemia. In 1999 the World Health Organization carefully reviewed the evidence and issued a statement saying that there was not enough evidence to support a link between vitamin K and childhood cancer. Research that combined data from six major studies that looked at the potential relationship between vitamin K and childhood cancer found no association between injectable vitamin K and any type of childhood cancer (Roman et al., 2002).

Nature's Tools

As parents it is important to be informed. Babies are low in vitamin K at birth but nature does provide the necessary tools to ensure a quick increase, otherwise we would never have survived as a race. Whilst a baby is travelling through the vagina and across the perineal area they ingest some of your body fluids, which contain the necessary natural bacteria that inoculate your baby's gut. Babies who breastfeed very soon after birth will also receive vitamin K from the breast milk. This can be improved by the mother having a high nutrient intake of vitamin K rich foods such as kale, alfalfa, spinach and other dark green leafy foods. This is also important in the last few weeks before birth.

If you blend these greens into a smoothie then the vitamin content increases immensely. You may read articles inferring that a healthy woman is unable to improve her levels of vitamin K with nutrition but the question I ask is what nutrition is being studied. The 'average' woman does not ingest super foods nor focus on a high raw food diet. The average 'healthy diet' does not contain high levels of dark green vegetables (for more information see the Nutrition Section).

So if you are choosing for your baby not to receive the vitamin K injection at birth my suggestions to increase baby's vitamin K levels as soon as possible are:

- throughout your pregnancy and daily leading up to birth, drink at least one dark green smoothie containing kale, spinach, alfalfa and any other dark green vegetables, adding watermelon, grapes and banana to taste. Blending vegetables and fruits provides a high absorbency level that turns them into super greens. You can buy Super Green formulas that can be added to your smoothie.
- if you can find vitamin K supplements then add these to your diet daily
- ensure you labour spontaneously and as naturally as possible
- ask not to be washed down with antiseptic wash during the delivery. This is routine in most hospitals and kills off necessary bacteria for your baby's gut inoculation.

- breastfeeding should begin at birth and continue every two hours or more often on demand. Although the volume of colostrum is not great, it is the perfect food for your baby during the first days and is very important to prevent classical vitamin K deficiency. If you supplement your diet with high vitamin K foods, levels in breast milk begin to rise almost immediately and are well increased by twelve hours (Frye, 1997).
- it is essential that you continue drinking vitamin K rich smoothies after the birth. Get your partner or support people to create smoothies for you daily. Nutribullet blenders are very popular now and available to purchase. See http://www.foodmatters.tv/ and other sites regarding raw food.

Cranial Osteopathy

I thoroughly recommend your baby undergo Cranial Osteopathy with a qualified osteopath or chiropractor following the birth to assist the reshaping of the baby's cranial bones back to their normal position and to assist with the ability to breastfeed. Cranial osteopathy is a refined and subtle treatment that encourages the release of stresses and tensions throughout the body, including the head. It is a gentle yet extremely effective approach.

The cranium is made up of twenty nine bones, each joined by various forms of joints. The most common form of joint is a suture, which can be compared to stitching, and allows yielding movement while at the same time binding the cranium tightly. The twenty nine bones join together to form a total of one hundred and two joints. Early anatomists believed that the sutures ossified after birth, but recently it has been confirmed that the cranial sutures should not ossify, but should allow a yielding movement. At birth, there are more than twenty nine cranial bones because many of the bones are formed by several parts which have not yet ossified together. This is an important point for the child's normal growth and development because if the bones ossify in a distorted manner this can affect the child's development and health.

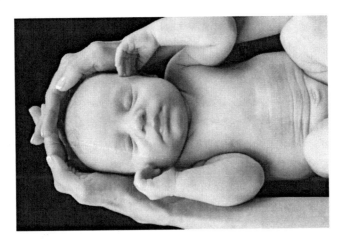

During birth these bones overlap so the baby's head can fit through the neck of the womb. This compression is normal and nature ensures the skull is flexible enough for it to happen. This same flexibility may lead to delicate bones being pinched or twisted during a long labour or complicated birth. Breech deliveries and intervention with forceps are even more traumatic and can give rise to long term problems which left untreated can last throughout life.

How does a newborn express that discomfort or pain? You may notice baby has difficulty in sucking, constant crying and crankiness, colic, reflux, sleep disorders, is very demanding. Alternatively, baby may be lethargic and unresponsive with no obvious cause or explanation. Cranial osteopathy therefore is an extremely relevant system of infant health care.

My eldest son was born via forceps delivery and, unbeknown to me, suffered headaches for many years until I learned about osteopathy. I took him for treatment where the practitioner explained to me that he could feel the dents from the forceps in his skull. After about six Osteopathic Release sessions my son's behaviour changed immensely where he became calm and relaxed. He stated that it felt like his head was as light as a balloon. Cranial osteopathy can assist with breastfeeding issues as well.

William Garner Sutherland is the pioneer of cranial osteopathy in America, where today most babies are routinely checked by an osteopath physician as a preventative measure to correct birth trauma. Unfortunately this is not so in Australia. Studies of the relationship between skeletal distortion during infancy and learning problems have found a direct link between the degree of cranial restriction and the child's problems. Many children are being diagnosed with ADD (Attention Deficit Disorder) and then being treated with unnecessary drugs, yet often this can be caused due to cranial membranes being slightly pinched at birth and results with osteopathy treatment are excellent. One study undertaken in 2000 of 1250 newborn infants found eighty eight percent had cranial bone dysfunction, whether the birth was normal or not. All benefited from osteopathy treatment. Cranial osteopathy is also successful in the treatment of Cerebral Palsy, epilepsy, learning and behavioural difficulties in older school age children.

Infant Male Circumcision

The World Health Organisation estimated in 2007 that fifty nine percent of males over the age of fifteen had been circumcised. Ten to twenty percent of Australian male babies are circumcised compared to sixty percent in the USA. Circumcision has a long history and has been practiced for religious reasons as a rite of passage in various societies. Egyptian male mummies dating back to 2300BC have been circumcised. Infant male circumcision is often performed without pain relief or anaesthesia.

As the foreskin is normal at this age, the procedure is performed for non-medical reasons. The foreskin firmly adheres to the glans penis and is designed to protect the head and maintain erotogenic sensitivity.

Sadly many parents still have this procedure carried out because of supposed health risks. These risks most likely date back to hygiene issues during the Victorian era, when circumcision was promoted as a way to desensitise the penis and so thwart masturbation. It was thought that masturbation could cause headaches, short-sightedness, paralysis, bed-wetting and insanity, just to name a few. Circumcision was placed more around morality than hygiene.

As Dr. Robert Darby pointed out, when hygiene was once limited there was a myth that the foreskin carried disease, whereas the foreskin can in fact protect against disease (Medical Journal of Australia, 2003). This myth grew during the sand wars of the first and second world wars. Research by Sir Duncan Stout, who wrote a chapter on military medicine in the tomb History of the Second World War, could not find any connection between disease and the foreskin. Sir Stout actually found quite the opposite and recommended circumcision not be performed.

The penis in the resting state, like the clitoris, is an internal organ. The penis is a uniquely specialised and sensitive functional organ of touch, it makes proteins that fight bacteria and viruses and produces a moisturiser that keeps the surface of the glans sensitive, soft and moist. The foreskin has more specialised nerve endings than any other part of the penis, and is as sensitive as the lips of the mouth.

Removing the foreskin makes as much sense as removing the eyelid to have a cleaner eyeball. Circumcision has a negative health ratio in that it causes morbidity/mortality and health care costs that are inappropriately expended. The pain of the infant is characterized by facial expression of brow bulging, creasing and furrowing. The eyes close, lips purse, the tongue is taut and the chin shivers. There are vigorous bodily movements with jerking, swinging of the arms, bicycling of the feet and thrusting of the limbs. The cry is compelling and meaningful.

A Danish study of men and their spouses (5552 participants altogether) found that circumcised men and their partners were more likely than uncircumcised men and partners to report frequent orgasm difficulties, more frequent sexual dysfunction and dyspareunia (painful sexual intercourse) (Frisch, Lindholm & Gronback, 2011).

Settling Baby

Every baby is as individual as you are with their own bio-rhythms. Time spent sleeping at night increases as they get older, especially if routines are established. The following is only an average assessment of the sleeping patterns of babies. Newborns tend to sleep six to eight times a day, each sleep lasting about two to three hours. Some babies may take up to an hour to feed at some feeds so it will feel like all you are doing in the early days is feeding, so get plenty of rest when your baby sleeps. By six weeks to two months, most have decreased to four to five sleeps, each lasting about two and a half to three hours. There will be longer waking periods where baby is happy to play by themselves.

Usually by about four months routines and breastfeeding have been well established and you as parents will be feeling confident as you and your baby have gotten to know each other. Your baby will usually have two longer sleeps (four to five hours), one of them usually at night, and three shorter sleeps (two to two and a half hours). Establishing a morning and afternoon sleep now will assist you to maintain this right up til about two years of age and can be a great sanity saver. Some babies by six months are sleeping eight to ten hours at night, but don't expect this as accepting your baby as individual is very important.

Tips for Settling Your Baby

Attachment

Babies need attachment both physically and emotionally. If your baby is crying, she needs you to go to her and care for her. The only way a baby can communicate its needs is by crying. Babies sleep for small amounts of time and frequently. Some babies will feed every couple of hours in the first few weeks. One of my sons fed two hourly until he was ten months old. This was his personality. In between feeds he was a very happy, chubby baby. Because his needs were met early in life he learned to trust the world. You cannot spoil a baby by doing this. A sling is very important and a wonderful sanity tool.

In the early months a baby needs to learn that her world is a safe place to be in, and that she can trust her carers to meet her needs. It has been my experience that the more a baby's needs are attended to in the early days the less likely they are to cry as they get older. However sometimes you may tick all the boxes on the tick list and still she will continue to cry. There may seem to be nothing wrong but at that time nothing seems to help her calm down. All you can do is sit and hold her and help her learn to cope with her own emotional distress, this is what we all must do in our life. Everyone has off days.

By providing cuddles and supports she will learn to trust and feel safe, which will have a large effect on her fear issues later in life. Over time many mums report that they are able to work out their baby's needs by the different types of crying the baby expresses. Obviously if you are able to stay calm then this will have a direct effect on the baby. If you are finding yourself feeling stressed, then seek out someone who can offer that calming support for the baby and to give you a rest. The calming freshness of someone else's arms can do the trick. Sometimes we all need time out from each other, even babies.

This is why sometimes when a baby is crying and you find you can't settle them, a knowing mother, midwife or grandmother takes the baby and it calms down simply because of the change in energy. It has nothing to do with your ability as a parent. It is no different to when we are an adult and are feeling upset. Some people who are not attached to the situation are able to help us feel more calm than others. Learn the signs that mean your baby is tired. You can then start settling the baby before he gets overtired.

Overtired babies can be irritable and harder to settle. Here are some signs that your baby is ready for sleep.

- yawning
- making jerking movements

- clenching fists
- fretting
- grimacing
- pulling at the ears
- rubbing eyes
- increased physical activity

Settling Notions

If baby has been fed, changed, cuddled and still won't settle you could:

- ensure the baby is wrapped up firmly in a bunny rug or sheet, this gives a sense of security
- walk with your baby or rock baby snuggled up close to your chest to hear your heartbeat, babies love movement, dance and rocking to music
- sing lullabies, hum a tune or croon to your baby
- carry baby in a sling or Mei Tai, your baby has been in your body for the past nine months and it can be quite a shock to be outside in the great big world
- tummy down across your lap - gently pat or rub your baby, this was my children's Nonna's suggestion and worked every time
- try taking baby for a walk outside in the fresh air or take them for a ride in the car this has been a time honoured solution. Many Dads have been known to be driving the block in the middle of the night.
- if you feel the need to use a pacifier do this only once breastfeeding has been well established and then only as a last option. I recommend using the pacifier to settle but once the baby is asleep remove the pacifier to prevent the baby from becoming attached to it and then later waking up looking for it.

The most important thing is to know your limitations and seek help and support if you find your patience is running thin. Don't try to be a hero, everyone needs time out and rest.

See your doctor, midwife, nurse or hospital straight away if your baby seems unwell. If in doubt seek professional help.

For more settling ideas go to the following website:
http://www.cyh.com/SubContent.aspx?p=102

Look After You

Establish a Routine

Babies love routine it helps them feel safe and secure. Establishing sleeping or resting times that are the same every day will ensure daytime naps continue as the baby gets older. Try not to go out in the evenings in the early days if this creates an unsettled baby. Establish a different routine in the evening, bath baby and put on night attire, reduce the noise stimulation, turn down the lights. Quietly feed before putting baby to bed even if you expect to be feeding again in a few hours, as this indicates to the baby that there is a change in energy as the evening draws to a close. As I have mentioned before some babies feed almost constantly in the evening, if you are able to allow your baby to feed as much as it wishes at this time it is more likely to sleep through later. I also encourage parents not to talk to their babies during the night, make the night time feeds as unstimulating as possible so that the baby learns to sleep through.

Relaxation

It is important that you are able to find ways to chill out and relax with or without your baby. When the baby sleeps you must sleep. Curl up together in the afternoon and have a nap together. Sleep your baby close to you, either with you or in a pram close to the bed at least in the first couple of months until you have established a routine. Mothers and babies breathe in tandem with each other and babies feel abandoned if placed too far away from the mother. This is why rooming in whilst in hospital has become the policy. There are many mother baby meditation or yoga groups that you may be able to join. Otherwise take time out to attend a meditation group for yourself.

Relationship

Babies are very aware of their surroundings and the energy of relationships around them. It is important to deal with any relationship issues you have if possible, as these will not only affect you but also the baby. Seek out a good friend or support person to discuss issues, expectations and parenting techniques with together. It is very important to maintain a good relationship separate to the baby if possible. Get a babysitter for a few hours as soon as you feel comfortable to leave your baby so that you can still maintain the feeling of being a couple. Having a good relationship as a couple will depend on how much time you invest in each other. Your baby is going to grow up and eventually leave home, though that may seem so far into the future.

Support

So many couples and single parents are going it alone without extended family. Establishing good friends who can truly support you if family is not available can be a great asset. Connect with other young parents so that you can help each other out. There are also community support systems available for parents going it alone, such as parenting groups or mother 's groups, which can provide a great space to share experiences and support breastfeeding. We humans generally thrive in a community atmosphere.

Fun

Find time to have fun. Babies thrive in a happy atmosphere. Forget the housework and go have fun. Watch a funny movie and don't forget to socialise.

Music

Soft music, rhythmic sounds or continuous machine noises (such as the noise made by the static of a radio off the channel) soothe some babies.

Parenting is sometimes not easy. Every parent or carer sometimes gets stressed. Although I must admit that those parents who do invest time and energy into their health before and during pregnancy do have easier postnatal experiences. Their babies settle more easily. So ensure you are taking those nutrients recommended for pregnancy in this book and continue to take them whilst breastfeeding .

No matter how you feel, never do anything that could hurt or frighten a baby. Try not to scream and shout.

You are better to leave, take a walk to calm down, than stay and risk harm.

NEVER shake a baby

Shaking can cause serious brain damage. The injuries can last forever, and some children die. Adults can easily hurt a baby by rough or angry handling. The more upset and angry you become the more upset your baby will become. It is very important to leave a baby in its cot crying and go seek out support or take a breather by walking outside rather than get upset with the baby. The baby does not understand adult behaviour. Walk away until you calm down. Phone a friend.

Touch/Massage

Just like us babies love to be touched and caressed. Rather than investing in a baby bath jump in the bath with your baby and allow them to float in the warm water and relax with you or your partner in the bath. When my children were very young my hubby would get in the bath when he came home from work and all three children jumped in with him, even the baby from a few days of age. This gave me a chance to catch my breath and relaxed and calmed the children ready for bed. It also offered a wonderful bonding time with Dad.

I thoroughly recommend undertaking a baby massage course or follow the reflexology suggestions ahead. Lavender is a wonderful relaxing oil and can be added to massage oil and massaged into your baby to help them relax. You can begin early in applying reflexology and massage techniques to newborn feet. No foot or body is too small to benefit from body therapy.

Touch is essential and imperative to life.

The touch needs to be gentle but firm so as to transfer a sense of confidence and trust to the child, so avoid tickling the child. Notably the feet and body are smaller so the touch must be adjusted accordingly. Keep a hand on each foot and let your fingers curl around the foot, pressing and squeezing gently to provide a sensation of security. Keep the session loose and playful. Each session needs only to be ten to fifteen minutes. Keep the feet bare to allow natural development especially whilst learning to stand and walk, do not squeeze feet into foot wear, this can do irreparable damage.

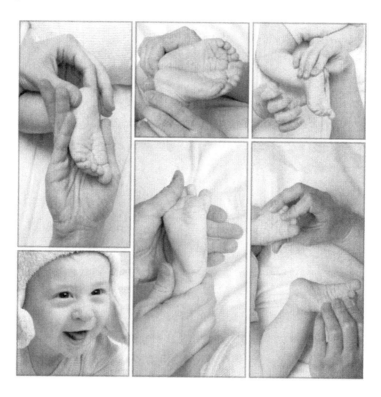

Reflexology Tips

Solar Plexus

This is a wonderful point to sedate and gently massage for colic or to settle the unsettled baby. The solar plexus reflex point is one of the most powerful points in foot reflexology. On the body, the solar plexus is found right in the middle of the upper half of the trunk of the torso, where the rib cage comes together at the stomach level in front of the diaphragm.

Psycho-somatically this is the area that represents your identity, the I Am. According to Theron Q. Dumont, author of The Solar Plexus or Abdominal Brain (2007):

> "its name, 'solar', was bestowed upon it by reason of
> (1) its central position
> (2) the fact that its filaments extend in all directions to the important abdominal organs, like the rays of the sun
> (3) the fact it is recognised as being the power-house, and great reservoir of 'life-force', just as the sun is the great power-house and reservoir of material energy of our solar system."

On the feet, it can be found if you draw an imaginary line from the second toe down, below the ball of the foot, right within that hollow. It can also be found if you gently squeeze the top of the foot inward. You should find a "little dimple space"- that's the solar plexus point. There is a very strong connection between the feet and the solar plexus.

You will find settling a baby easy by relaxing and sedating this point on the feet. A group of newborn premature babies were given two hourly massages from birth and their speed of growth was almost twice that of the non-massaged group (Field, 2001).

Constipation

Reflexology points along the Gut and Colon can be stimulated to help elimination.

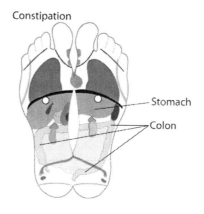

Hiccoughs

Use the points above but also bring in the ear points as shown here. Press in the middle of the inner ear (diaphragm zone) to stop hiccough spasm.

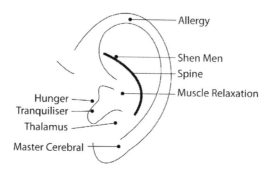

Breastfeeding & Postnatal Care

Breastfeeding Best for Baby

Breastfeeding helps create a close and loving bond between you and your baby and can be a deeply satisfying experience for you both.

Breastfeeding provides for baby:

- a personalised balance of nutrients and fluids specifically created and which changes according to your baby's needs
- provides and creates a strong immune system for life
- protection against the risk of allergy and food intolerance
- protection against obesity, heart disease and related conditions, diabetes and some cancers later in life
- emotional connection.

Breastfeeding exclusively for the first six months or more helps protect your baby against:

- ear infections
- gastro-intestinal infections
- chest infections
- urine infections
- childhood eczema
- obesity.

Breastfeeding is beneficial for mothers:

- convenient, cheap and readily available
- fresh, clean and safe
- encourages the flow of normal hormones that help the uterus return to normal more efficiently after childbirth as well as assisting in fat burning
- research indicates it provides protection against breast cancer and encourages the absorption of calcium for bone density,

preventing osteoporosis later in life, especially if sustained for over six months

- ensures mother and baby have quality time during feeds.

An Australian study of nearly 2200 children who were followed to age six years showed that giving infants breast milk and nothing else for at least four months after birth reduced the risk of developing asthma. Babies who were introduced to milk other than breast milk before four months were twenty five percent more likely to develop asthma and fourty percent more likely to develop a wheeze (British Medical Journal 319, as reported in Nursing Times, Vol. 95 No. 40, 1999).

Breastfeeding provides a range of benefits for an infant's growth, immunity and development. Exclusive breastfeeding to around six months of age gives the best nutritional start to infants and is recommended by the Australian Government Department of Health and Ageing, the World Health Organization (WHO) and other health authorities. Breastfeeding benefits maternal health and contributes economic benefits to the family, health care system and workplace.

> "Human breast itself is capable of something the formula industry will never be able to duplicate: adjusting the contents of milk to suit a baby's daily, even hourly needs."
>
> Rita Laws. Midwifery Today
> April 2000 (Issue 2:15).

The Demise of Breastfeeding

> "The technology of engineering an artificial feed of cow's milk in a bottle with a rubber teat literally initiated an unprecedented event in human history. Human mothers are the only mammals who have a choice about whether or not to give their own milk to their infants. The decision to use cow's milk was not based on any scientific investigation to compare the suitability of other mammals' milk for human consumption. Expediency was the priority and cow's milk became the substitute of choice mostly for

economic reasons, as there was at least one cow available in every village farm. During the first thirty to forty years of the twentieth century, cow's milk was diluted with water, and sugar was added to make it palpable to the infant. Because the proportion of the basic constituents of cow's milk are inappropriate to human needs (large amount of protein and small fat content with no long chain fatty acids), constructing a safe formula using cow's milk as a breast milk substitute became the subject of intense medical scientific investigation."

Breastfeeding Nemesis, by Susanne Colson

Midwifery Today, 2000: 2(15).

Even though infant mortality rates soared the emphasis was not placed on improving mother's ability to feed but rather time and money was invested to create milk formulas from cow's milk to replace nature's perfect formula. Human beings for all their intelligence often behave quite stupidly.

Of course the science world at this time was dominated by males who would have found the thought of breastfeeding to be primitive and tribal so to find an alternative milk substitute that could be given through a bottle would be a great scientific feat. So now to put things right we have created a science out of breastfeeding, putting breast milk to the test. However tests are still so inadequate that many of the beneficial nutrients and properties found in breast milk are yet to be discovered.

Rather than women expecting breastfeeding to be a natural progression following birth they ask the question 'should I breast feed?' Many women express a belief that breastfeeding may not happen at all, or it will be very difficult, setting themselves up for a difficult time.

Midwives and breastfeeding supporters face the challenge of changing this thinking, to bring breastfeeding back to it's rightful place in society. For the majority of women, if they follow their natural instincts and allow themselves to learn through trial and error, breastfeeding will be a very pleasant and rewarding experience.

Suggestions to Help Breastfeeding

Preparation

Massage natural crèmes and oils into the breasts in a nurturing and loving way. Honour your breasts for they are about to sustain another life. Roll the nipples between thumb and first finger, gently extending the nipple. This helps you to become used to handling the breast. Practice putting baby to the breast using a doll or teddy. An excellent book and instructional video to use as a guide is "Breastfeeding I can do that!" Sue Cox, Lactation Consultant.

Inverted Nipple

A nipple that inverts or appears to move inwards to the breast instead of pointing outwards when stimulated is regarded as inverted. Stimulation of the nipple may help to change the direction or wearing a breast shield can be effective in encouraging the nipple to come out.

Women who are pregnant for the first time may find the nipple does not protrude fully. Some degree of inversion will occur in about one third of mothers, but as the skin becomes more elastic during pregnancy, only about ten percent will still have some inversion by the time their baby is born. Inversion tends to become less with each subsequent pregnancy.

Most inverted or flat nipples will not cause problems during breastfeeding. This is because your nipple becomes like a teat and is not actively involved with milk production. Also breast attachment by your baby occurs on the surrounding breast tissue, not the nipples. Nipples may be so flat or inverted that they do cause problems as the baby is unable to get hold of the breast tissue around the nipple.

There are steps you can take to help correct the problem both before and after the baby is born.

Hoffman Technique

Start at the beginning of the seventh month of pregnancy

1. draw an imaginary cross on the breast with the vertical and horizontal lines crossing at the nipple.
2. place the thumbs or the forefingers opposite each other at the edge of the areola (the darkened circular area behind the nipple) on the imaginary horizontal line. Press in firmly then pull the thumbs (or fingers) back and forth to stretch the areola.
3. in the vertical position, pull the thumbs or fingers upwards and downwards.

Repeat procedure about five times each morning. The nipple will become erect and easier to grasp, so that it can be slowly and gently drawn out.

Reflexlogy Points to Work:

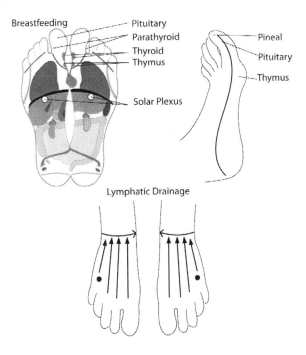

First Feed

The first feed will most likely occur within a short time of birth, even after a Ceasarean, unless there have been complications or the baby is affected by drugs. Babies are born with a natural desire to seek out the breast. The video 'Self-Attachment' shows very clearly babies born without drugs naturally crawling to the breast and self attaching within twenty minutes of birth.

It is best to stay relaxed. Have the baby in skin to skin contact, chest to chest, close to the breast, mouth in line with the nipple. You can gently touch baby's lips with your nipple to encourage your baby's mouth to open wide. This ensures the baby takes the entire nipple and as much as possible of the areola (the darker area around the nipple) into its mouth. It is best if mother attempts to attach baby. The midwife can assist by supporting the baby's head, leaving mum's hand free to assist her baby.

Ensuring baby is in the correct position will reduce nipple trauma. Expect an unusual feeling at first, a feeling that has been described as a strong pulling on the nipple with a stretchy feeling along with needles and pins in the breast. A baby positioned correctly for breastfeeding should not hurt you.

Successful breastfeeding relies on being relaxed about when and how often you feed. Try not to judge your baby's needs by the clock. Babies feed erratically in the first few weeks until they develop their own patterns of feeding. Most babies will feed every couple of hours in the first few days until the full milk supply comes in. Then they will usually settle into three to four hourly feeding times.

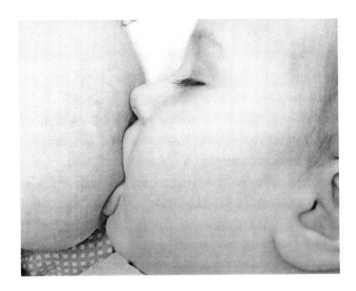

Some feeds may take twenty minutes, others longer. I suggest allowing your baby to feed well from the first breast until satiated unless they are particularly hungry or restless, then move to the next breast. Some mothers produce enough milk to feed their babies from one breast at each feed. Forcing baby to feed from each breast at each feed can cause over feeding and lots of reflux. Watch, observe and learn what your baby does. I had such a great supply I fed all my babies one breast at a time at each feed. We are designed to feed twins. Breastfeeding is a feedback mechanism - stimulation equals production.

Ensure you feed overnight. Do not be tempted to give baby a bottle so you can sleep, this will definitely lead to low milk supply and the beginning of feeding problems.

REMEMBER YOUR BREASTS CREATE MILK IN RESPONSE TO YOUR BABY'S NEEDS.

Your body adjusts to breastfeeding. Breastfeeding mothers fall into a deep sleep immediately between feeds, ensuring they receive adequate REM sleep, another benefit of breastfeeding. When not breastfeeding it can take some time to fall into deep sleep.

Tips in the first days of Breastfeeding:

- allow baby to have skin to skin contact as much as possible
- allow baby to attach and feed as frequently as baby wishes, keep feeds short and frequent
- your baby will only be receiving 3-5 mls of highly nutritious colostrum at each feed, sucking for too long can damage the nipple and create feeding problems
- stimulate nipple erection with a cool face washer, ice and manual stimulation before baby attaches
- express a small amount of colostrum onto the nipple at the beginning of each feed
- get comfortable, support your back and arms
- keep visitors to a minimum
- keep your baby with you as it learns to bond
- try different positions
- your baby will naturally prefer one breast over the other

Nipple Care

Many women experience sore nipples in the first few weeks. Like any part of the body that has been dormant, it takes time to create suppleness and flexibility. Very sore nipples are usually caused by the baby not taking the nipple into its mouth properly due to poor positioning. The problem can be corrected by the mother being shown how to attach correctly. It is important for a new mum to have positioning checked by an experienced midwife in the first few days to prevent long term problems.

Expressing small amounts of milk onto the nipples and massaging into them between feeds will help with suppleness and preventing infections. Avoid any product that will dry the nipple. However, there are some lubricated crèmes available that are good for nipples. Break the suction with the little finger before attempting to take the baby off the breast.

Exposing the nipples to the sun for ten to twenty minutes each day can help immeasurably, but of course this relies on sunshine!

Cracked Nipples

Cracked nipples usually develop from sore nipples that are abraded by the baby attaching onto the end of the nipple rather than applying the jaw behind the whole nipple. Often the first sign is a sharp pain on attachment.

- it is important to dry the nipples thoroughly after feeds and ensure breast pads are dry, otherwise the cracks can develop into more painful cracks where bleeding can occur
- change the feeding position on that beast to relieve pressure. Try twin feeding, where baby tucks under your armpit and feeds from the side.
- once the positioning of the baby is corrected the nipple will heal quickly, usually within a day or so. If the crack is quite severe then resting of that breast will benefit.
- be sure to express well so as not to lose supply and try to only rest it for one or two feeds. The best advice you can seek is from an experienced midwife, lactation consultant or Nursing Mum.
- homeopathic remedy - Phytolacca and sepia
- diets high in sugars and yeast tend to aggravate nipple soreness so it may be advisable to remove these from the diet.
- ensure adequate nutrition, especially omega 3s, zinc found in oily fish, nuts (not peanuts) and seeds.

If the problem gets worse sometimes a soft pliable nipple shield can be worn to rest the nipple for a few feeds. It's best not to use nipple shields for too long as they can decrease the supply.

Thrush on Nipples

Take high doses of probiotics orally. Make a paste by mixing powdered probiotic with water or breastmilk and place on nipples before the next feed so baby absorbs the probiotic aswell. You can also give your baby specific infantile probiotics.

Homeopathic remedy - Borax

Managing Breast Engorgement

Engorgement mostly occurs in the first few days after birth, particularly around day three. The extra blood developed in your system now reroutes to the breasts to build hormone levels ready to initiate breast milk production. This can create heat and engorgement before the milk comes in. Lack of good attachment and feeding technique can create further problems so be sure to check and re-check attachment.

- feed baby frequently
- when the supply is copious you may find one side feeding beneficial as baby will fill up on one breast, not needing the second
- express a small amount off the breast before the feed to help baby attach, use a warm washer or shower which will help get the milk flowing. Be careful not to over express as this will just create more milk compounding the problem.
- soaking engorged breasts in Epsom salt can soften the breasts and allow better flow. Mix one teaspoon Epsom salts in one cup (250ml) warm water. Mix well, soak a face washer in mixture then place the washer on the breasts. Better still, if you have a bath add two tablespoons Epsom salts to your bath and hop in with baby.

I have found placing cold packs on the breasts as soon as the mother feels the breasts becoming warm (indicating that the blood flow is increasing ready for the incoming supply of milk) helps engorgement. Cold packs between feeds can help with the venous engorgement but generally aren't of great benefit once the blood flow has settled and the breasts are mainly full of milk. After feeding, place cool washed cabbage leaves from the refrigerator on the breasts. These leaves have been found to contain properties that help relieve engorgement. Change the leaves frequently when warm.

- you may find it more comfortable to place a towel around the breast in the first few days rather than a bra. When wearing a bra make sure the bra is well fitted and remove completely before feeding.
- use different positions when feeding to help drain the whole breast and avoid blockages.

Sometimes babies need encouragement to get them to attach, even when they have been feeding for a few days. I have found this technique to be beneficial. Very gentle breast massage during feeding enhances milk flow, helps empty clogged ducts and makes higher calorie milk available to the baby. Once the baby has latched well, pay attention to the pauses in sucking. At this time gently press the milk ducts on one part of the breast towards the baby's mouth. If the baby pauses again, rotate the position of your fingertips and press another quadrant of the breast. It is a gentle massage around the breast, helping to ensure all milk ducts are emptied, preventing blocked ducts. Changing position at feeds also helps drainage.

Blocked Ducts
Sometimes occur when there is a pressure build up and lack of emptying in one or two of the ducts.

Prevention:

- ensure your baby is attaching well to your breasts and is feeding well
- don't sleep too long in one position as any pressure in one place on the breast can cause a damming effect
- ensure you keep breasts free, avoid ill fitting or tight bras
- massage breasts gently daily to encourage good milk flow

- changing positions is very important as this helps to drain different ducts around the breast
- avoid pressing a finger on the breast whilst feeding. This can happen if you have larger breasts and are trying to see what your baby is doing by pushing the breast away to see, inadvertently blocking a duct.

The faster you treat a blocked duct the better to prevent it becoming mastitis

- breastfeed as often as your baby wants to feed, beginning each feed from the affected breast
- keep the affected breast empty as much as possible
- avoid missing or putting off feeds
- if a breast becomes uncomfortably full, wake your baby for a feed. If your baby is not interested in feeding express a small amount for comfort.
- rest as much as you can
- avoid giving your baby any other fluids except your breast milk, unless medically advised to
- if the breast becomes warm apply cold packs between feeds and apply heat just before a feed to assist the duct to drain
- massage the breast towards the nipple whilst your baby feeds to encourage good flow
- see your medical adviser if these measures do not clear the blockage within 12 hours, or if you develop a fever or feel unwell.

** Make sure your medical practitioner has experience as some will suggest weaning and this is the very thing you must not do.

Mastitis

Mastitis is an inflammation within and around a milk duct. It is generally caused through a blockage in the duct resulting in milk being forced into the surrounding tissue. This creates an inflammatory response.

The first signs of Mastitis can be sudden where the breast is sore, hot and inflamed. You may also feel suddenly quite ill. Mastitis can also come on slowly with the first signs being flu like symptoms such as sudden changes in body temperature, feelings of hot and cold, shivers and aches and pains in your body.

What you can do

As soon as you sense that something is not quite right follow the treatments for blocked duct (above).

- gently massage the breast, also massage the blocked duct to encourage it to drain. This may be quite uncomfortable.
- you must feed from this breast frequently as emptying now is essential. If you are considering weaning at this time, DO NOT. Your breast must be kept empty as much as possible and feeding is the easiest way to do this. Drain the milk ducts either through feeding or expressing. If your breasts feel full and your baby won't feed often hand express before, after and between feeds.
- hand expressing under a warm shower can also assist as sometimes your baby may refuse to feed from this breast as the milk can taste salty
- your milk is perfectly safe for your baby as it is the tissue that is inflamed not the milk
- feed frequently from this breast and begin each feed on this breast, but still ensure you are draining the other breast as well to avoid the same problem
- apply heat just before a feed to encourage the let-down
- cold packs after a feed may help relieve pain and reduce swelling, do not use heat between feeds
- do make sure you are 'letting down' at each feed, check for the let-down feeling and for signs of milk flow and swallowing by your baby
- change feeding positions at each feed and massage the breast towards the nipple to assist the flow

- talk to your lactation consultant or an Australian Breastfeeding Association counsellor for ideas on other feeding positions
- go to bed, taking your baby with you, or rest as much as possible
- take homeopathic Phytolacca, Bryonia alternating with Belladonna and maybe add in some Silica.
- ensure high intake of superfoods
- natural anti-inflammatories such as Kaprex (Healthworld) may assist

The faster you treat the problem the less likely it is to develop into an infection or abscess.

Homeopathics for Breastfeeding

Take remedies in 30c doses. Take not more than three doses a day for acute cases, or once a day for three days for a less intense problem. Seek assistance if no improvement after three days.

Cracked or sore nipples – Phytolacca, Castor Equus

Engorgement - Phytolacca

Mastitis or pain or discomfort in the breasts – Phytolacca, Bryonia alternating with Belladonna and maybe add in some Silica.

Candida / Thrush – Borax is excellent when there is candida overgrowth resulting in thrush.

Sepia officianalis is often referred to as the woman's remedy. It is beneficial for all manner of female emotional and physical ailments. Particularly good for the strong independent woman who finds herself restricted by life's events. Some women may find it difficult to assert their independence, or feel they are being moulded into a role outside of their control such as breastfeeding and early parenting. Parenting can feel stifling at times, leaving a woman feeling that her needs go unmet. This can result in feelings of resentment towards the obligations represented by her partner or children. Sepia is a great remedy when mum is feeling worn out, negative, resentful, impatient and fearful.

Physically mum may display a general chilliness and sensitivity to cold air, she may lack appetite and may have low libido during and after pregnancy. She may feel congested in the abdomen or the rectum, a tendency towards constipation and may have an intolerance to tight clothing around her waist.

Breast Engorgement - Bella Donna is used when there is a sudden onset of heat, redness or hard throbbing pain indicating a block, abscess or mastitis. Good one to have on hand as mastitis can occur quite quickly and the faster you respond the more rapid the effect.

Milk supply - Urtica Urens (stinging nettles) helps balance milk supply. Drink as a herbal tea or take as a homeopathic remedy.

Low supply

- Lac decfloratum increases milk supply if there seems to be an extended low supply, feeling chilly, exhausted or if there is diabetes involved
- Agnus Castus is good for low milk supply when there is retained placenta or depression
- Lac humanun when the supply is very low or having difficulty with the milk coming in at all. Can be used if an abscess occurs but if this is the case please seek practitioner advice immediately

Over supply

- Lac Caninum is great for an over abundance of milk, particularly if associated with anxiety and low self-esteem.

Emotional Response

- Ignatia increases milk supply when associated with sadness, grief and crying, good for third day blues
- Nat Mur also great for over supply associated with sadness and grief

Weeping and emotion whilst breastfeeding - Pulsatilla

Breast abscess with cheesy pus - Hepar sulph

Breast pale and hot with pain on movement - Bryonia

Encouraging a Good Supply

A baby who has six to eight wet nappies a day, is gaining weight, is alert when awake and settles reasonably well is getting enough.

The following may help to increase supply and maintain feeding:

- having baby close, especially when young, encourages the normal bonding hormones to be strong. Using a baby sling allows baby to be close to you, creating a flow of natural mother-baby energy. You cannot spoil a baby with too much attention.
- giving baby a cuddle before feeding allows each of you to relax and settle before feeding
- try not to let baby cry for long or become distressed
- create privacy if you need until you feel confident, draw the curtains or go to another room

- massage your breasts in the shower, allowing the milk to flow naturally
- prioritise your feeding above all else - this is the most important job you will ever do, the housework can wait
- rest when your baby rests - remember you are restocking while baby sleeps so do not overdo it between feeds. Allow baby to sleep with you and feed at will, especially in the afternoon.
- drink high energy fluids rather than tea or coffee and ensure plenty of water
- continue to take the nutrients you were taking in pregnancy
- homeopathic remedy - Pulsatilla and Urtica Urens
- let baby feed as often as it wishes. There will be times when baby feeds frequently, especially every six to eight weeks when baby will be increasing your supply to meet its growth.
- I have found that Fenugreek and fennel seeds are excellent for increasing supply and eating cashews whilst drinking stout has brought good results for some mums
- make night feeds uneventful, do not talk to your baby, keep the lighting low and after a couple of weeks you will find it unnecessary to change your baby's nappy at night. This way they will learn to sleep through, realising night time is fairly boring. They will not expect to be entertained and hopefully begin to sleep longer sooner. Stimulate during the day.

Nutrition

- eat globe artichoke, carrots, aniseeds, barley, cashews
- almond milk drink - cover almonds and raw cashews with barley water and puree, drink this formula to produce more nutritious milk
- almond milk instead of cows milk may be given to the baby as a substitute for breast milk if you need to supplement your feeds or are going out
- take high nutrition Superfoods.

Successful Breastfeeding Tips

1. Nipple pain is not to be expected! Pain is a signal that something is wrong.
2. Toughening nipples with 'preparations' containing alcohol or spirit or soaps does not help. These products will cause damage rather than help.
3. Creams or ointments will not prevent/cure sore nipples.
4. Women with lighter nipple colouring are not more susceptible to nipple pain and trauma.
5. Sore nipples are not caused by over-feeding. If baby is attached correctly, time spent feeding will not cause pain. Leaving a baby unsettled will cause pain.
6. Milk supply does not run out even after feeds. Production is continuous. Babies usually only drink about 40-60% of the milk in the breasts. Stimulation is the only way to make more milk.
7. Milk supply does not diminish as the day progresses. Every baby is individual and will have unsettled times, however universally this tends to be around 4-6 pm.
8. You cannot tell how much milk is in the breasts by the feel of them. Breasts return to normal within a few weeks and invariably become smaller. The milk production becomes efficient and the breasts feel quite soft most of the time.
9. Breast milk is never too weak. Nutrients will be supplied to breast milk ahead of other areas of the body. It is nature's way of ensuring the future of the race.
10. Drinking (cow's) milk does not make milk. Although cow's milk is an excellent source of calcium there are many other foods that provide just as many nutrients. During the first six months of feeding baby takes most of the calcium for its own growth. During the second six months the mother increases bone density in her bones which later reduces her risk of low bone density and osteoporosis. Breastfeeding assists both.

11. When a baby sucks on the breast it is satisfying many of its innate needs, nutrition, sucking and touching. The breast is the most natural place for a baby to go. The sucking action stimulates the production of prolactin ensuring its food supply.

12. Low milk supply is not usually the cause of an unsettled, crying baby. Babies cry for many reasons.

13. Baby does not need extra fluids in hot weather. Breast milk changes consistency to meet a baby's demands. In hot weather a baby will feed more frequently to receive the liquid it needs.

14. You cannot spoil a baby with too much attention. Babies who are the most happy are often those whose needs are met quickly. Some researchers suggest that a baby is best treated as though totally dependant on their mother for at least nine months, as if still in the womb. Crying is not good, it indicates a baby is unhappy. Babies learn to cry more when their needs are not met.

15. You cannot rely on breastfeeding to protect against pregnancy. If your baby is totally breastfed, receiving eight to ten feeds a day without going longer than four hours between feeds at night up to six months of age, and you haven't had a period the chance of pregnancy is less than two percent. Don't take the risk, use condoms. Remember, you ovulate before having a period, thus you can fall pregnant before ever having a period.

The Parents

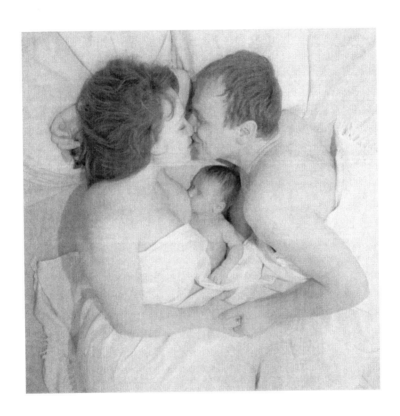

Postnatal Emotions

Emotions often run high after birth and can vary from great joy to fear and sadness. You may have times when you feel a little flat. You are no longer pregnant, but your body is not as it was before you became pregnant. There are many body changes after the birth of a child, hormone levels can be chaotic and your body may feel sore and tender as it begins the journey back to your non-pregnant beautiful self.

With a good diet, exercise and adequate rest your body will return to normal. Pelvic muscles will regain tone and breastfeeding will assist excess fat to go. As your libido and your desire for sexual activity returns, sex can be resumed gently within a couple of weeks of birth, but only when you feel ready. Experiment with different positions that do not put pressure on your perineum if it feels tender. If the tenderness continues after a few weeks be sure to see your medical practitioner. Everything should be back to normal by about six weeks. Your sexual relationship will be different as you now have a baby to contend with, and babies seem to have a wonderful knack of crying for a feed just when you are enjoying a passionate moment. The best thing you can have here is a good sense of humour!

With the birth of your first baby new roles are acquired and new relationships formed. It is not surprising that along with the joys of new parenthood come confusion and anxiety. Your new baby may not be like the baby you had imagined. The demands of your baby, the obligation baby brings and the loss of your single self may come as a shock to you. So may the occasional lack of maternal reactions you experience in response to those demands. All this may lead to guilt as you realise that you cannot live up to the image you had of yourself as the perfect parent. Allow yourself to truly express and feel your emotions, this allows healing and acceptance to occur. Be gentle with yourself. Thus you may find that before you can fully accept your new baby you need to grieve the loss of your fantasy baby, your single self and the concept of yourself as the 'perfect' parent so you can accept and celebrate who you truly are.

Grief may be a response to a birth which was not as the you expected, such as an emergency caesarean instead of a vaginal delivery, a medically-aided birth instead of a home birth or a painful or traumatic birth. Parents may need to grieve for their lost ideal birth and accept the reality of the actual birth.

There are 3 Identifiable Mood Changes That can Occur at This Time

1. **Baby blues** - Eighty per cent of all women who have given birth experience a feeling of emotional distress and tearfulness during the first week after birth. This condition usually passes within a few days.

2. **Postnatal depression** - Postnatal depression, or PND, is an illness, it can happen to any woman after any pregnancy. Postnatal depression affects one in eight women after delivery of a child and in some cases may be the continuation of a pre-existing depression that began during pregnancy (antenatal depression) and continues to develop postnatally. It can present:

   - as the result of, or a worsening of, an existing antenatal depression
   - suddenly after the birth
   - suddenly in the weeks after birth
   - or slowly over the months after birth.

Postnatal depression is much more than 'feeling unhappy' or 'feeling depressed', and is beyond the woman's control.

3. **Postpartum psychosis** - is the most acute postnatal illness, affecting one in five hundred women, usually in the first fourteen days after giving birth. Postnatal psychosis requires urgent medical help and a hospital stay, preferably in a Mother-Baby Unit. It has an excellent recovery rate.

Baby Blues

The blues are a very common emotion that arises in the first two weeks (usually from day three to day five) after childbirth.

The symptoms may be:

- feeling flat or depressed
- mood swings
- irritability
- feeling emotional (eg. crying easily)
- tiredness
- insomnia
- lacking confidence (eg. in bathing and feeding the baby)
- aches and pains (eg. headache)

The third day blues as they are coined don't generally occur on the third day but anytime in the first weeks of pregnancy. Many women can become worried about the feelings they are having and may feel they are heading for postnatal depression.

A couple of days of feeling sensitive, easily crying or experiencing emotional highs and lows, is well within normal limits. Sometimes these emotional swings may be experienced over a couple of hours or daily for a week or two and then settle. Other times you may not experience them at all.

The important thing is to be able to talk the feelings through. It is also a common occurrence to have feelings of tiredness or exhaustion where you just need to escape the baby and have time out. These are all perfectly normal and do not mean you are an inadequate mother.

Recognising your needs foremost makes for more balanced relationships and inevitably teaches your child how to be healthily selfish. When you are happy those around you can be too.

Isolation is a problem in our society, especially following the excitement and nurturing following the birth of a child. After a few weeks the excitement calms and many mothers find themselves in ever-increasing times of aloneness. Few women are ever really prepared for the demands of motherhood. The lack of sleep and worry of caring for another human being can be very stressful, especially if you have been an organised person prior to the birth of your baby.

Organisation and babies do not go hand in hand. Babies come with the word 'chaos' attached to them. The more stress a woman experiences, the more likely she is to develop symptoms of postnatal depression. Stress is a heavy task master on the nutritional needs of the body (see the section on <u>Stress</u>) . Lack of nutrients at this time will lead to postnatal complications. You must have adequate levels of phytonutrients for your baby's continuing brain development whilst breastfeeding. This is why I recommend continuing with the <u>nutritional superfoods</u> for as long as possible following the birth. Since introducing phytoplankton to my clients I have not had one client report postnatal depression. It is also imperative to continue with regular reflexology or body care.

What is the Outcome?

Fortunately 'the blues' are a passing phase and last only a few days. It is important to get plenty of help and rest until they go away and you feel normal. Bush flower remedies are excellent for clearing emotional blocks (see <u>Depression</u> and <u>Stress</u>).

What Should You do?

All you really need is encouragement, phytonutrients and support from your partner, family and friends, so tell them how you feel.

- avoid getting overtired, rest as much as possible
- talk over your problems with a good listener, perhaps another mother with a baby.

Accept help from others in the house.

- allow your partner to take turns getting up to attend the baby.

- get out and take your baby for a walk, the exercise is excellent for you and the fresh air wonderful for encouraging sleep for the baby.
- give yourself permission to have reflexology or a massage.

The biggest mistake new mums make is trying to be 'Super Mum'. Don't be a martyr, ask for help, let others know what your needs are. Your role at this time is to feed your baby above everything else. Rest when your baby rests. Go out and enjoy the company of other mums and friends.

If your partner is around get them to do tasks that they can with the baby whilst allowing you free time to indulge in those little luxuries such as a bubble bath.

Get help before the crisis hits. Hopefully during your pregnancy you have developed a good support system with family or friends. Get a nappy service if you can afford it or if someone asks you what gift you would like suggest this one. Have your house cleaned if you can.

For support people and partners, if the mother is beginning to be overwhelmed or finding even the simplest task difficult then she is on the verge of postnatal depression so please seek help. A mother who has lost her sense of humour and has no joy for life is particularly vulnerable.

Remember partners can also experience postnatal depression, the changes to them are just as confronting.

http://www.beyondblue.org.au/index.aspx?link_id=94.1468

http://www.panda.org.au/

Postnatal Depression

Why Feel This Way?

Mood changes are common after childbirth and vary from very mild to very severe. The onset seems to involve the variations in hormone levels and the physical, psychological and social changes which occur around the time of birth. Homeopathic remedy sepia may help at this time. A woman in a sepia state may show a lack of interest in their families, irritability and lack of energy.

Symptoms of Postnatal Depression

The severity of the illness depends on the number of symptoms, their intensity and the extent to which they impair normal functioning.

- mood change, low, or fluctuating from high to low
- sleep disturbance unrelated to baby's needs, sudden waking, bad dreams, early morning waking, inability to sleep even when the baby is asleep, oversleeping
- appetite disturbance, loss of appetite, forgetting to eat, overeating
- chronic exhaustion or hyperactivity
- crying or wanting to cry without knowing why
- feeling unable to cope
- obsessive cleaning
- irritability, tension and anxiety
- sensitivity to noise
- anxiety, hyperventilation, panic attacks, hot and cold flushes, heart palpitations, dizziness, feeling as if 'you are not there'
- negative, obsessive or morbid thoughts
- feeling that life has no meaning
- loss of concentration
- loss of memory
- loss of sexual interest
- loss of self confidence and self esteem
- unrealistic feelings of guilt, inadequacy
- fear of being alone
- fear of social contact
- a feeling that you cannot cope with life (eg hopelessness, helplessness)
- feeling a failure as a mother.

As compiled by the Post & Ante Natal Depression Association (PaNDa).
http://www.panda.org.au/

Some women develop a very severe depression within the first six months (usually in the first six months) after childbirth. They seem to get 'the blues' and cannot snap out of it.

What is the Outcome?

This is a very serious problem if not treated, and you cannot shake it off by yourself. There is a real risk of a marriage or relationship breakdown because you can be a very miserable person to live with, especially if your partner does not understand what is going on.

If it is severe, there is a risk of suicide and a risk of hurting the baby.

What Should You Do?

You must be open and tell everyone how you feel.

- you need help
- take your baby to the Baby Health or Parent Centre for review
- it is most important to consult your doctor and explain exactly how you feel
- your problem can be treated and cured with antidepressant medicine.

I have successfully assisted the condition with nutritional medicine, counselling, reflexology and emotional release work.

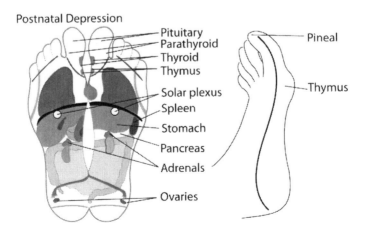

Postnatal Depression

Postnatal Depression: How Can Family Help?

It is no-one's fault and the causes are not certain. Postnatal depression has been documented for two centuries, but has been overlooked in recent decades. Keep in mind that the condition is temporary and that with support the mother will recover. Recovery may take some time and support for the duration is essential.

Postnatal depression doesn't develop in any one personality type and is not a sign of weakness. Although it is thought to be triggered by hormonal imbalance, some symptoms are similar to general depression, which is why naturopathic, homeopathic and nutritional medicine treatments are so effective.

Please do not make statements such as 'snap out of it'. Try to accept that postnatal depression is an illness which responds to treatment and support. At times, the mother may not be able to be alone and will need company. She may find everyday domestic activities challenging at times, others may need to help with shopping, with the baby, other children and housework. She may be unable to keep appointments and may need babysitting or driving assistance to do so. She is not being lazy, she will do these activities again when she feels able.

It is very important to just listen, allow her space to express, cry and let it out. Then again, she may not feel up to talking about how she feels, don't take her silence as personal rejection. Just let her know 'you are there'.

If you want to help, you can regularly put frozen casseroles in the freezer, offer to baby-sit and help with the housework and shopping, to support as much as needed. As postnatal depression settles the woman will want to do more, but needs support. FrequenSea is highly recommended now.

In her book, 'The New Mother Syndrome', Carol Dix (1985) says:

> "Although PND is one of the major causes of marital stress and divorce, it is a topic that most are reluctant to talk about."

Dorothy Scott (1992) says:

> "Some people argue that support from a husband is critical when one has a baby. It may not be that a difficult marriage causes depression, rather that a depression can cause problems in the marital relationship."

It can be suggested that when someone is depressed their needs can become so great that even the most supportive partners cannot meet their needs. It is important with postnatal depression not to take the irritability personally and react. While that is difficult, with postnatal depression it is a collection of symptoms, not a personal reaction.

She may be easily tired and both of you may feel angry at the illness. Many women who have recovered from postnatal depression say that the support they received from family brought relationships closer and they feel great gratitude which they couldn't at the time. The road to recovery will involve good and bad days, patience is so important.

Preventing Postnatal Depression

A large study by Surrey University (UK) looked at the correlation between mineral supplementation, postnatal recovery and baby health. Eight hundred women were tested for zinc and magnesium levels prior to the birth of their baby and immediately following the delivery of the placenta. The study involved both full term and premature births. One half were supplemented with zinc and magnesium, whereas the other half were not. All the placentas were tested for mineral levels with all in the supplemented group returning very high levels of zinc and magnesium.

The supplemented group had high levels of minerals prior to birth and these levels continued immediately after birth. By eight months the levels were still well within normal range.

The supplemented group experienced:

- less birth complications
- **None** experienced postnatal depression
- babies were settled
- breastfeeding was successful for all the mums

The unsupplemented group had low levels of zinc and magnesium. Levels dropped markedly following the delivery of the placenta and took an average of eight months to recover normal range. The unsupplemented group experienced:

- high number of birth interventions
- postnatal depression was very common in this group
- babies were irritable
- there were many feeding problems.

The study concluded that supplementation of therapeutic doses of multi-vitamins, magnesium, zinc and EPA/DHA was clearly indicated in preventing complications of labour and postnatal healing.

Research by the National Institute of Health found that new mothers have lower than normal levels of a stress-fighting hormone that earlier studies found help to combat depression (Magiakou et al., 1996). When we are under stress, the hypothalamus secretes corticotrophin-releasing hormone(CRH). Its secretion triggers a cascade of hormones that ultimately increases the amount of cortisol in the blood. Cortisol raises blood sugar levels and maintains normal blood pressure, which helps us perform well under stress.

During the last trimester of pregnancy the placenta secretes a lot of CRH. The rise of CRH levels in the maternal bloodstream increases threefold. Researchers devised that this was the way the body was able to cope with the stress of labour and birth. However following the birth, once the placenta is delivered, all women had low levels of CRH. Those women with very low CRH levels suffered the most from depression. Cortisol requires approximately two hundred more nutrients to metabolise than when the body is in a normal relaxed state. Supplementation of nutrients assists this process immensely.

There are traditional cultures who, following the birth, eat the placenta over several weeks, therefore ingesting there own Cortisol and nutrients. Unfortunately for most people the thought of eating your own placenta would be abhorrent, so supplementation of cortisol would be the next best idea.

Cortisol is not readily available as a supplement therefore many traditional midwives are now freeze-drying the placenta, grinding it into a powder then placing into capsules so the mother can take them. This appears to be an excellent way of ensuring correct nutrients post-delivery (Discover Magazine, December 1995).

Statistically, homebirth midwives have significantly less postpartum depression in their case loads than hospital based midwives. This leads to the theory that hospital is far more stressful on both mother and baby compared to the supportive nurturing environment of home. Breastfeeding is linked with less postnatal depression as well, possibly because it assists natural hormonal balance.

My Story – Vicki Delpero

Justin's Birth

Even though I have always had a sense that something far greater exists other than our immediate physical world, it was following the birth of my first son, Justin, in 1984 that I truly began to explore the concept of the 'souls journey'. Up until this time I was working as a registered nurse on the paediatric ward at the local hospital. I knew very little about pregnancy and birth, but had a considerable amount of knowledge regarding babies and breastfeeding. Much of my pregnancy was spent talking to other peers about what I should or shouldn't do in relation to the medical management of the birth.

My peers referred me to the best obstetrician in town, who at the time was renowned for being excellent in an emergency. After all I believed it was important to have the best care in case something went wrong. I was frightened and could not for the life of me understand how this ever increasing bundle developing in my abdomen was going to fit through such a small opening. I attended childbirth classes with a local physiotherapist who tended to favour the medical management of birth rather than allowing things to take their natural course.

I didn't read many books except to see how my baby was progressing, growth wise and spent the majority of my pregnancy in blissful ignorance, after all I was a nurse wasn't I? I could not face the concept of birth, so chose ignorance. I did not have access to support systems of other women who had birthed well or midwives who could have allayed my fears.

Fear is possibly a woman's worst enemy in pregnancy as it places stress on the body emotionally and physically. If you are pregnant and have fears, regardless of how small, seek out someone whom you can discuss and work through these fears with.

As a consequence of working late into the pregnancy hypertension (high blood pressure) developed at around 36 weeks pregnancy and I seemed to be very large and swollen. For someone who was normally very strong willed I seemed to have lost all sense of direction and just followed what ever my doctor told me to do. At one physiotherapy class, I recall we were all propped up on pillows practicing our breathing and pushing technique, I found myself over-come with dizziness. On expressing concern to the physiotherapist she promptly told me to go straight to my doctor as I could have an eclamptic fit at any time. In reality I was just over-breathing.

I left in panic, enough to give anyone high blood pressure. As the doctor was not available when I arrived at the surgery, the receptionist / midwife took my blood pressure and noting it was on the high side suggested I go to the hospital to be checked. On examination they decided to admit me for observation and rest. The next week was spent in rest, embroidering and chatting to nursing friends. My doctor had gone away for the weekend and the registrar in the hospital took over my care. She seemed to be very sensible and not in a hurry to induce me as my body was not ready yet. My blood pressure remained stable so I was discharged.

I now know that the blood pressure was most likely a result of the fear and nervousness I was experiencing due to my naivety, hence its response to rest and relaxation. The rest would have made little difference if I had been suffering from a clinical condition. Blood pressure can be assisted immeasurably with reflexology, medicinal nutrition, homoeopathic and support, all of which are explored in this book.

Justin was not due until the 24th November, 1984 but on the 6th November I felt tightenings, what I know now were Braxton Hicks' contractions. They seemed to be forming a pattern and I became all excited thinking I was going into labour. Lino, my husband, was suffering from the flu and was feeling very miserable. He was attempting to sleep whilst I was up and about trying to make these contractions/tightenings get stronger. I was basically talking myself into believing I was in labour, the mind is a powerful tool. Had I gone to bed and attempted to rest they would have most likely subsided.

Being impatient and naively wanting to get things happening more quickly I woke Lino around 4 am and told him I thought I was in labour. He believed me, after all I was the nurse, I should know. We rang the hospital and spoke to one of the midwives in labour ward. She tried to ascertain how progressed I was and I guess because I was so anxious to get on with it I convinced her I was in labour so she told me to come in and be checked. We arrived at 5 am, but by the time I reached hospital I did not have any more contractions and the Cardiotocograph (CTG) did not pick any signs of labour up.

Under normal circumstances I would have been sent home following false labour, a common experience for many women. Unfortunately for what ever reasons this did not happen and my doctor was called. After some discussion, I was given a shot of morphine to ensure my blood pressure did not rise. I was told he would be in to break my waters (artificially rupture the membranes) and induce labour using synthetic Oxytocin as I was in the hospital anyway, so may as well get on with it. The morphine totally zapped me and I fell into a drug-induced sleep.

At 8am my doctor arrived to get things going. I transferred into a labour room with apricot floral curtains and trimmings. I have never forgotten. Even after I began working in the labour ward later this room always held strong memories for me. The vaginal examination conducted by my doctor was abnormally very distressing as my cervix was so high and unripe (not soft and low), a strong sign I was not ready to birth.

A Drew Smyth instrument (a long curved metal device) was used to create a hole in the membranes behind the baby. A rare intervention used when the head is high in order to release pressure from behind the baby and force the baby onto the cervix. With the knowledge I now have it is obvious that all the signs were present that my baby was not ready to enter the world yet. I should have been sent home. Fortunately it is very rare that this technique is used now and I must say I have never experienced it with any of the labours I have worked with as a midwife over the past twenty six years.

A drip of Syntocinon (a synthetic form of Oxytocin) was instigated to get me contracting. Lino sat by my side totally lost in all that was happening feeling miserable and confused, but leaving it all up to the 'experts'. Hospitals and the medical system are a totally alien world to him. I began to contract and every now and then I would exclaim "wow that was a big one". Only to be told by a very 'off the cuff' midwife 'oh my dear, if you think that was a contraction then you don't t really know what a contraction feels like, you have it all to come'. This served to induce the fear-pain cycle even more. I did not get up and move around but lay on the bed like a beached whale, only getting up every now and then to go to the toilet.

Around 11am the doctor returned to re-examine me. Luckily my body had responded under extraordinary circumstances and the baby's head had descended well into the pelvis. I was two centimetres dilated, quite an achievement under the circumstances. But still the Dr. broke my fore waters to get things moving more quickly, which it did. I received another shot of morphine just for good measure. I can't remember much from that point on as I was experiencing a state of powerful drug induced contractions complicated by a drug-induced stupor. I remember at one stage thinking I was floating out the window. The morphine did not reduce the pain, only reduced my ability to cope with it. Lino sat by my side patiently reading and attending to any need I had but he expressed later how useless he felt. I do recall watching the Melbourne cup at around 3pm to distract myself from the experience.

At 4pm I received another dose of morphine and continued on my drug induced journey. By 5pm I was becoming overwhelmed by the continual loss of control and pain inflicting my body. I know that the majority of this was due to fear and lack of understanding about what my body was doing. An epidural, a drug slowly injected into the dural space near the spinal cord creating numbness from waist down, was suggested. In walked a doctor in white overalls looking like the local painter. He sent Lino out of the room, which distressed me no end. Lino thought he was some sort of worker; he had no idea who he was.

He probably introduced himself but I have no recollection, although I know who he is and have worked with him many times. An epidural was inserted, during a difficult time of trying to curl up into a ball whilst contracting and doing my best to remain still. Finally the epidural was in with a drip in my hand and a catheter in my bladder as the numbness had resulted in a loss of bladder control. I felt as though I had tubes coming out of me everywhere. Lino was very disturbed and confused. He had never been anywhere near hospitals before and thought at any moment I was going to die, this was certainly not how we envisaged birth to be. The epidural only mainly worked on the right-hand side of my body, which seemed to make things worse not better. The pain I was experiencing on the left hand side became intense like my muscles were on fire. The midwives did everything they could to get the block to happen but it didn't.

On I went contracting every two minutes with machines ticking away. One pumping Syntocinon into my body another recording the baby's heartbeat and me with tubes coming out of what felt like everywhere lying on the bed. At one stage I had a sense of standing and watching as everyone else was controlling the birth of my baby as if it had nothing to do with me, I was just the vessel. My baby was being extracted from my body.

I have little recollection of the next few hours until at 10 pm the same midwives who had admitted me the morning before returned for their night shift. I remember one of them examining me and saying, 'she is fully delighted, we had better call the doctor'. I gathered they meant I was fully dilated, meaning the cervix had gone and I was ready to push. My attempts at pushing were very feeble due to not being able to feel contractions, a common complication for women who have epidurals, but against all the odds my baby had managed to get through the pelvis on his own accord.

At midnight the doctor arrived and I recall his words 'she is exhausted, we had better give this baby a hand out'. Up I went into stirrups, my bottom propped on the end of the bed and out came the Neville Barnes forceps. Not the smallest of forceps. I was given a very large episiotomy and my baby was dragged from my body and placed on my tummy at 0055hrs am.

I do recall looking into his bruised eyes from the forceps, counting his toes and fingers thinking he is ok and falling back on the pillows exhausted. I did attempt to breast feed Justin as I knew this was so important but he was so drugged he did not wake up. He was wrapped and handed to Lino to hold, who was overcome with emotion at the sight of his child alive and well. The next step for me was to be given Ergometrine (a strong synthetic drug that causes a sudden contraction) to deliver the placenta. I felt my body go into spasm and shock, all I wanted to do was vomit and luckily I was given a bowl, otherwise it would have been on top of my doctor's head. This was a traumatic experience and luckily one women no longer experience due to new drug formulations. Of course it is always better when a women can deliver her own placenta unaided by drugs, explained when we explore the third stage of labour.

After all the drama was over Lino sat holding Justin whilst I slept. Lino was so overawed by the intense feelings he was experiencing and so disappointed in my apparent lack of interest. Eventually, the midwives came, gave me a wash and transferred me upstairs to my room. Because I was hospital staff I did get the best room in the house. I did not see Lino or Justin again until the morning. At around 8 am a midwife brought my baby to me. I had to trust her as I held no recognition for this precious child in my arms. I just knew he was my son and the bruising around the eyes was familiar. Lino came in with a dozen red roses totally in awe of what I had been through. He had not slept a wink. As the day wore on I fell madly and deeply in love with my beautiful son whom remains particularly special to me today because of all he went though.

Justin did not wake for two days. He was heavily affected by the drugs and could not open his eyes because they were so badly bruised by the forceps. I did not realise how badly he was bruised until I later became a midwife and saw what babies looked like after a normal healthy birth. He was force fed Condensed Milk 1 part to 6 parts water, the treatment of the day for low blood sugar levels, which did work well for him. He brightened after this and thankfully went to the breast and fed well. Feeding him was easy and as a baby he mainly slept and fed. At times my love for him was overwhelming, I could not imagine loving another human being in the way I loved him. He did however exert his personality at about eighteen months of age and then did he rebel. My healing took quite a long time. It has only been the last few years, now twenty eight years later, that I have finally reconciled to the experience. I took my own stitches out of a very painful episiotomy scar around four weeks after the birth, as I could not sit down without incredible discomfort. They were meant to dissolve but didn't. For years I had difficulty with the scar in my perineum, it got infected. Maybe I held onto this at a subconscious level as a way of remembering so I would remain centred on helping prevent other women having similar experiences. Since letting go of the issues in the tissues it has healed.

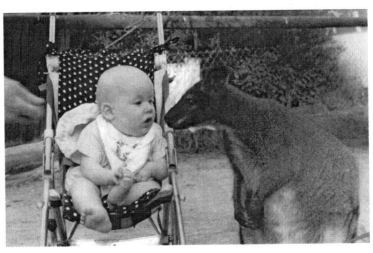

Justin aged five months (below), meeting his first wallaby.

When Justin was eighteen months old I began my midwifery training and by the end of the first day of class I learned how everything that had happened to me was totally unnecessary. I was very angry. I asked my friend who worked in records to get my medical records so I could read what had happened. After I read them I was even angrier. There was nothing in the notes to indicate the type of management I received. My blood pressure was not even that high to warrant intervention. The rage inside of me was turned to passion as I decided I had to help other women. I have a special relationship with my beautiful son and give thanks for his courageous journey. For without his lesson to me I would not have the passion to help others. I was a passionate student midwife throughout my training and experienced memories every time I walked into that labour room or had to work with the people involved with my birth. It took me a long time to forgive.

Martin's Birth

Near the end of my training I found I was pregnant again. This threw me into a panic. Even though I was informed and knew the system well, I did not trust anyone. All my fears surfaced. But luck was on my side when a homebirth midwife came to speak to our class about the experience of birthing at home. I nudged my friend and said, 'This is what I have been looking for'.

This is amazing in its self, considering only two years ago I was denouncing homebirth as dangerous and for the extremist. I raced home and asked Lino what he thought about homebirth. His response was to burst into emotion and express the pain he had been carrying since Justin's birth. He expressed how painful it was to sit by and watch the person he loved being poked and prodded. The thought of a private homebirth was wonderful to him. I was taken by complete surprise, I had no idea he harboured such resentment, he had never spoken of it to me since the birth. It showed me what men go through and that they need nurturing and direction too. I cannot tell you the difference of Martin's birth compared to Justin's. All through the pregnancy I read everything I could find on natural birth and home birth. I found and located a supportive doctor. Many people tried to tell me I was risking mine and my baby's life especially after everything that had happened the first time. I tried to tell them that it wasn't my body. If I had been left alone to get on with it, I would not have experienced what I did and the fact that Justin managed to still get through against all the odds meant I could birth easily if left alone to do so.

I enrolled in natural birth classes, learning about how important nutrition is to a healthy pregnancy and birth outcome. These classes were positive and empowering, instilling a sense of confidence. I just knew I could do this even though at times I had concerns about how I would cope considering I could not cope with the pain the first time. I was reassured that the pain of a natural labour is very different than induced labour pain.

Boy were they right! There is no comparison. I spent time with positive people who had experienced wonderful homebirths. I learned to visualise and affirm the birth daily. My midwife was supportive and encouraging, I found myself becoming more and more involved with the homebirth association. My life was transforming because I was opening to the life force within me. I was learning to trust my intuition because I was treated as the expert by those around me.

Martin was due on July 8. My doctor examined me about a week before, at my request to see what was happening, as I felt like I was beginning labour. I was already 3-4 cm dilated without experiencing any pain. He did tell me that some women walk around with this sort of dilation for some time before going into labour. On the first of July, 1987, I rang Lino feeling a bit off colour and asked if he could come home early as I felt I needed his company. He bought take-away for dinner and at around 5pm whilst eating I felt and heard this very strange popping sensation. I exclaimed 'Oh my god I am wetting my pants' and raced to the toilet.

I realised when I got there that my waters had broken and almost immediately I started to strongly contract and it felt so good, so different. We rang our midwife and friend who were going to support us through this and organised for Justin to be picked up by my sister. I quietly walked around contracting every 3-5 minutes strongly. I kept saying 'this can't be labour it isn't hurting like it did with Justin', but my midwife reassured me I was progressing very well. So well in fact by 9 pm I began to feel the effects of transition and chose to take a shower to help me through. This was the most intense part of labour as I felt so many sensations running through my body. The contractions were consuming and I began vomiting, urinating and poohing, all at the same time, classic signs of transition, where the last of the cervix sheers away readying the uterus for birth. A time when all dignity goes out the door. It's a good idea to be in the shower during this time. I remember seeing my midwife friends smiling with that knowing look of it won't be long now and all I could do was grimace. I began to feel like pushing, a sensation I had not experienced with Justin. It is the most incredible overwhelming urge that feels so fantastic. Your body just does it naturally, all you can do is go with it.

I walked to the living room and squatted between Lino's legs as I had chosen this position so I could use a mirror to guide the birth. This was the most intense time due to the perineal scarring from the first birth and I had not felt the stretching of the perineum with Justin due to the epidural so this was like a first birth to me. At times it was hard to focus and became overwhelming but by using the mirror to watch the progress I was able to work with the contractions and guide my baby out. Maybe because I was a midwife this made it easy, I don't know, it was however a very powerful experience for me.

After one or two pushes he was out and I was holding him close. He was so alert, eyes watching and locking with mine. I cannot believe the love I felt at that moment. He breastfed straight away and I did not cut the cord attached to the placenta until after I had delivered the placenta myself about ten minutes following the birth. It is so hard to express the difference of how I felt. I was awake, alert, and full of energy, not tired like after Justin's birth and it had only taken all of three hours from beginning to end. I wanted to climb to the top of the mountain and cry out 'I have done it'. I think I spent the first day telling everyone I knew about my wonderful birth experience. I couldn't stop talking about it. It was such a special feeling to cuddle up in our big bed the three of us after the midwives had left. It felt very strange to be totally responsible for this new life but also so wondrous.

After this experience I became very passionate about homebirth. I became a great advocate and assisted with the organising of the National Homebirth conference in Hobart where I met so many inspirational people. I began teaching natural birth classes with the homebirth group and eventually set up a class through adult education with another passionate advocate. We stirred the pot and vowed to improve maternity services for women in Tasmania. It was during this time that we decided that homebirth was too exclusive and felt that it was very important to include all women no matter what their choice of birth setting. All women deserved to be given the opportunity to birth naturally first before requiring medical intervention. A group of us created the Natural Birth Association, with the aim of acting as advocates for women. I was strongly involved for over ten years. This time also resulted in the setting up of the Hobart birth centre, the Know Your Midwife scheme (KYM) and the acceptance of homebirth as a safe alternative. Birthing was revolutionised in Tasmania and women began to have a choice.

Vanessa's Birth

In 1989 I delivered my beautiful daughter one week past her due date. This birth was very different and again a wonderful learning experience for me. I was much more complacent about this pregnancy, working many shifts at the maternity unit and looking after two boys under the age of four. Because I was teaching antenatal classes and had done it all before, I thought I would be fine so was not as diligent with my diet and preparation.

I experienced false labour every evening on and off for nearly two weeks prior to the birth of Vanessa, which was very exhausting. On the 24th August, heavily pregnant, I was running a childbirth class with Elizabeth Bowden, a wonderful local Reflexologist. Elizabeth's role was to teach the group how to massage their feet for health in pregnancy and birth. During the second half of the session she massaged my feet diligently for over an hour, knowing I was overdue and wanting to stimulate labour. I felt the contractions every time she worked the uterine point and by 10pm I felt the contractions pick up pace and continue on.

At home we rang our midwife around 11pm when I began to experience strong contractions. The contractions were far more intense this time because I was experiencing a low haemoglobin level. Prior to labour my haemoglobin level was only 10.7, very low compared to my normal level of 13.5 at Martin's birth. I was anaemic and my doctor had warned me two weeks before that if I didn't increase my haemoglobin level to above 10.5, I would not be permitted to birth at home. So I ate macrobiotic food, thanks to my wonderful midwife friend Sue, along with all sorts of supplements high in iron managing to get to 10.7. Though an acceptable level this was still very low for me, which meant I was extremely tired with a low pain threshold.

This labour, though short, was like one long contraction from beginning to end. I did not get the respite that I had with Martin nor did my uterus work as well. It proved to me how important nutrition really is. I spent the whole of the labour in Lino's arms using his energy to get through. It was a great bonding for us both. Finally I began to consider having some form of pain relief even though I knew it was most likely ineffective and required transferring into hospital, but I was feeling desperate and asked to be examined. Helen my intuitive midwife asked me to visualise how dilated I thought I was. I closed my eyes and visualised the cervix. I could see what I interpreted as around 8 cm dilated. On vaginal examination this proved to be true. Because I was so advanced I resolved to continue on. I took a shower and felt the pressure get stronger and stronger.

Eventually my membranes ruptured and I thought 'this is great not long to go now'. The intensity increased immeasurably due to the natural progression of the babies head onto the cervix. I did not feel like pushing and asked my midwife why and she once again intuitively asked me to visualise and ask myself. On visualisation I saw there was a small amount of cervix still to go, commonly known as a 'lip'. So I worked hard at relaxing and going with the contractions, not an easy task. All of a sudden I felt an amazing urge to push, nothing I had ever felt before. I raced to lean over the couch as I had an overwhelming need to be on all fours, natural instinct is incredible. With one uncontrollable push out came my baby, unravelling from her cord as she almost fell to the ground and was caught by Sue. We were all a little shocked at the speed of delivery, especially Vanessa who took a little while to breathe and adjust to the world.

After about a minute Helen suggested I gently caress my fingers up her spine at the same time expressing a welcome to her to the world. As I did this she awakened and looked into my eyes. I had a daughter! At about this time Justin (almost five years old) walked out of his bedroom and said in a matter of fact way 'hello Vanessa, it is about time you got here I've been waiting for you', kissed and cuddled us both, walked back to his room and went back to sleep. He had told everyone whilst I was pregnant that Vanessa would be born on Friday, 25th August at 2 am and she was. He knew something we didn't. My family was now complete.

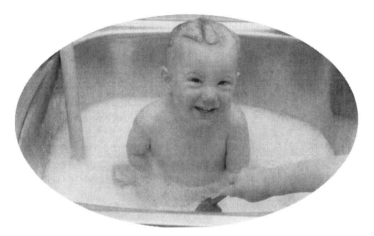

Vanessa, age ten months, enjoying a bath in the laundry sink.

Appendix

Nutritional Superfoods

You can find out more about the nutritional superfoods recommended throughout this book by clicking on the name to follow the link, or type the URL into your web browser.

FG Express
http://casadelsole.fgxpress.com/farmers-market/

FrequenSea
http://casadelsole.fgxpress.com/farmers-market/

PURE
http://casadelsole.fgxpress.com/farmers-market/

A.I.M.
http://casadelsole.fgxpress.com/farmers-market/

Pulse-8
http://casadelsole.fgxpress.com/farmers-market/

Azul
http://casadelsole.fgxpress.com/farmers-market/

Metagenics Patient Order System

Call 1800 777 648, Quote 4999X and place your order. Ask for a patient order form so you have a list of all the products for future orders. To see the full range of products go to;

http://www.healthworld.com.au/metagenics.html

Where on the Web

Birth Choices - Information and Services

http://www.casadelsole.com.au/ Vicki Delpero, Casa Del Sole

http://www.homebirthaustralia.org/ Homebirth Australia

www.midwiferytoday.com/homebirth.htm Midwifery Today - on homebirth, Medical literature on the safety of homebirth

http://www.pregnancy.com.au/ Pregnancy, birth and beyond by Jane Palmer, Midwife/Childbirth Educator (NSW)

www.moonlily.com/obc Online Birth Centre (USA based) midwifery, pregnancy, birth and breastfeeding information

http://evidencebasedbirth.com/home/ Evidence Based Birth

http://www.birthrites.org/ Birth after Caesarean homepage of Birthrites - Healing after Caesarean (WA)

www.childbirthsolutions.com Childbirth Solutions, preconception, pregnancy, birth, postpartum, dads

www.sheilakitzinger.com Sheila Kitzinger's homepage

www.aims.org.uk/aims.htm Association for Improvements in Maternity Services (AIMS UK)

http://www.motherfriendly.org/MFCI/ Ten steps of the 'Mother Friendly Childbirth Initiative'

www.waterbirth.org Water birth International

www.unassistedchildbirth.com Unassisted Birth, natural pregnancy, sensual birth by Laura Shanley

www.homebirth.org.uk Homebirth Reference Site (UK)

www.changesurfer.com/Hlth/homebirth.html Dr J Hughes Changesurfer Consulting

Birth Centres In Australia

http://www.pregnancy.com.au/birth-choices/birth-centres/australian birth centres.shtml

Midwifery Information Sites

www.midirs.org MIDIRS, Midwifery Digest homepage. An authoritative resource for midwifery information.

www.who.int/reproductive-health/index.htm Reproductive Health and Research (World Health Organisation and others)

www.aitex.com.au/joy.htm Joy Johnston's Midwifery and Lactation page

http://www.breechbirth.ca/Welcome.html Coalition for Breech Birth

Books

http://www.hencigoer.com/betterbirth/ 'The Thinking Woman's Guide to Better Birth' by Henci Goer

http://www.hencigoer.com/obmyth/'Obstetric Myths vs. Research Realities' by Henci Goer

Breastfeeding Information

https://www.breastfeeding.asn.au/ Australian Breastfeeding Association

http://www.waba.org.my/resources/lam/index.htm l Family Planning - Lactational Amenorrhea Method

http://www.unicef.org.au/Discover/What-We-Do/Baby-Friendly-Hospital-Initiative.aspx Baby friendly hospital initiative (successful breastfeeding)

http://worldbreastfeedingweek.org/ World Breastfeeding Week Information

Parenting Sites

www.bygpub.com/natural/attachment-parenting.htm   Attachment Parenting

www.awareparenting.com Aletha Solter's Aware Parenting

www.continuum-concept.org Jean Liedloff's Continuum Network home page

http://positiveparenting.com/BePositive/ Positive Parenting

www.naturalchild.org The Natural Child Project

www.infantmassage.com Baby Massage

Support and/or Community Action Groups

http://www.panda.org.au/ Post and Antenatel Depression Association Inc.

http://www.beyondblue.org.au/index.aspx? Beyond Blue

www.lalecheleague.org/links.html LaLeche League

http://www.gval.com/ Vaccination Awareness League

www.nocirc.org Circumcision debate information

http://www.motherfriendly.org/ Coalition for Improvements to Maternity
Services (CIMS)

http://www.stillbirthfoundation.org.au/ Stillbirth Foundation Australia

References & Bibliography

Abbott, J (1833) *The Mother at Home; or The Principles of Maternal Duty.* New York, USA: American Tract Society.

Akilen, R, Tsiami, A, Devendra, D & Robinson N (2010) 'Glycated haemoglobin and blood pressure-lowering effect of cinnamon in multi-ethnic Type 2 diabetic patients in the UK: a randomized, placebo-controlled, double-blind clinical trial'. *Diabetic Medicine,* 27(10): 1159-1167.

American Institute of Ultrasound Medicine (1988) *Bioeffects Report.* American College of Obstetricians.

Austin, P (1999) 'Forget the newborn bath!' *Midwifery Today E-News,* 1(40).

Australian College of Midwives (2012)' Media release: Insurance and collaborative arrangements.'

Bahasadri S, Ahmadi-Abhari S, Dehghani-Nik M & Habibi G (2006) Subcutaneous sterile water injection for labour pain: a randomised controlled trial, *Australian and New Zealand Journal of Obstetrics and Gynaecology,* Apr;46(2):102-6.

Balaskas, J & Gordon, Y (1997) *The Encyclopaedia of Pregnancy and Birth.* London: Little Brown & Co.

Balch, P A, Rister, R (2002) *Prescription for Herbal Healing: An Easy-to-Use A-Z Reference to Hundreds of Common Disorders and Their Herbal Remedies.* New York: Avery Trade.

Banks, M (1998) *Breech Birth, Woman Wise.* Hamilton NZ: Birth Spirit Books Ltd.

Banks, M (2000) *Homebirth Bound, Mending the Broken Weave*. Hamilton NZ: Birth Spirit Books Ltd.

Barker, D (2004) The Developmental Origins of Adult Disease, *Journal of the American College of Nutrition*, December 23(6): 588S-595S.

Barker, D (2011) 'The Nine Months That Made You' <http://www.youtube.com/watch?v=51_E4hc2_JM>.

Barrett, J F R et al. (1992) 'Randomized trial of amniotomy versus the intention to leave membranes intact until the second stage'. *British Journal of Obstetrics and Gynaecology*, 94: 512-517.

Baxter, L (2006) 'What a difference a pool makes: Making choice a reality' *British Journal of Midwifery*, 14(6): 368-372.

BBC Video (2011) 'The Human Body' < http://www.bbc.co.uk/programmes/b0110f51>.

Beliomo, G (1999) 'False Hypertension Linked With Cesareans', *Midwifery Today E-News*, 1(44). Midwifery Today, 1999 (Issue 44).

Bendich, A & Keen CL (1996) 'Influence of maternal nutrition on pregnancy outcome'. *Public Policy Issue, NY, USA*.

Blais, R (2002) 'Are home births safe?' *Canadian Medical Association Journal*, 166(3): 335-336.

Body Ecology (2012) 'Autism on the Rise: What Mothers and Expectant Mothers Need to Know' <http://bodyecology.com/articles/autism-on-the-rise-what-mothers-and-expectant-mothers-need-to-know>.

Bone ME, Wilkinson DJ, Young JR, McNeil J & Charlton S (1990) 'Ginger root -- a new antiemetic. The effect of ginger root on postoperative nausea and vomiting after major gynaecological surgery'. *Anaesthesia*, 1990:45(8): 669-71.

Brackbill, Y (1979) 'Effects of obstetric drugs on human development'. *Paper presented at the conference Obstetrical Management and Infant Outcome arranged by the American Foundation for Maternal and Child Health, New York*.

Bradford & Chamberlain (1998) *Pain Relief in Childbirth*. London: Harper Collins.

Brewer, T (1983) 'The Brewer Diet Plan'

British Medical Journal (1999) 'Babies delivered in water: Perinatal mortality is no higher'. *British Medical Journal*, 319:7208.

Broughtin Pipkin, F (2001) 'Risk factors for pre-eclampsia'. *New England Journal of Medicine*, 344:925-926.

Brown, L. (1998) 'The tide has turned: Audit of water birth.' *British Journal of Midwifery*, 6(4):236-243.

Buckley, S (2002) 'Ultrasound scans - cause for concern.' *Nexus Magazine* 9(6).

Burns, D (2014) <http://feelinggood.com/>

Busfield, S, Samuel R, McNinch A & Tripp J H (2013) Vitamin K deficiency bleeding after NICE guidance and withdrawal of Konakion Neonatal: British Paediatric Surveillance Unit study, 2006-2008.< http://www. ncbi.nlm.nih.gov/pubmed/23148314>.

Callahan, R (2012) Thought Field Therapy (TFT) Tapping <http://www. rogercallahan.com/index2.php>.

Castro, M (1992) *Homoeopathy for Mother and Baby*. London: Macmillan.

Chamberlain, D (1989) 'Babies Remember Pain.' *Pre- and Perinatal Psychology Journal*, Vol 3(4) Summer.

Childbirth Forum (1997) *Stress and pregnancy abnormalities*. Summer, UK.

Colson, S (2000) 'Breastfeeding Nemesis.' *Midwifery Today*, 2(15).< http:// www.midwiferytoday.com/enews/enews0215.asp>

Dabroski, R (2012) 'Clamping update to be delivered.' *Royal College of Midwives*, <http://www.rcm.org.uk/midwives/news/clamping-update-to-be-delivered/ >.

Devoe, L D & Scholl, J S (1983) 'Postdates pregnancy. Assessment of fetal risk and obstetric management.' *The Journal of Reproductive Medicine*, 28(9): 576-80.

Dick-Read, G (1984) *Childbirth Without Fear, the Original Approach to Natural Childbirth*. New York: Harper Collins.

Dix, C (1985) *The New Mother Syndrome: Coping with Postpartum Stress and Depression*. Doubleday.

Dougans, I & Ellis, S (1992) *The Art of Reflexology, a Totally New Approach Using the Chinese Meridian Theory, A Step by Step Guide*. Dorset: Element Books.

Dumont, T (2007) *The Solar Plexus or Abdominal Brain*. New York, USA:Cosimo Inc.

Dunn, P (1986) 'Nutrition Helps Children With Mental Problems',< http://americannutritionassociation.org/newsletter/ nutrition-helps-children-mental-problems>

Edmunds, J (2000), 'Quote of the Week', *Midwifery Today* 2(2).

Egoscue, P & Gittines, R (2000) *Pain Free: A Revolutionary Method for Stopping Chronic Pain*. USA: Random House

Ekdahl, L & Petersson, K (2010) 'Acupuncture treatment of pregnant women with low back and pelvic pain- an intervention study' *Scandinavian Journal of Caring Sciences*, 24(1): 175-182.

Enkin, M, Keirse, M, Renfrew, M, & Neilson, J (1996) *A Guide To Effective Care In Pregnancy and Childbirth, 2nd Ed*. Oxford UK: Oxford University Press.

Enzer, S (2000) *Reflexology a Tool For Midwives*. Hornsby, NSW: Snap Printing.

Enzer, S (2002) *Maternity Reflexology Manual*. Sydney, NSW: Soul to Soul Reflexology.

Eriksen, L (1992) 'Using reflexology to relieve chromic constipation, Chairman of the FDZ Research Committee' < http://www.reflexologyresearch. net/ReflexologyConstipationResearch2.shtml>.

Eriksson M, et al.(1996) 'Warm tub bath during labor.A study of 1385 women with prelabor rupture of the membranes after 34 weeks of gestation'. *Acta Obstet Gynecol Scand*, 75:642-4.

Fontaine, P & Adam, P (2000) 'Intrathecal narcotics are associated with prolonged second-stage labor and increased oxytocin use'. *The Journal of Family Practice*, 49(6): 515-520.

Feral, C (2000) *Wisdom of the Midwives: Tricks of the Trade Vol 2*. A Midwifery Today Book.

Field, T (2001) 'Massage therapy facilitates weight gain in preterm infants'. *Current Directions in Psychological Science*, 10: 51-54.

Flocco, W. & Oleson, T (1993) 'Randomized controlled study of premenstrual symptoms treated with foot, hand and ear reflexology'. *Obstetrics and Gynaecology*, 82:906-911.

Franks, S. P (1990) 'A randomized trial of amniotomy in active labour'. *Journal of Family Practitioner*, 30: 49-52.

Fraser, W. D (1988) 'A randomized controlled trial of the effect of amniotomy on labour duration'. *MSc thesis. Alberta, Canada: University of Calgary.*

Fraser, W. D et al. (1991) 'The Canadian multicentre, RCT, of early amniotomy'. *Journal of Perinatal Medicine*, 2.

Frisch, M, Lindholm, M & Gronback, M (2011) 'Male circumcision and sexual function in men and women: A survey-based, cross-sectional study in Denmark'. *International Journal of Epidemiology*, 40(5):1367-1381.

Frye, A (1995) *Holistic Midwivery Vol I*. Portland: Labrys Press.

Frye, A (1997) 'Vitamin K Deficiency Bleeding and the Breastfed Infant from Understanding Diagnostic Tests in the Childbearing Year'. *Midwifery Today*, 6(1997).

Funkhouser, L. & Bordenstein, S R (2013). 'Mom Knows Best: The Universality of Maternal Microbial Transmission'. <http://www.plosbiology.org/article/info%3Adoi%2F10.1371%2Fjournal.pbio.1001631>

Gaskin, I M (2010) in Robyn Sheldon's *The Mama Bamba Way: The Power and Pleasure of Natural Childbirth*. South Africa: Findhorn Press.

Gibb D (1995) *Your Natural Pregnancy, A Guide to Complimentary Therapies*. London: Eddison Sadd Editions.

Gilbert, R & Tookey, P (1999) *Perinatal mortality and morbidity among babies delivered in water: surveillance study and postal survey*. BMJ 1999;319:483

Goer, H (1995) *Obstetric Myths versus Research Realities: A Guide to the Medical Literature*. Westport, USA: Bergin & Garvey.

Golding, J, Greenwood,R, Birmingham, K & Mott, M (1992) Childhood cancer, intramuscular vitamin K, and pethidine given during labour. <http://www.ncbi.nlm.nih.gov/pubmed/1392886>

Graham, D (1997) *Episiotomy, Challenging Obstetric Interventions*. Oxford UK: Blackwell Sciences.

Haire, D (1994)*Obstetric Drugs and Procedures: Their effect on Mother and Baby*. Paper presented at the Future Birth Conference, Australia.

Hanna, T (1988) *Somatics - Reawakening the Minds Control of Movement, Flexibility and Health*. Cambridge, USA: De Capo Press.

Hannah, M E, et al. (2000) 'Planned caesarean section versus planned vaginal birth for breech presentation at term: A randomised multicentre trial'. *The Lancet,* 356: 1375-183.

Hannah, M, Hannah, J & Willan, A (2000) Term Breech Trial < http://www.thelancet.com/journals/lancet/article/PIIS0140-6736(05)71323-4/fulltext>.

Harper, B (1999) *Gentle Birth Choices.* Vermont, Canada: Healing Arts Press.

Hay, L. <http://www.louisehay.com/>

Henderson, C (1990) 'Artificial Rupture of The Membranes' in Alexander, J, Levy, V, & Roch, S (eds.) *Intrapartum Care-A Research Based Approach.* Hampshire: Macmillan Education.

Herrerra J A (1993) 'Nutritional factors and rest reduce pregnancy-induced hypertension and pre-eclampsia in positive roll-over lest primigravidas'. *International Journal of Gynaecology and Obstetrics,* 41(1): 31-5.

Hines M (2010) 'Sex-related variation in human behaviour and the brain'. *Trends in Cognitive Sciences,* 14(10):448-56.

Jacobson B, Eklund G, Hamberger L, et al. (1987) 'Perinatal origin of adult self-destructive behavior'. *Acta Psychiatrica Scandinavia,* 1987;76(4): 364-71.

Jakobsson, H,et al., (2014) ' Decreased gut microbiota diversity, delayed Bacteroidetes colonisation and reduced Th1 responses in infants delivered by caesarean section.' *Gut* Apr;63(4):559-66.

Jameson, S (1993) 'Zinc Status in Pregnancy: The effect of zinc therapy on perinatal mortality, prematurity, and placental ablation'. *Annals of the New York Academy of Sciences,* 678: 178-92.

Janov A (1984) *Imprints: The Lifelong Effects of the Birth Experience.* New York, USA: Putnam Publishing Group.

Jowitt, M (2003) *Childbirth Unmasked.* United Kingdom: Peter Wooller.

Kaplan, L (2000) 'Love is the Heart of Labour'. *Midwifery Today,* 2(24).

Kaplan Shanley, L (2000) 'Love is the heart of labor'. *Midwifery Today,* 2:24.

Kashanian, M & Shahali, S (2009) 'Effects of acupressure at the Sanyinjiao point (SP6) on the process of active phase of labor in nulliparas women'. *Iran University of Medical Sciences, Department of Obstetrics & Gynaecology.*

Keen G L et al. (1993) 'Primary & secondary zinc deficiency as factors underlying abnormal CNS development'. *Annals of the New York Academy of Sciences,* 678: 37-47.

Kerr, C E, Sacchet, M D, Lazar, S W, Moore,C I & Stephanie R Jones (2013) 'Mindfulness starts with the body: somatosensory attention and topdown modulation of cortical alpha rhythms in mindfulness meditation. ' <http://www.frontiersin.org/Human_Neuroscience/10.3389/fnhum.2013.00012/abstract>

Kirksey, A & Wasynczuk, A Z (1993) 'Morphological biochemical and functional consequences of vitamin B6 deficits during central nervous system development'. *Annals of the New York Academy of Sciences,* 168: 62-80.

Kitselman, A (2013) *E-Therapy.* Cork, Ireland: Masterworks International.

Klein, M C et al., (1994) 'Relationship of episiotomy to perineal trauma and morbidity, sexual dysfunction, and pelvic floor relaxation.' *American Journal of Obstetrics and Gynecology,* 171(3):591-8.

Kuhnert, Groh-Wargo, Webster Erhard & Lasebuik (1992) 'Smoking alters the relationship between maternal zinc Intake and biochemical indices of foetal zinc status'. *The American Journal of Clinical Nutrition,* 55(5): 981-4.

Lagercrantz, H & Slotkin, T (1986) 'The stress of being born'. *Scientific American,* 254(4): 100-107.

Lake, D & Wells, S (2009) 'EFT and the Role of Energy in Therapy' <http://www.eftdownunder.com/about.html>.

Landau, D (1953) 'Hyaline membrane formation in the newborn: Hematogenic shock as a possible etiologic factor'. *Missouri Med,* 50:183.

Lawrence Beech, B (1999) 'Drugs in labour: What effects do they have 20 years hence?' *Midwifery Today,* 1999.

Laws, R (2000) Midwifery Today, April 2000 (Issue 2:15), < http://www.midwiferytoday.com/enews/enews0215.asp>

Leboyer, F (1975) *Birth Without Violence.* Healing Arts Press.

Lehrner J et al., (2000) 'Ambient odor of orange in a dental office reduces anxiety and improves mood in female patients.' *Physiology & Behaviour,* Oct 1-15;71(1-2):83-6.

Lieberman, A (1992) Easing Labour Pain. Boston, Massachusetts: Harvard Common Press.

Lonsdorf, N, Butler, V & Brown, M (1999) *A Woman's Best Medicine*. New York: Jeremy P Tarcher.

Luminare-Rosen, C (2000) *Parenting Begins Before Conception*. Rochester, Vermont: Healing Arts Press.

Mac-Coll, M (2009) *The Birth Wars*. Brisbane, Australia: University of Queensland Press.

Magiakou, M A et al. (1996) 'Hypothalamic corticotropin-releasing hormone suppression during the postpartum period: implications for the increase in psychiatric manifestations at this time'. *The Journal of Clinical Endocrinology and Metabolism*, 81(5): 1912-7.

Makela, C (1998) 'My Unassisted Home Birth'. http://traditionalmidwife. com/unassistedbirth.html>.

Marsh, Geoffrey N & Renfrew, M J (Eds) (1998)*Community-based Maternity Care*. UK: Oxford University Press.

Mason, L, Glenn, S, Walton, I & Appleton, C (1999) ' The prevalence of stress incontinence during pregnancy and following delivery'. *Midwifery*, 15(2): 120-128.

Metagenics Practitioner's Seminar Series (1995) *Maternal Nutrition and Pregnancy*. Brisbane: Health World Ltd.

Midwifery Today E-News (2000) 'Electronic fetal monitoring'. *Midwifery Today*, 2(42).

Midirs (1996) 'High vitamin A in early pregnancy was associated with birth defects'. *Midwifery Digest, December 1996*.

Midirs (1997) 'Magnesium sulphate in the treatment of pre-eclampsia and pre-eclampsia'. *Midwifery Digest, June 1997: 177*.

Midirs (1997) 'Meta-analysis: Calcium supplementation reduces blood pressure and pre-eclampsia during pregnancy'. *Midwifery Digest, March 1997: 54*.

Midirs (1997) 'Effect of calcium supplementation on pregnancy-induced hypertension and pre-eclampsia: a meta-analysis of random controlled trials'. *Midwifery Digest, June 1997: 178*.

Midirs (1997) 'Constipation in pregnancy, is your advice on diet effective'. *Midwifery Digest March 1997: 36.*

Midirs (1997) 'What does it feel like?' *Midwifery Digest, 1997: 36-66.*

Midwifery Today (1999) 'Postnatal Depression' <http://www. midwiferytoday.com/enewsenews0113.asp>.

Miller, R K, Faber W et al. (1993) 'The role of the human placenta in embryonic nutrition: Impact of environmental and social factors'. *Annals of the New York Academy of Sciences,* 678: 92-107.

Motha, G, Swan MacLeod, K (2004) *The Gentle Birth Method: The Month-by-Month Jeyarani Way Programme.* Hammersmith, London: Thorsons.

Motha, G (1994) 'The Magic of Reflexology in Pregnancy' <http://www. reflexologyuxbridge.co.uk/phdi/p1.nsf/imgpages/3404 reflexionartdrmotha.pdf/$file/reflexionartdrmotha.pdf>.

Motz, C, Roth, H P & Kirchgessmer, M R (1995) 'Changes in zinc status and some side-effects on long-term diuretic therapy in growing rats'. *Institute of Nutrition Physiology, Technical University Munich, Freising-Weihenstephan, Germany.*

Movnihan, R (1998) *Too Much Medicine.* Sydney, Australia: ABC Books.

Müller, H (2011) Psychosomatic Breakthrough, Certificate III, PSYCHO1A.

Müller, H (2003) *Face to Face With Facts, Personality Potential.* Trafford Publishing.

Murphy, J (1963) *The Power of Your Sub-Conscious Mind.* London: Prentice Hall.

Naisch, F & Roberts, J (1999) *The Natural Way to Better Pregnancy.* NSW: Doubleday.

Naisch, F & Roberts, J (2000) *The Natural Way to Better Birth and Bonding.* NSW: Doubleday.

National Childbirth Trust (1989) *Rupture of the Membranes in Labour: Women's Views.* London: National Childbirth Trust Publishing Ltd.

Noble, E (1988) 'Channel for a New Life, The Outdoor Water Birth of Carsten Noble Sorger', DVD Release < http://elizabethnoble.com/file/DVDs.html>.

Nogier, P (1957) 'Auricolotherapy' <http://www.torquerelease.com.au/Auriculotherapy-Seminar-Brochure.pdf>.

Norman L (1988) *The Reflexology Handbook*. London: Piaktus.

Nursing Times (1999) 'Anxiety leads to low birth weight babies'. *Nursing Times, 4(1)*.

Odent, M (1999) *The Scientification of Love*. London: Free Association Books Ltd.

Odent, M (1997) 'Can water immersion stop labour?' *Journal of Nurse-Midwifery*, 42(5):414-416.

Odent, M (2000) 'A landmark in the history of birthing pools'. *Midwifery Today, Int Midwife*. Summer (54):17-8, 69.

Olsen, O (1997) 'Meta-analysis of the safety of home birth'. *Birth*. 24(1):4-13.

Ott, J (1990) *Health and Light*. York, United Kingdom: Ariel Press.

Owens, P (2000) 'Disease Triggered in Womb.' <http://www.pregnancystages.com.au/pregnancy-stages-articles/2000/11/3/disease-triggered-in-womb/>

Pearce J C (1992) *Evolution's End: Claiming the Potential of Our Intelligence*. San Francisco: Harper San Francisco.

Peltonen, T (1981) 'Placental transfusion – advantage and disadvantage'. *European Journal of Pediatrics*, 137(2)L 141-146.

Perri, S (2003) 'Water and pregnancy, part 1'. *Midwifery Today*, 5(21).

Phelps, J Y. Higby, K, Smith M H, Ward J A, Arredondo, F & Mayer A R (1995) 'Accuracy and intraobserver variability of simulated cervical dilatation measurements.' http://www.ncbi.nlm.nih.gov/pubmed/7573274?dopt=Abstract&holding=f1000,f1000m,isrctn

Piantino, E (2009) *Midwifery Today*, 9:3, 2009.

Rachan, S (2000) *Lotus Birth*. Victoria, Australia: Greenwood Press.

Rajan, L (1994) 'The impact of obstetric procedures and analgesia/anaesthesia during labour and delivery on breast feeding'. *Midwifery*, 10(2): 87-103.

Raw For Beauty (2103) < http://rawforbeauty.com/blog/?s=The+cells+in+your+body+react+to+everything+that+your+mind+says.+Negativity+brings+down+your+immune+system.>,

Reid, E & Enzer, S (1997) *Maternity Reflexology, a Guide for Reflexologists*, Fast Books, NSW, Australia: Pymble.

Reid, E & Enzer, S (1997) *Maternity Reflexology, Born to be Free*, NSW, Australia: Pymble.

Roberts, J (1998) *Zinc, Its Role in Achieving Optimal Reproductive Outcomes*. Metagemics Practitioner's Seminar Notes. Brisbane: Health World Ltd.

Robertson, A (1994) *Empowering Women, Teaching Active Birth in the 90's*. Camperdown, NSW: Ace Graphics.

Robson, K M and Kumar, R (1980) 'Delayed onset of maternal affection after childbirth'. *The British Journal of Psychiatry*, 136: 347-353.

Roger, J & McWilliams, P (1986) *You Cant Afford The Luxury of a Negative Thought*. Los Angeles: Prelude Press.

Rodier, H (2006) 'An Investigation into reversing metabolic syndrome with an integrated nutrition protocol'. *University of Utah Medical School*.

Roman E et al. (2002) 'Vitamin K and childhood cancer: analysis of individual patient data from six case-control studies.' British Journal of Cancer 86(1): 63-69.

Roseboom, T (2009) 'The Dutch famine cohort study' *Academic Medical Centre, Amsterdam*.

Sandstead, H (1994) 'Understanding zinc: Recent observations'. *The Journal of Laboratory and Clinical Medicine, September*, 124(3): 322-7.

Sandstead, H (1991) 'Zinc deficiency, A public Health Problem'. *American Journal of Diseases of Children, August*, 145(8): 853-9.

Scott, D (1992) 'Early identification of maternal depression as a strategy in the prevention of child abuse'. *Child Abuse and Neglect*, 16(3): 345-358.

Shafei, H F, AbdelDayem, S M & Mohamed, N H (2012) 'Individualized homeopathy in a group of Egyptian asthmatic children'. *Homeopathy, October*, 101(4):224-30.

Shearer, M. J. (2009). 'Vitamin K deficiency bleeding (VKDB) in early infancy.' *Blood Rev* 23(2): 49-59.

Shepherd, A, Cheyne, H, Kennedy, S, McIntosh, C, Styles, M &Niven, C (2010) 'The purple line as a measure of labour progress: a longitudinal study' <http://www.readcube.com/articles/10.1186/1471-2393-10-54?locale=en>

Simontacchi, C & Tarcher, J (2007) *The Crazy Makers: How the food industry is destroying our brains and harming our children.* USA: Jeremy P Tarcher.

Smart, J L, Massey, R F, Nash S C & J Tonkiss (1987) 'Effects of early-life undernutrition in artificially reared rats: Subsequent body and organ growth'. *British Journal of Nutrition,* 58(2):245-255.

Smith, C & Dahlen, H (2009) 'Caring for the pregnant woman and her baby in a changing maternity service environment: The role of acupuncture'. *Acupuncture Medicine, Sep* 27(3): 123-5.

Somier, E (1993) *Nutrition for Women, the Complete Guide.* Melbourne: Bookman Press.

Stapleton, R (1994) *Lead is a Silent Hazard.* USA: Walker Publishing Co.

Steinhorn, R (1998) Prenatal ultrasonography: first do no harm? *The Lancet,* 352(9140):1568-1569.

Stewart, P (1982) 'Spontaneous labour, when should the membranes be ruptured?' *British Journal of Obstetrics and Gynaecology,* 99: 5-10.

Stine, S (1999) "Vitamin K Deficiency" *Midwifery Today,* 1(41).

Stormer, C (1995) *Reflexology, the Definitive Guide.* London: Hodder & Stoughton.

Sutton, J & Scott, P (1995) *Understanding and Teaching Optimal Foetal Positioning.* NZ: Birth Concepts.

Sweha, A, Hacker, T W & Nuovo, J (1999) 'Interpretation of the electronic fetal heart rate during labor'. *American Family Physician,* 1(59)L 2487-2500.

Tallman, N & Hering, C (1998) 'Child abuse and its effects on birth'. *Midwifery Today,* 45: 19-21.

Tennant, J (2006)'Tennant Institute of Integrative Medicine' < http://www. tennantinstitute.com/>.

Tew, M (1985) 'Place of birth and perinatal mortality'. *Journal of the Royal College of General Practitioners,* 35: 390-94.

The American College of Obstetricians and Gynaecologists (2013) *Special tests for Monitoring Fetal Health* <http://www.acog.org/~/media/ For%20Patients/faq098.pdf?dmc=1&ts=20140528T2110104176

The Clinical Research Resource for Cellular Nutrition & Trace Mineral Analysis (2013) "Tin – Health Effects" <http://www.acu-cell.com/tin.html>

Thomas, P. (1996) *Every Woman's Birthrights*. London: Thorsons.

Thomson, A M & Hillier, V F (1994) 'A re-evaluation of the effect of pethidine on the length of labour'. *Journal of Advanced Nursing*, 19(3): 448-456.

University of Maryland Medical Centre (2012) 'Ginger'< http://www.umm.edu/altmed/articles/ginger-000246.htm#ixzz25Xesk4oQ>.

Vadas, P, Wai, Y, Burks, W & B Perelman (2001) 'Detection of Peanut Allergens in Breast Milk of Lactating Women'. *Journal of American Medical Association* 285(13): 1746-1748.

Luminare-Rosen, C (2000) *Parenting Begins Before Conception*. Rochester, Vermont: Healing Arts Press.

rosenVirtue, D & Virtue, G (2010) 'Your Power Words, Expressions that Affirm and Heal'< http://www.healyourlife.com/author-doreen-virtue-and-grant-virtue/2010/11/wisdom/inspiration/your-power-words>

Wagner, M (1994) *Pursuing The Birth Machine*. Camperdown, NSW: Ace Graphics.

Wagner, M (2000) 'Technology in Birth: First do no Harm'. *Midwifery Today*.

Wainer, N (2001) 'A butcher's dozen'. *Midwifery Today*, 57, Spring.

Wainer Cohen, N & Estner, L (1983) *Silent Knife: Cesarean Prevention and Vaginal Birth After Cesarean, Vbac*. South Fadley, MA: Bergin & Garvey Publishers.

Wardlaw, R & Insel, P (1993) *Perspective in Nutrition*. USA: McGraw-Hill.

Weed, S (1986) *Wise Woman Herbal for the Childbearing Year*. Woodstock, NY: Ash Tree Publishing.

Weiss, R F (1999) 'Herbal preparations and dosage guidelines'. *Midwifery Today E-News* 1(44).

Wesson, N (2000) 'Quote of the Week' . *Midwifery Today E-News* 2(24).

Wetrich, D W (1970) 'Effect of amniotomy upon labour. A controlled study'. *Obstetrics and Gynaecology*, 35: 800-806.

Wilberg, G (1992) *Preparing For Birth and Parenthood, Awareness Training and Teaching Manual For Childbirth Professionals.* Oxford: Butterworth-Heinermann, Ltd.

Woelk, H (2000) 'Comparison of St John's wort and imipramine for treating depression: Randomised controlled trial' *British Medical Journal*, 2000:321:536.

World Health Organisation (2000) 'Breastefeeding' <http://www.who.int/topics/breastfeeding/en/>.

World Health Organisation (2006) 'International Regulatory Cooperation for Herbal Medicines ' <http://www.who.int/medicines/areas/traditional/en/>.

World Health Organisation (2007) 'Male Circumcision: Global Trends and Determinants of Prevalence, Safety and Acceptability' < http://whqlibdoc.who.int/publications/2007/9789241596169_eng.pdf>.

Yerby, M (1996, May) 'Managing pain in labour Part 3: pharmacological methods of pain relief'. *Modern Midwife*, 22-25.

Image credit: <a href='http://www.123rf.com/photo_8579520_portrait-of-a-smiling-baby-sitting-wearing-a-chef-hat-sitting-inside-a-large-cooking-stock-pot-surro.html'>gallerykempton / 123RF Stock Photo</a> page 43

Image credit: <a href='http://www.123rf.com/photo_12195322_happy-family-mother-father-and-baby-isolated-on-white-background.html'>gallerykempton / 123RF Stock Photo</a>page 351

Image credit: <a href='http://www.dreamstime.com/paha_l_info'>Pavel Losevsky</a>

Image credit © <a href='http://www.dreamstime.com/ia64_info'>Ia64</a> | <a href='http://www.dreamstime.com/'>Dreamstime.com</a>

Acknowledgements

This book has been through a long gestation with many masters and finally the universe said it is time and sent me the perfect midwife, Karen Collyer (editor and desktop publisher). It has been her depth of commitment and energy that has seen it through its labour of love to be birthed finally to the world. I am forever grateful.

I would also like to acknowledge:

- ❖ All the couples who have put their faith and trust in my midwifery hands in assisting them to bring new life on to this earth and for their contribution in photos and stories.
- ❖ The Australian College of Midwives group of colleagues who have been a great inspiration in continuing to improve maternity services for women and their families.
- ❖ All I have met at the many Natural Therapy seminars and trainings who have motivated me to keep on following my dream.
- ❖ The Reflexology Association of Australia who gave me training, grounding and support throughout those early years of stepping into something completely new.
- ❖ Hermann & Marie Müller, the founder of the AIMBAPT and the Psychosomatic Family who have supported and guided me home to me.
- ❖ All the students who come to my trainings with enthusiasm and openness to learn.

- ❖ My wonderful circle of friends who have tirelessly sat over a red wine, listened, debriefed and given constructive input to the creation of this baby.
- ❖ Most of all to my beautiful husband Lino, who patiently supported me with encouragement when I chose to have a homebirth, who has looked after and cared for our three beautiful children when I was off training or teaching somewhere in the world, and for his wonderful humour that has kept me sane all these years.
- ❖ To my three beautiful children, who chose me as their mother, giving me the beautiful birthing experiences I have had so that I may then go on to assist others, and to their partners who have inspired me with their input along the way.

Index